Respiratory Diseases: Role of Dietary and Metabolic Factors

Respiratory Diseases: Role of Dietary and Metabolic Factors

Editor: Sansa Holly

AMERICAN
MEDICAL PUBLISHERS
www.americanmedicalpublishers.com

AMERICAN
MEDICAL PUBLISHERS
www.americanmedicalpublishers.com

Cataloging-in-Publication Data

Respiratory diseases : role of dietary and metabolic factors / edited by Sansa Holly.
p. cm.
Includes bibliographical references and index.
ISBN 979-8-88740-436-3
1. Respiratory organs--Diseases. 2. Respiratory organs--Diseases--Nutritional aspects.
3. Respiratory organs--Diseases--Diet therapy. 4. Respiratory organs--Metabolism--Disorders.
5. Respiratory infections. I. Holly, Sansa.
RC731 .R473 2023
616.2--dc23

© American Medical Publishers, 2023

American Medical Publishers,
41 Flatbush Avenue,
1st Floor, New York,
NY 11217, USA

ISBN 979-8-88740-436-3 (Hardback)

This book contains information obtained from authentic and highly regarded sources. Copyright for all individual chapters remain with the respective authors as indicated. All chapters are published with permission under the Creative Commons Attribution License or equivalent. A wide variety of references are listed. Permission and sources are indicated; for detailed attributions, please refer to the permissions page and list of contributors. Reasonable efforts have been made to publish reliable data and information, but the authors, editors and publisher cannot assume any responsibility for the validity of all materials or the consequences of their use.

Trademark Notice: Registered trademark of products or corporate names are used only for explanation and identification without intent to infringe.

Contents

Preface

Respiratory diseases are a group of pathological conditions that affect parts of respiratory system and lungs. These diseases can be classified into three categories, namely, obstructive lung disease, restrictive lung diseases and chronic respiratory disease. Obstructive lung diseases are respiratory conditions characterized by obstruction of air flow. They include diseases like chronic bronchitis, asthma, chronic obstructive pulmonary disease (COPD) and bronchiectasis. Restrictive lung diseases are diseases classified by a loss of pulmonary compliance. Idiopathic pulmonary fibrosis, sarcoidosis, muscular dystrophy and amyotrophic lateral sclerosis are some common restrictive lung diseases. Chronic respiratory diseases (CRDs) are a group of long-term diseases that affect the structures and airways of lungs. CRDs include diseases like occupational lung diseases and pulmonary hypertension. Diet and nutrition play a major role in the management of respiratory diseases. The intake of fruits and vegetables rich in antioxidants, vitamins, minerals, fiber and phytochemicals has potential advantages in the management of respiratory conditions. The various advancements in study of respiratory diseases are glanced at and the role of dietary and metabolic factors is looked at in detail within this book. It will provide comprehensive knowledge to the readers.

Significant researches are present in this book. Intensive efforts have been employed by authors to make this book an outstanding discourse. This book contains the enlightening chapters which have been written on the basis of significant researches done by the experts.

Finally, I would also like to thank all the members involved in this book for being a team and meeting all the deadlines for the submission of their respective works. I would also like to thank my friends and family for being supportive in my efforts.

Editor

1

Nutritional Interventions to Improve Asthma-Related Outcomes through Immunomodulation

Lieve van Brakel [1], Ronald P. Mensink [1], Geertjan Wesseling [2] and Jogchum Plat [1,*]

[1] Department of Nutrition and Movement Sciences, NUTRIM (School of Translational Research in Metabolism), Maastricht University Medical Center, 6200 MD Maastricht, The Netherlands; lieve.vanbrakel@maastrichtuniversity.nl (L.v.B.); r.mensink@maastrichtuniversity.nl (R.P.M.)

[2] Department of Respiratory Medicine, Maastricht University Medical Center, 6200 MD Maastricht, The Netherlands; g.wesseling@mumc.nl

[*] Correspondence: j.plat@maastrichtuniversity.nl

Abstract: Asthma is a chronic inflammatory disease of the airways, characterized by T-helper (Th) 2 inflammation. Current lifestyle recommendations for asthma patients are to consume a diet high in fruits and vegetables and to maintain a healthy weight. This raises the question of whether other nutritional interventions may also improve asthma-related outcomes and whether these changes occur via immunomodulation. Therefore, we systematically reviewed studies that reported both asthma-related outcomes as well as immunological parameters and searched for relations between these two domains. A systematic search identified 808 studies, of which 28 studies met the inclusion criteria. These studies were divided over six nutritional clusters: herbs, herbal mixtures and extracts ($N = 6$); supplements ($N = 4$); weight loss ($N = 3$); vitamin D3 ($N = 5$); omega-3 long-chain polyunsaturated fatty acids (LCPUFAs) ($N = 5$); and whole-food approaches ($N = 5$). Fifteen studies reported improvements in either asthma-related outcomes or immunological parameters, of which eight studies reported simultaneous improvements in both domains. Two studies reported worsening in either asthma-related outcomes or immunological parameters, of which one study reported a worsening in both domains. Promising interventions used herbs, herbal mixtures or extracts, and omega-3 LCPUFAs, although limited interventions resulted in clinically relevant results. Future studies should focus on further optimizing the beneficial effects of nutritional interventions in asthma patients, e.g., by considering the phenotypes and endotypes of asthma.

Keywords: asthma; nutrition; immune system; inflammation; lifestyle

---

1. Introduction

Asthma is a chronic inflammatory disease of the respiratory system, which affects over 300 million people worldwide [1]. The inflammation is characterized by infiltration of immune cells into the airways, among others the T-helper (Th) cells. In asthma patients, these cells predominantly secrete the Th2 cytokines interleukin (IL) 4, IL-5 and IL-13 [2]. The release of these cytokines activates a cascade of reactions, including mast cell activation and immunoglobulin E (IgE) production. Ultimately, airway inflammation leads to symptoms such as wheezing, cough and shortness of breath [2]. The Global Initiative for Asthma (GINA) provides treatment steps to determine the type of treatment [3]. Frequently, asthma patients have prescribed a combination of short-acting β2-agonists for short-term relief and inhaled corticosteroids in order to suppress the airway inflammation, thereby preventing exacerbations. Compliance to inhaled corticosteroids is generally low and was previously estimated to be between

22% and 63%, whereas short-acting β2-agonists are often used too frequently [4,5]. Noncompliance to inhaled corticosteroids could lead to a gradual worsening of the airway and even systemic inflammation in asthma patients over time [4,6]. This does not only worsen asthma severity, but long-term continuous low-grade systemic inflammation may also contribute to the simultaneous development of disorders related to low-grade inflammation, such as cardiovascular diseases [7]. Therefore, asthma patients could benefit from acceptable and easily applicable strategies in conjunction with pharmacological treatment to decrease airway inflammation and asthma symptoms.

In recent years, there has been a growing interest in the effects of lifestyle and, more particularly, nutrition in the prevention of noncommunicable diseases [8–10]. For example, the importance of nutrition in the prevention of common lifestyle-related diseases such as diabetes and cardiovascular diseases is well known and has been described in various reviews and meta-analyses [10–13]. The role of nutrition in relation to asthma has also been studied extensively. Over the past decades, numerous nutrients, foods, diets or even dietary patterns have been suggested to lower exacerbation rates, improve lung function and asthma control, or even decrease inflammatory markers [14,15]. According to several reviews and meta-analyses, vitamin D [16], omega-3 long-chain polyunsaturated fatty acids (LCPUFAs) [17], and increased fruit and vegetable intake [18] are promising interventions for asthma patients. In line with these observations, the current GINA guidelines state that the use of non-pharmacological strategies on top of asthma medication could contribute to the improvement of asthma control [3]. These guidelines advise clinicians to recommend their asthma patients to follow a healthy lifestyle. More specifically, they recommend to quit smoking [19,20], lose weight in case of obesity (with [21,22] or without [23] bariatric surgery), and consume a diet high in fruit and vegetables. Furthermore, regular physical activity is recommended to reduce cardiovascular disease risk [24] and improve quality of life [25]. However, as mentioned above, asthma severity may be reduced by many more dietary approaches than just by increasing the intake of fruit and vegetables. Moreover, it is relevant to emphasize that most of these interventions potentially affect the immune system, which could explain the decrease in inflammation of the respiratory system and the consequent reduction in asthma complaints. An example is a suggestion made in a review that vitamin D could have a direct effect on the immune system, since a variety of immune cells involved in asthma pathology express the vitamin D receptor [26]. However, despite promising results of vitamin D interventions [16], data are inconsistent. This may at least partly be related to the different doses of vitamin D supplemented in the various studies [26,27]. Therefore, a better understanding of mechanisms underlying the immunomodulatory effects of nutritional components is needed to support dietary approaches to improve asthma control. However, a systematic evaluation of randomized controlled trials studying these effects is missing. Therefore, the aim of this review is to provide an overview of nutritional interventions in asthma patients and reported asthma-related outcomes as well as immunological parameters and to search for possible relations.

2. Materials and Methods

2.1. Search Strategy

The preferred reporting items for systematic review and meta-analyses (PRISMA) checklist was used to structure this systematic review [28]. The aim of the search was to find controlled intervention studies in which the effects of a dietary intervention on asthma-related outcomes as well as on immunological parameters in asthma patients were reported. Three databases (Medline, Embase and the Cochrane Controlled Register of Trials) were used to conduct the search strategy. The abstracts of papers present in these databases were searched in August 2019 without any restriction on publication date. The following search string was used: asthma and immune system or immune function or immunology or inflammation or inflammatory or immunity and trial or clinical study or intervention or RCT and nutrition* or food or diet* or supplement* or micronutrient* or antioxidant*.

2.2. Selection of Studies

After the removal of duplicates, two researchers (LvB and JP) screened the articles that were retrieved from the databases. The screening consisted of two rounds. First, titles and abstracts were screened to determine potential eligible papers. Second, all these papers were read and included in the systematic review if they met all inclusion criteria. Relevant papers present in the reference lists of selected articles were screened as well. The following inclusion criteria were used: (1) randomized-controlled trials, (2) written in English, (3) scientific papers, (4) publication in a peer-reviewed journal, (5) used a nutritional intervention, (6) the subjects used medication for allergic asthma, (7) at least one immunological parameter was reported, (8) at least one asthma-related outcome was reported. Studies were excluded if they did not have a control group or were not randomized. Additionally, conference abstracts or posters were excluded. Differences in selection by the two researchers were solved by discussion. If two articles referred to the same study, both were included in the review, provided that both articles presented either different asthma-related outcomes or immunological parameters. Data of articles describing the same study were merged and presented as one study in tables. In this systematic review, this occurred twice and has been mentioned as a footnote of the corresponding table.

2.3. Data Extraction

After the second screening, data were extracted from the eligible papers and transferred to Excel. The following characteristics were extracted: (1) study information (first author, year of publication, study design, duration, subgroups, intervention, type of asthma, participants' health status, medication use, dietary requirements during the study) (2) baseline characteristics (number of subjects, gender, age, body mass index (BMI)), (3) immunological parameters measured, and (4) asthma-related outcomes measured. For each paper, data were extracted for the experimental and control groups separately. If outcome parameters were only presented in a figure, corresponding means or medians were estimated using a pixel ruler [29]. If not presented in the paper, within-group changes were calculated by subtracting the mean or median outcome of the baseline measurement from the mean or median of the final measurement in that group for both parallel and crossover studies [30–32].

For asthma-related outcomes, a wide variety of parameters was reported. Therefore, we decided that the three most reported questionnaires (asthma control test (ACT), asthma control questionnaire (ACQ) and asthma quality of life questionnaire (AQLQ)) and the three most reported lung function parameters (forced expiratory volume in one second (FEV_1), forced vital capacity (FVC) and peak expiratory flow (PEF)) were the focus of this review. Moreover, a study was classified to result in improved asthma-related outcomes if at least one of these parameters was significantly improved as compared to control treatment. For immunological outcomes, there was an even wider variation in outcome parameters. Therefore, we decided to focus on markers that were reported by at least five different studies. A study was classified to result in improved immunological outcomes if at least one of these five parameters was significantly improved as compared to control treatment. If a study did not report one of the three most used asthma questionnaires or lung function parameters, results were still included in the systematic review and listed under the heading "other" in the corresponding tables. The same applies to studies that only used immune markers that were not measured in five or more studies. Interventions that observed statistically significant changes in both asthma-related outcomes and immunological parameters were used to search for possible relations between these two outcome domains.

FEV_1 and FVC were reported as the percentage of the predicted value unless the original paper only reported these outcomes in liters. If FEV_1 or FVC were reported in milliliters, the unit was transformed into liters. PEF was also reported as the percentage of the predicted value unless the original paper reported PEF in L/min. The total score of the AQLQ was calculated from domain scores if the total score was not presented in the original paper. Units for the immunological parameters IgE, IL-10 and C-reactive protein (CRP) were transformed into IU/mL, pg/mL and mg/L, respectively.

Units for eosinophils in blood were transformed into 10^9 cells/L unless the original paper reported eosinophils as a percentage of total leukocytes.

2.4. Methodological Quality Assessment

The methodological quality of the trials was assessed by calculating the Jadad score [33]. Studies received a total score ranging from 0 to 5 based on methodological aspects, including randomization, blinding and description of withdrawals. Outcomes are described in Supplemental Table S1.

3. Results

The search resulted in 808 records, and six other papers were identified through other sources. In the end, 30 articles were included in this review after removal of duplicates, the title and abstract screening (first screening round) and the full-text screening (second screening round) (Figure 1). These articles described 28 individual studies.

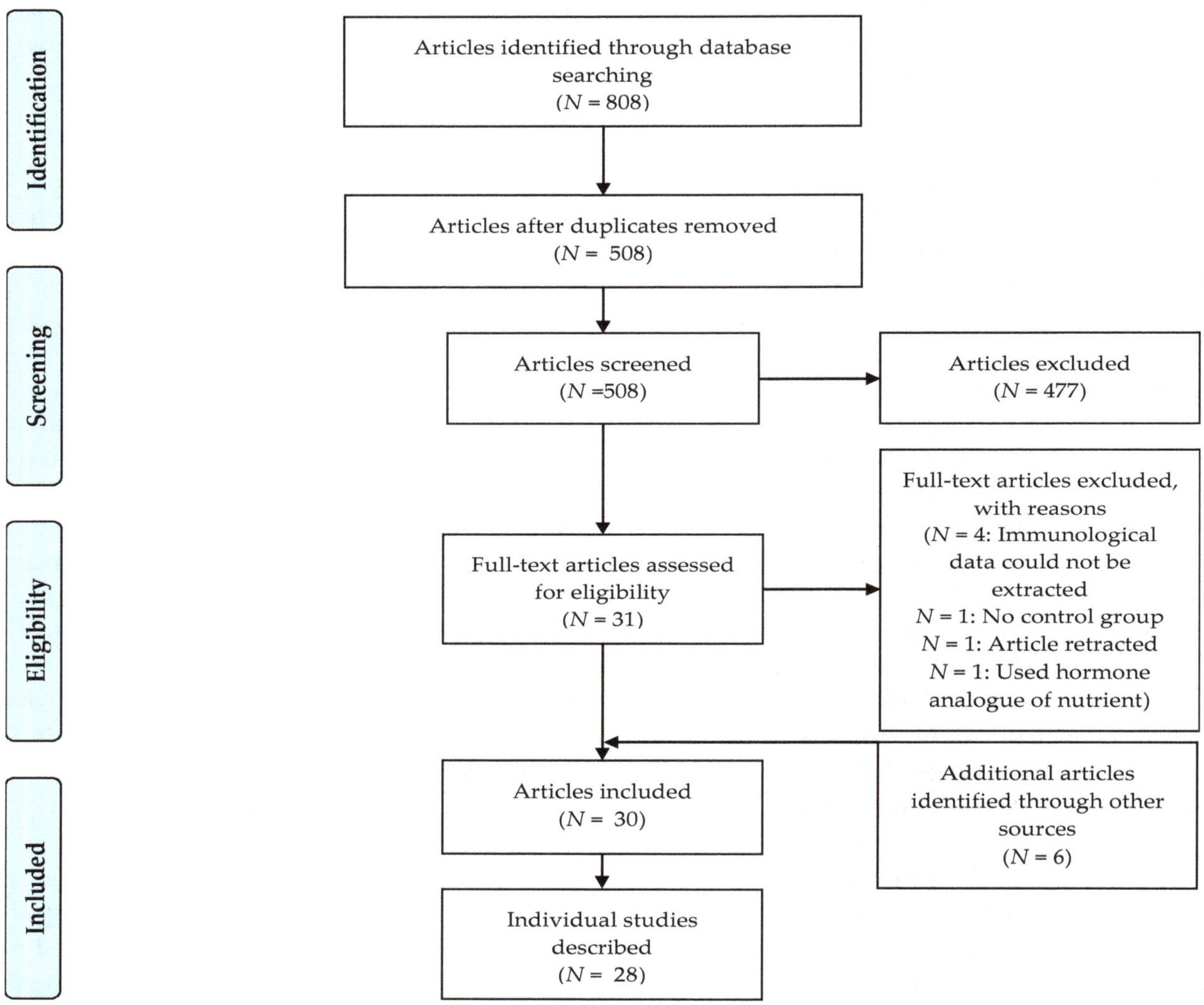

Figure 1. PRISMA flow diagram of study selection. In total, 30 articles describing 28 studies were included in the review.

These 28 studies were clustered based on the nutritional interventions used. The following six clusters (with their respective number of articles) were formed: herbs, herbal mixtures and extracts ($N = 6$); supplements ($N = 4$); weight loss ($N = 3$); vitamin D3 ($N = 5$); omega-3 LCPUFAs ($N = 5$); and whole-food approaches ($N = 5$). An overview of the clusters and selected studies with their characteristics is presented in Table 1.

Table 1. Study characteristics.

Cluster	First Author (Year)	Study Design	Population	Asthma Diagnosis	Intervention and Dose [##]	Study Duration	*n*	Age (Years)	Male (%)
Herbs, herbal mixtures and extracts	Barlianto (2017) * Barlianto (2018) * [34,35]	Parallel	Children with asthma	GINA guidelines	*Nigella sativa* oil 15–30 mg/kg/day	8 weeks	28	9 [#]	39 [#]
	Hosseini (2018) ** Zilaee (2019) ** [36,37]	Parallel	Adults with mild-to-moderate asthma	GINA guidelines	Saffron 100 mg/day	8 weeks	76	41 [#]	63 [#]
	Khayyal (2003) [38]	Parallel	Adults with mild-to-moderate asthma	National Institutes of Health and GINA guidelines	Aqueous extract of propolis 13% solution, equivalent to active constituents in 2 mL of aqueous extract of propolis per day	2 months	46	Range: 19–52	78 [#]
	Koshak (2017) [39]	Parallel	Adults with asthma	GINA guidelines and ACT score	*Nigella sativa* oil 1 g/day	4 weeks	80	41 [#]	41 [#]
	Salem (2017) [40]	Parallel, 3 arms	Adults with asthma	Previous physician's diagnosis and National Institutes of Health criteria	*Nigella sativa* (low dose) 1 g/day *Nigella sativa* (high dose) 2 g/day	12 weeks	76	38 [#]	34 [#]
	Yugandhar (2017) [41]	Parallel	Adults with bronchial asthma	Previous physician's diagnosis	Extract of *B. serrata gum* resin and *A. marmelos* fruit 200 mg/day	56 days	29	39 [#]	41 [#]
Supplements	Ghaffari (2014) [42]	Parallel	Children with moderate asthma	Previous physician's diagnosis	Vitamin E 50 mg/day	8 weeks	240	9 [#]	54 [#]
	Pearson (2004) [43]	Parallel	Adults with asthma	Previous physician's diagnosis and medication use	Vitamin E 500 mg/day	6 weeks	72	48	46
	Smith (2015) [44]	Parallel	Children and adults with asthma	Previous physician's diagnosis, symptoms and medication use	Soy isoflavone 100 mg/day	6 months	386	36	34
	Wood (2008) [45]	Crossover, 3 arms	Adults with stable asthma	Previous physician's diagnosis, symptoms and airway hyper-responsiveness	Tomato extract 45 mg lycopene/day Tomato juice 45 mg lycopene/day	7 days	22	52	36
Weight loss	Dias-Junior (2014) [46]	Parallel	Obese adults with severe asthma	Previous physician's diagnosis and treatment according to GINA guidelines	Low-calorie intake, use of sibutramine (10 mg/day) and use of orlistat (max. 120 mg/day)	6 months	33	43 [#]	6 [#]
	Jensen (2013) [47]	Parallel	Obese children with asthma	Previous physician's diagnosis	Energy reduction (−500 kcal/day) and counseling sessions	10 weeks	28	12 [#]	61 [#]
	Toennesen (2018) [1] [48]	Parallel, 4 arms	Adults with asthma	ACQ score and positive diagnostic test	High protein and low glycemic index diet Combination of diet and exercise	8 weeks	125	40 [#]	31 [#]
Vitamin D3	Bar Yoseph (2015) [49]	Parallel	Children with mild asthma	Previous physician's diagnosis, positive methacholine challenge test	Vitamin D3 14.000 IU/week	6 weeks	39	13 [#]	64 [#]
	Castro (2014) [50]	Parallel	Adults with symptomatic asthma	Previous physician's diagnosis, evidence of bronchodilator reversibility or airway hyper-responsiveness	Vitamin D3 100.000 IU once, followed by 4000 IU/day	28 weeks	408	40 [#]	32 [#]

Table 1. *Cont.*

Cluster	First Author (Year)	Study Design	Population	Asthma Diagnosis	Intervention and Dose ##	Study Duration	*n*	Age (Years)	Male (%)
	de Groot (2015) [51]	Parallel	Adults with nonatopic asthma	Evidence of bronchodilator reversibility or airway hyper-responsiveness	Vitamin D3 (cholecalciferol) 400.000 IU single dose	9 weeks	44	56 #	59 #
	Kerley (2016) [52]	Parallel	Children with uncontrolled asthma	Previous physician's diagnosis and medication use according to GINA guidelines	Vitamin D3 2000 IU/day	15 weeks	39	8 #	62 #
	Martineau (2015) [53]	Parallel	Adults with asthma	Previous physician's diagnosis, evidence of bronchodilator reversibility	Vitamin D3 (Vigantol oil) 120.000 IU/2 months	1 year	250	48 #	44 #
Omega-3 LCPUFA	Emelyanov (2002) [54]	Parallel	Adults with mild-to-moderate atopic asthma	American Thoracic Society asthma definition	Lipid extract of the New Zealand green-lipped mussel 200 mg/day EPA + DHA	8 weeks	46	39 #	26 #
	Hodge (1998) [55]	Parallel	Children with asthma and a history of episodic wheeze in the last 12 months and airway hyperresponsiveness to histamine	Symptoms and airway hyper-responsiveness	Omega-3 fatty acid-rich diet and omega-3 fatty acid supplementation 1200 mg/day EPA + DHA	6 months	39	10 #	41 #
	Mickleborough (2013) [56]	Crossover	Adults with mild-to-moderate persistent asthma	Previous physician's diagnosis	Marine lipid fraction PCSO-524™ 400 mg/day omega-3 LCPUFA, of which 120 mg/day EPA + DHA	3 weeks	20	23	60
	Moreira (2007) [57]	Parallel	Adults with stable, persistent asthma	Previous physician's diagnosis and use of inhaled corticosteroids	N-3 PUFA 780 mg/day EPA+DHA 10 mg/day vitamin E	2 weeks	20	38 #	0
	Schubert (2009) [2] [58]	Parallel	Adults with asthma and house dust mite allergy	Unknown	N-3 PUFA-enriched fat blend 750 mg/day (of which 630 mg/day EPA + DHA)	3 weeks	23	24 #	43 #
Whole food approaches	Bseikri (2018) [59]	Parallel	Obese adolescents with asthma	Previous physician's diagnosis and ACQ score	Nutrient-dense bar (CHORI-bar) 2 bars/day	2 months	56	15 #	55 #
	Papamichael (2019) [60]	Parallel	Children with mild asthma	Previous physician's diagnosis and GINA guidelines	Two meals with fatty fish per week as part of the Greek Mediterranean diet	6 months	64	8 #	52 #
	Sexton (2013) [61]	Parallel, 3 arms	Adults with symptomatic asthma	Previous physician's diagnosis, bronchodilator reversibility or PEFR variability during run-in	High-intervention: encouraged to adopt a Mediterranean diet and received intensive initial advice and 41 h of consultation sessions with a dietitian Low intervention: received less intensive advice and spent 2 h with a dietitian	12 weeks	35	38 #	29 #
	Sudini (2016) [62]	Parallel	Adults with asthma and a positive skin test to an indoor allergen	Previous physician's diagnosis	Broccoli sprouts 100 g/day	3 days	40	34 #	40 #
	Wood (2012) [2] [63]	Parallel	Adults with stable asthma	Previous physician's diagnosis, symptoms and airway hyper-responsiveness	High antioxidant diet	14 days	137	57 #	42 #

Abbreviations: ACT = asthma control test; ACQ = asthma control questionnaire; DHA = docosahexaenoic acid; EPA = eicosapentaenoic acid; GINA = Global Initiative for Asthma; IU = international unit; (LC)PUFA = long-chain polyunsaturated fatty acid; PEFR = peak expiratory flow rate; [1] = exercise arm not included in this review; [2] = not all data of this article could be extracted; */** = articles were based on the same study; # = calculated; ## = habitual intake and reference data for nutritional interventions is presented in Supplemental Table S2.

3.1. Herbs, Herbal Mixtures and Extracts

Asthma-related outcomes: The results for the cluster "Herbs, Herbal Mixtures and Extracts" are shown in Table 2. Lung function parameters were reported in five studies in the "herbs, herbal mixtures or extracts" cluster. Saffron, *Nigella sativa* or an extract of *B. serrata* gum resin and *A. marmelos* fruit caused an increase in these parameters as compared to the control group [36,40,41]. In contrast, no effect of *Nigella sativa* was found on airway function in another study [39]. Only within-group changes were reported in a study using an extract of propolis. Therefore, no statement could be made if the change of the intervention group differed significantly from the change in the control group [38]. Improvements in asthma control as measured via the ACT were reported in three studies using *Nigella sativa* [35,39,40]. Furthermore, an extract of *B. serrata* gum resin and *A. marmelos* fruit improved asthma-related quality of life [41].

Immunological parameters: *Nigella sativa* oil did not change fractional exhaled nitric oxide (FeNO) [40] but caused a decrease in the number of eosinophils in blood [39].Th1 cytokines were reported in four studies. *Nigella sativa* and an extract of *B. serrata* gum resin and *A. marmelos* fruit increased interferon-γ (IFN-γ) [34,40,41]. Th1 cytokines were reported in a study using an extract of propolis, but between-group changes were not presented. Therefore, no statement could be made if the change of the intervention group differed significantly from the change in the control group [38]. Th2 cytokines or IgE were reported in four studies. *Nigella sativa* and an extract of *B. serrata* gum resin and *A. marmelos* fruit caused decreases in these parameters [34,41]. In contrast to the *Nigella sativa* intervention by Barlianto et al. (2017) [34], two other *Nigella sativa* interventions did cause a significant effect on Th2 cytokines or IgE [39,40]. Treg cytokines were analyzed in two studies. *Nigella sativa* had no effect on these parameters [40]. Only within-group changes were reported in a study using an extract of propolis [38]. Proinflammatory markers were reported in three studies and only decreased after saffron supplementation [36]. *Nigella sativa* did not change these markers [40]. Only within-group changes were reported in a study using an extract of propolis [38].

Overlap between both domains: Five out of six studies from this herb, herbal mixture, or extract cluster showed significant improvements in both asthma-related as well as immunological parameters, compared to the control group [34–37,39–41]. *Nigella sativa* ($N = 3$) increased ACT score in children with 1.9 points [34,35], and in adults with 1.3, 1.4 [40] or 2.1 points [39]. It also increased PEF variability with 8.2 and 5.8 L/min in adults, depending on the dose used [40]. *Nigella sativa* also increased IFN-γ with 7.8 pg/mL in children [34,35] and with 0.5 or 0.9 pg/mL in adults [40]. It decreased IL-4 with 0.3 pg/mL in children [34,35] and eosinophils in blood with 65 cells/µL in adults. Saffron ($N = 1$) increased FEV_1 with 5% and FVC with 1% and decreased CRP with 37.5 ng/mL in adults [36,37]. A mixture of *B. serrata* gum resin and *A. marmelos* fruit ($N = 1$) improved PEF with 46.2 L/min, the AQLQ score with 0.5 points, increased IFN-γ with 7.6 pg/mL and decreased IL-4 with 0.4 pg/mL in adults [41].

3.2. Supplements

Asthma-related outcomes: The results for the cluster "Supplements" are shown in Table 3. All six studies that used supplements as intervention reported lung function parameters. Soy isoflavone supplementation decreased FVC [44]. Using vitamin E, tomato juice, or a tomato extract did not cause changes in lung function [43,45]. Another study with vitamin E supplements only reported within-group changes. Therefore, no statement could be made if the change of the intervention group differed significantly from the change in the control group [42]. No effects were found of soy isoflavones on ACT score [44] or a tomato extract or juice on ACQ score [45].

Table 2. Changes in asthma-related outcomes and immunological parameters as compared to the control group for the herbs, herbal mixtures and extracts cluster.

First Author (Year)	Jadad Score ***	Intervention and Dose	Asthma-Related Outcomes						Immunological Parameters				
			Lung Function			Asthma Control	QoL						
			FEV1	FVC	PEF	ACT	(P)AQLQ	FeNO	Cells (Sputum, Blood)	Th1	Th2, IgE	Treg	Pro-Inflammatory Markers
Barlianto (2017) * Barlianto (2018) * [34,35]	2	*Nigella sativa* oil 15–30 mg/kg/day				↑ [1]				↑	↓		
Hosseini (2018) ** Zilaee (2019) ** [36,37]	5	Saffron 100 mg/day	↑	↑					=				↓
Khayyal (2003) [38]	2	Aqueous extract of propolis 13% solution, equivalent to active constituents in 2 mL of aqueous extract of propolis per day	N/A	N/A	N/A					N/A		N/A	N/A
Koshak (2017) [39]	5	*Nigella sativa* oil 1 g/day	=		=	↑			↓		=		
Salem (2017) [40]	3	*Nigella sativa* (low dose) 1 g/day	=	=	↑	↑		=		↑	=	=	=
		Nigella sativa (high dose) 2 g/day	=	=	↑	↑		=		↑	=	=	=
Yugandhar (2017) [41]	4	Extract of *B. serrata gum* resin and *A. marmelos* fruit 200 mg/day	=		↑		↑			↑	↓		

Abbreviations: FEV_1 = forced expiratory flow in one second; FVC = forced vital capacity; PEF = peak expiratory flow; ACT = asthma control test; (P)AQLQ = (pediatric) asthma quality of life questionnaire; FeNO = fractional exhaled nitric oxide; Th = T helper cell; IgE = immunoglobulin E; Treg = regulatory T cell; QoL = quality of life; ↑ = significant increase as compared to the control group; ↓ = significant decrease as compared to the control group; = = no change as compared to the control group; N/A = between-group changes not reported; * = based on the same study; ** = based on the same study; *** = Jadad score was calculated to assess the methodological quality of the RCTs. The calculation of the Jadad score can be found in Supplemental Table S1; [1] = both articles presented ACT data; only between-group changes are shown here since comparing changes results in less bias than comparing scores at the final time point. Quantitative data showing the within-group changes is presented in Supplemental Tables S3–S7.

Table 3. Changes in asthma-related outcomes and immunological parameters as compared to the control group for the supplements cluster.

First Author (Year)	Jadad Score *	Intervention and Dose	Asthma-Related Outcomes						Immunological Parameters		
			Lung Function			Asthma Control					
			FEV_1	FVC	PEF	ACT	ACQ	FeNO	Cells (Sputum, Blood)	Th2, IgE	Pro-Inflammatory Markers
Ghaffari (2014) [42]	3	Vitamin E 50 mg/day	N/A	N/A						N/A	
Pearson (2004) [43]	5	Vitamin E 500 mg/day	=	=	=					=	
Smith (2015) [44]	5	Soy isoflavone 100 mg/day	=	↓	=	=		↑	=		=
Wood (2008) [45]	3	Tomato extract 45 mg lycopene/day	=	=			=	=	↓; =		
		Tomato juice 45 mg lycopene/day	=	=			=	=	↓; =		

Abbreviations: FEV_1 = forced expiratory flow in one second; FVC = forced vital capacity; PEF = peak expiratory flow; ACT = asthma control test; ACQ = asthma control questionnaire; FeNO = fractional exhaled nitric oxide; Th = T helper cell; IgE = immunoglobulin E; ↑ = significant increase as compared to the control group; ↓ = significant decrease as compared to the control group; = = no change as compared to the control group; N/A = between-group changes not reported; * = Jadad score was calculated to assess the methodological quality of the RCTs. The calculation of the Jadad score can be found in Supplemental Table S1. Quantitative data showing the within-group changes is presented in Supplemental Tables S3–S7.

Immunological parameters: Two studies reported the effect of their intervention on FeNO, but no effects were reported for a tomato extract or tomato juice [45]. Soy isoflavone supplementation even worsened FeNO concentrations [44]. The number of immune cells in sputum or blood was reported by two studies. Tomato extract and tomato juice decreased the number of immune cells in sputum [45]. Soy isoflavones had no effect [44]. Two studies reported Th2 cytokines or IgE, and one study reported proinflammatory markers. Vitamin E did not change IgE levels [43]. Another study using vitamin E supplements only reported within-group changes. It is unknown if the change of the intervention group differed significantly from the change in the control group [42]. Soy isoflavones did not change proinflammatory markers [44].

Overlap between both domains: None of the studies reported improvements in both asthma-related outcomes and immunological parameters. In adults, soy isoflavones worsened both asthma-related outcomes and immunological outcomes, as FVC was decreased by 0.1 L and FeNO increased with 4.9 ppb compared to the control group [44].

3.3. Weight Loss

Asthma-related outcomes: The results for the cluster "Weight Loss" are shown in Table 4. Lung function parameters were reported in all three studies of the weight loss cluster. Low caloric intake combined with weight loss medication (sibutramine and orlistat) caused a reduction in BMI of 5.3 kg/m^2 in the intervention group and improved FVC compared to the control group [46]. A high protein and low glycemic index diet, high-intensity interval training, or a combination of this diet and high-intensity interval training caused weight losses of 2.3 kg, 1.0 kg and 3.1 kg, respectively [48]. Combining energy restriction and counseling sessions resulted in a weight loss of 3.4 kg and a reduction in BMI z-score of 0.2 [47]. No changes were found in lung function parameters in these two studies [47,48]. Additionally, asthma control was evaluated in all studies. Low caloric intake combined with weight loss medication and energy restriction together with counseling sessions improved asthma control [46,47]. The study evaluating diet and high-intensity interval training reported an improvement in asthma control in the group that combined the diet with high-intensity interval training [48]. Asthma-related quality of life was increased after this same diet combined with high-intensity interval training [48], but not after energy reduction combined with counseling sessions [47].

Immunological parameters: FeNO was reported as an immunological outcome in all studies, but no significant improvements were found. The number of immune cells was also evaluated by all three studies. Energy reduction, combined with counseling sessions, decreased sputum lymphocyte numbers [47]. The other interventions did not change immune cell numbers [46,48]. Low caloric intake, combined with weight loss medication, did not change IgE levels [46]. Proinflammatory markers were reported in all studies. Only energy reduction in combination with counseling sessions decreased CRP [47].

Overlap between both domains: Energy reduction in combination with counseling sessions in children significantly decreased ACQ score by 0.6 points, decreased sputum lymphocyte numbers with 0.1×10^6 cells/mL, and decreased CRP with 1.1 mg/L compared to the control group [47].

3.4. Vitamin D3

Asthma-related outcomes: The results for the cluster "Vitamin D3" are shown in Table 5. Lung function parameters were evaluated in four out of five studies from the vitamin D3 cluster, but no significant improvements were found [50–53]. The effect of vitamin D3 on asthma control was also evaluated in four studies, but none found significant improvements [50–53]. The effect of vitamin D3 on asthma-related quality of life was reported in two studies, although no changes were reported [51,52]. Finally, Bar Yoseph et al. (2015) did not find an effect of vitamin D3 on the provocative dose causing a 20% fall in FEV_1.

Table 4. Changes in asthma-related outcomes and immunological parameters as compared to the control group for the weight loss cluster.

First Author (Year)	Jadad Score *	Intervention and Dose	Asthma-Related Outcomes					Immunological Parameters			
			Lung Function		Asthma Control		QoL				
			FEV_1	FVC	ACT	ACQ	(P)AQLQ	FeNO	Cells (Sputum, Blood)	Th2, IgE	Pro-Inflammatory Markers
Dias-Junior (2014) [46]	3	Low-calorie intake, use of sibutramine (10 mg/day) and use of orlistat (max. 120 mg/day)	=	↑	↑	↓		=	=	=	=
Jensen (2013) [47]	3	Energy reduction (−500 kcal/day) and counseling sessions	=	=		↓	=	=	↓; =		↓; =
Toennesen (2018) [48]	3	High protein and low glycemic index diet	=	=		=	=	=	=		=
		Combination of diet and exercise	=	=		↓	↑	=	=		=

Abbreviations: FEV_1 = forced expiratory flow in one second; FVC = forced vital capacity; ACT = asthma control test; ACQ = asthma control questionnaire; (P)AQLQ = (pediatric) asthma quality of life questionnaire; FeNO = fractional exhaled nitric oxide; Th = T helper cell; IgE = immunoglobulin E; QoL = quality of life; ↑ = significant increase as compared to the control group; ↓ = significant decrease as compared to the control group; = = no change as compared to the control group; * = Jadad score was calculated to assess the methodological quality of the RCTs. The calculation of the Jadad score can be found in Supplemental Table S1. Quantitative data showing the within-group changes is presented in Supplemental Tables S3–S7.

Table 5. Changes in asthma-related outcomes and immunological parameters as compared to the control group for the vitamin D3 cluster.

First Author (Year)	Jadad Score *	Intervention and Dose	Asthma-Related Outcomes							Immunological Parameters				
			Lung Function			Asthma Control		QoL						
			FEV_1	FVC	PEF	ACT	ACQ	(P)AQLQ	Other	FeNO	Cells (Sputum, Blood)	Th2, IgE	Treg	Pro-Inflammatory Markers
Bar Yoseph (2015) [49]	4	Vitamin D3 14.000 IU/week							= [1]	=	=	=		=
Castro (2014) [50]	5	Vitamin D3 100.000 IU once, followed by 4000 IU/day	=			=					=			
de Groot (2015) [51]	4	Vitamin D3 (Cholecalciferol) 400.000 IU single dose	=				=	=		=	↓ [2]	=		
Kerley (2016) [52]	3	Vitamin D3 2000 IU/day	=	=		=		=					=	↑
Martineau (2015) [53]	5	Vitamin D3 (Vigantol oil) 120.000 IU/2 months	=		=	=				=				

Abbreviations: FEV_1 = forced expiratory flow in one second; FVC = forced vital capacity; PEF = peak expiratory flow; ACT = asthma control test; ACQ = asthma control questionnaire; (P)AQLQ = (pediatric) asthma quality of life questionnaire; FeNO = fractional exhaled nitric oxide; Th = T helper cell; IgE = immunoglobulin E; Treg = regulatory T cell; QoL = quality of life; ↑ = significant increase as compared to the control group; ↓ = significant decrease as compared to the control group; = = no change as compared to the control group; * = Jadad score was calculated to assess the methodological quality of the RCTs. The calculation of the Jadad score can be found in Supplemental Table S1; [1] = provocative dose causing a 20% fall in FEV_1; [2] = significant difference after correction for baseline. Quantitative data showing the within-group changes is presented in Supplemental Tables S3–S7.

Immunological parameters: FeNO was reported in three studies, but no changes were found [49,51,53]. Only a single dose of 400.000 IU vitamin D3 decreased sputum eosinophilia after adjustment for baseline values [51]. Other interventions did not change the number of eosinophils in sputum [50] or blood [49]. Th2 cytokines and IgE were reported twice [49,51], as well as Treg cytokines [49,52]. No changes in these parameters were reported. Two studies reported proinflammatory markers. One study using a daily dose of 2.000 IU vitamin D3 reported an increase in CRP [52], whereas no effect on CRP was found in another study using the same dose of vitamin D3 [49].

Overlap between both domains: None of the vitamin D3 interventions resulted in improvements in both asthma-related outcomes and immunological parameters.

3.5. Omega-3 LCPUFAs

Asthma-related outcomes: The results for the cluster "Omega-3 LCPUFAs" are shown in Table 6. Lung function parameters were evaluated in all five studies of the omega-3 LCPUFA cluster [54–58]. PEF increased after using a lipid extract of the New Zealand green-lipped mussel [54,56]. Omega-3 LCPUFA supplementation, an omega-3 LCPUFA rich diet or an omega-3 LCPUFA enriched fat blend did not improve lung function parameters [55,57,58]. ACQ score did not change after omega-3 LCPUFA supplementation [57].

Immunological parameters: FeNO was reported by three studies and decreased after using an extract of the New Zealand green-lipped mussel and a fat blend enriched with omega-3 fatty acids [56,58]. Another study did not find any changes [57]. Furthermore, the number of sputum eosinophils was not changed after increasing omega-3 LCPUFA intake [55,58]. Finally, Emelyanov et al. showed that an extract of the New Zealand green-lipped mussel decreased exhaled H_2O_2 [54].

Overlap between both domains: Two studies that used lipid extracts of the New Zealand green-lipped mussel as intervention found significant improvements in asthma-related outcomes as well as immunological parameters in adults, compared to the control group [54,56]. Combined morning and evening PEF increased with 21.8 L/min and FeNO decreased with 9.9 ppb in one study [56], whereas morning PEF increased with 80.4 L/min and exhaled H_2O_2 decreased with 0.1 uM in the other study [54].

3.6. Whole Food Approaches

Asthma-related outcomes: The results for the cluster "Whole Food Approaches" are shown in Table 7. Lung function parameters were reported in all five studies using a whole-food approach intervention [59–63]. Consuming a high antioxidant diet increased FEV_1 and FVC [63]. The other interventions did not change lung function parameters. Additionally, asthma control was evaluated in all studies. However, no changes in ACT or ACQ score were found. The Mediterranean diet did not improve asthma-related quality of life [60,61].

Immunological parameters: FeNO was reported in four studies [59,60,62,63]. Consuming two meals with fatty fish per week as part of the Mediterranean diet decreased FeNO [60]. A nutrient-dense bar [59], broccoli sprouts [62] and a high antioxidant diet [63] did not have an effect on FeNO concentrations. The Mediterranean diet and a high antioxidant diet did not change Th1 cytokines [61,63]. In the same study on the Mediterranean diet, no changes in Treg cytokines and immune cell count were found [61]. Using a nutrient-dense bar or broccoli sprouts did not change Th2 cytokines or IgE [59,62]. Proinflammatory markers were not changed after using a nutrient-dense bar, the Mediterranean diet, a high antioxidant diet or broccoli sprouts as an intervention [59,61–63].

Table 7. Changes in asthma-related outcomes and immunological parameters as compared to the control group for the whole-food approach cluster.

First Author (Year)	Jadad Score *	Intervention and Dose	Asthma-Related Outcomes						Immunological Parameters					
			Lung Function			Asthma Control		QoL						
			FEV_1	FVC	PEF	ACT	ACQ	(P)AQLQ	FeNO	Cells (Sputum, Blood)	Th1	Th2, IgE	Treg	Pro-Inflammatory Markers
Bseikri (2018) [59]	2	Nutrient-dense bar (CHORI-bar) 2 bars/day	=	=		=			=			=		=
Papamichael (2019) [60]	3	Mediterranean diet	=	=	=		=	=	↓ [1]					
Sexton (2013) [61]	2	Mediterranean diet (high intervention) [2]	=	=			=	=		=	=		=	=
		Mediterranean diet (low intervention) [2]	=	=			=	=		=	=		=	=
Sudini (2016) [62]	4	Broccoli sprouts 100 g/day	=	=		=			=			=		=
Wood (2012) [63]	3	High antioxidant diet	↑	↑			=		=	=	=			=

Abbreviations: FEV_1 = forced expiratory flow in one second; FVC = forced vital capacity; PEF = peak expiratory flow; ACT = asthma control test; ACQ = asthma control questionnaire; (P)AQLQ = (pediatric) asthma quality of life questionnaire; FeNO = fractional exhaled nitric oxide; Th = T helper cell; IgE = immunoglobulin E; Treg = regulatory T cell; QoL = quality of life; ↑ = significant increase as compared to the control group; ↓ = significant decrease as compared to the control group; = = no change as compared to the control group; * = Jadad score was calculated to assess the methodological quality of the RCTs. The calculation of the Jadad score can be found in Supplemental Table S1; [1] = significant difference after correction for baseline; [2] = High-intervention: encouraged to adopt a Mediterranean diet and received intensive initial advice and 41 h of consultation sessions with a dietitian. Low intervention: received less intensive advice and spent 2 h with a dietitian. Quantitative data showing the within-group changes is presented in Supplemental Tables S3–S7.

Table 7. Changes in asthma-related outcomes and immunological parameters as compared to the control group for the whole-food approach cluster.

First Author (Year)	Jadad Score *	Intervention and Dose	Asthma-Related Outcomes						Immunological Parameters					
			Lung Function			Asthma Control		QoL						
			FEV_1	FVC	PEF	ACT	ACQ	(P)AQLQ	FeNO	Cells (Sputum, Blood)	Th1	Th2, IgE	Treg	Pro-Inflammatory Markers
Bseikri (2018) [59]	2	Nutrient-dense bar (CHORI-bar) 2 bars/day	=	=		=			=			=		=
Papamichael (2019) [60]	3	Mediterranean diet	=	=	=		=	=	↓ [1]					
Sexton (2013) [61]	2	Mediterranean diet (high intervention) [2]	=	=			=	=		=	=		=	=
		Mediterranean diet (low intervention) [2]	=	=			=	=		=	=		=	=
Sudini (2016) [62]	4	Broccoli sprouts 100 g/day	=	=		=			=			=		=
Wood (2012) [63]	3	High antioxidant diet	↑	↑			=		=	=	=			=

Abbreviations: FEV_1 = forced expiratory flow in one second; FVC = forced vital capacity; PEF = peak expiratory flow; ACT = asthma control test; ACQ = asthma control questionnaire; (P)AQLQ = (pediatric) asthma quality of life questionnaire; FeNO = fractional exhaled nitric oxide; Th = T helper cell; IgE = immunoglobulin E; Treg = regulatory T cell; QoL = quality of life; ↑ = significant increase as compared to the control group; ↓ = significant decrease as compared to the control group; = = no change as compared to the control group; * = Jadad score was calculated to assess the methodological quality of the RCTs. The calculation of the Jadad score can be found in Supplemental Table S1; [1] = significant difference after correction for baseline; [2] = High-intervention: encouraged to adopt a Mediterranean diet and received intensive initial advice and 41 h of consultation sessions with a dietitian. Low intervention: received less intensive advice and spent 2 h with a dietitian. Quantitative data showing the within-group changes is presented in Supplemental Tables S3–S7.

Overlap between both domains: None of the studies from this whole-food approach cluster found improvements in asthma-related outcomes and immunological outcomes simultaneously.

3.7. Effect Sizes in the Context of Minimal Clinically Important Difference

Eight studies found changes in asthma-related outcomes as well as in immunological parameters, which may indicate a link between immunological parameters with asthma-related outcomes. The magnitude of changes in asthma-related outcomes in comparison to the minimal clinically important difference is shown in Figure 2. In three of these eight studies, the changes as compared to those of the control group had an effect size that exceeded the minimal clinically important difference. These three interventions were part of the following clusters: herbs, herbal mixtures and extracts ($N = 1$), weight loss ($N = 1$) and omega-3 LCPUFAs ($N = 1$) and showed effects on PEF (extract of *B. serrata* gum resin and *A. marmelos* fruit; lipid extract of the New Zealand green-lipped mussel), ACQ (energy reduction combined with counseling) and AQLQ (extract of *B. serrata* gum resin and *A. marmelos* fruit). A minimal clinically important difference of FVC could not be found in the literature.

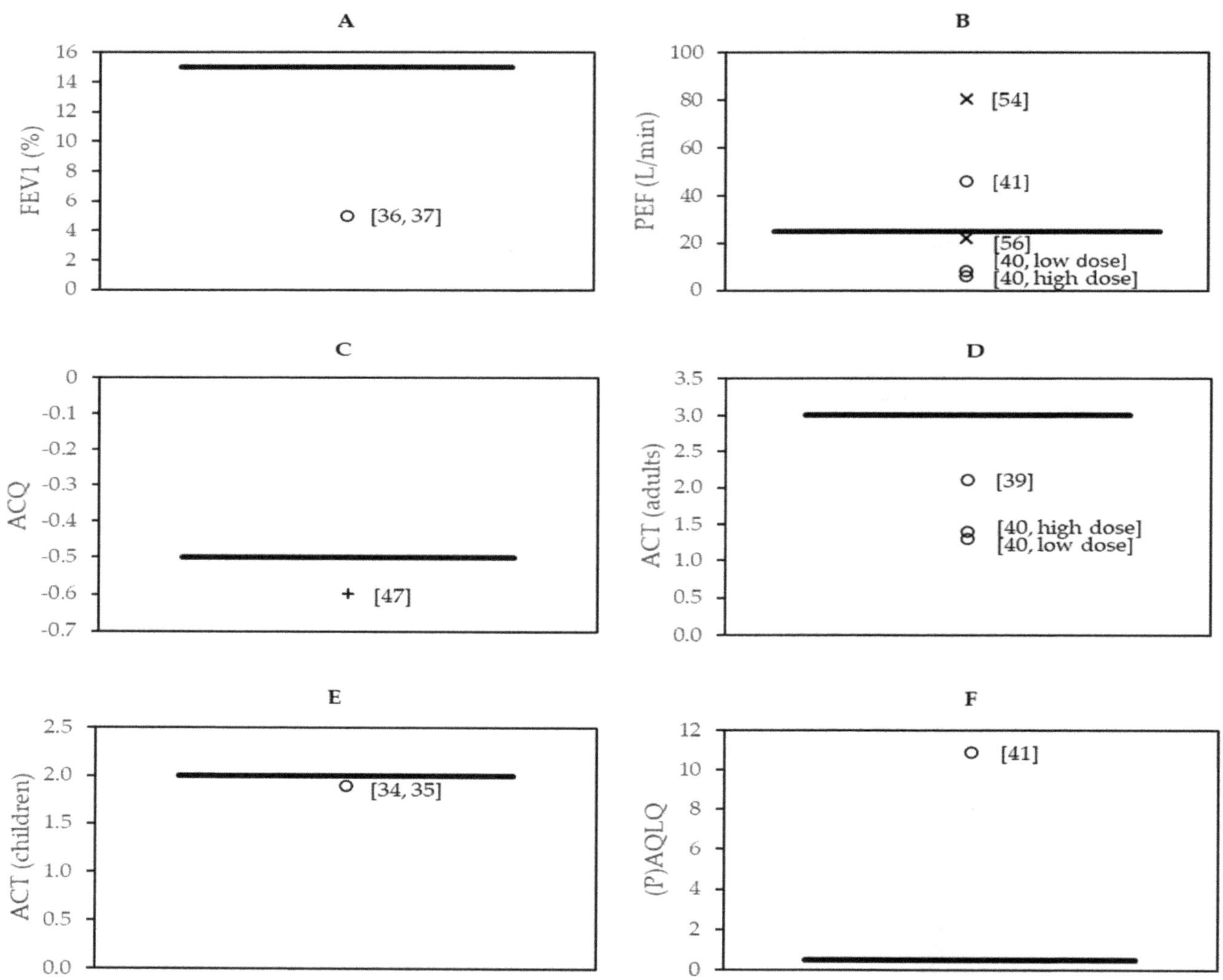

Figure 2. The magnitude of changes in asthma-related outcomes compared to the minimal clinically important difference for (**A**) FEV1; (**B**) PEF; (**C**) ACQ; (**D**) ACT for adults; (**E**) ACT for children; and (**F**) (P)AQLQ. The symbols (○ = herbs, herbal mixtures and extracts; x = omega-3 LCPUFA; + = weight loss) represent individual studies, and the line (–) indicates the minimal clinically important difference. Reference numbers for individual studies are noted next to the corresponding symbol.

4. Discussion

The aim of this systematic review was to provide an overview of studies that examined the effects of nutritional interventions in asthma patients on both changes in asthma-related outcomes as well as immunological parameters and search for possible relations. The reason for this approach was that we hypothesized that nutritional interventions might affect asthma severity via modulation of the immune system. Therefore, interventions that improved asthma-related outcomes, as well as immunological parameters, were considered as indications of a link between these two outcome domains, without claiming causality. Current guidelines for asthma patients do contain lifestyle recommendations, but only to a limited extent. It is only advised to increase fruit and vegetable intake and to maintain a healthy weight in order to improve asthma-related outcomes. Based on the results of our systematic review, it may be interesting to consider whether these lifestyle recommendations could be extended in the future. As shown in Tables 2–7, fifteen out of 28 controlled dietary intervention studies reported an improvement in at least one asthma-related outcome or immunological parameter. However, also two studies reported a worsening in one of the domains, of which one study using soy isoflavones observed a worsening in both domains. With respect to our hypothesis that nutritional interventions likely affect asthma severity via modulation of the immune system, we identified eight studies that showed a simultaneous improvement in asthma-related outcomes and immunological parameters. These studies used *Nigella sativa* ($n = 3$), saffron ($n = 1$), an extract of *B. serrata* gum resin and *A. marmelos* fruit ($n = 1$), energy reduction in combination with counseling sessions ($n = 1$) or a lipid extract of the New Zealand green-lipped mussel ($n = 2$) as an intervention. Regarding the clinical relevance of these results, we showed in Figure 2 that three out of the eight studies were able to find clinically relevant changes in asthma-related outcomes. Clinically relevant changes were found in lung function parameters, asthma control and quality of life.

In the context of identifying nutritional interventions that improve asthma-related outcomes via immunomodulation, the "herbs, herbal mixtures and extracts" cluster showed the most consistent and promising results. When interpreting the effects of this cluster, however, it should be noted that exact concentrations of the active compounds of herbal extracts are not always known, and concentrations of extracts could be variable. The use of *Nigella sativa* resulted in an improvement in asthma control and PEF, which was accompanied by a reduction in eosinophils numbers in blood, an increase of IFN-γ and an increase in IL-4 [34,35,39,40]. An intervention with saffron increased FEV_1 and FVC and simultaneously decreased CRP levels [36,37]. An increase in PEF and asthma-related quality of life was observed after using an extract of *B. serrata* gum resin and *A. marmelos* fruit. These changes in asthma-related outcomes occurred simultaneously with an increase in the Th1 cytokine IFN-γ and a decrease in the Th2 cytokine IL-4 [41]. These results suggest that the improvement in asthma-related outcomes after using these herbal interventions is mediated by affecting the Th1/Th2 balance, thereby dampening the Th2 driven pathological process. Since the Th1/Th2 balance in asthma is disturbed as asthma is characterized by Th2 mediated inflammation, asthma patients could benefit from interventions that increase Th1 activity, thereby contributing to restoring the Th1/Th2 balance [64]. Based on mouse models, it has been suggested that increased production of Th1 cytokines, such as IFN-γ, could contribute to a decrease in immune cell infiltration in the lungs and eventually to a decrease in local inflammation [64–66]. This suggested mechanism is supported by the findings in this review and is in accordance with previous research. For example, the main constituent of *Nigella sativa* oil, thymoquinone, stimulates IFN-γ production and decreases IL-4 production in animal models of asthma [64,67,68]. Moreover, lowering Th2 cytokine concentrations is part of the suggested mechanism underlying the effects of crocin, which is the main active component of saffron [69]. However, there are additional pathways that can be modulated by thymoquinone [70] and crocin [71], which indicates that herbal interventions could reduce asthma-related complaints via several mechanisms.

The second cluster that showed promising results was the omega-3 LCPUFA cluster. Two studies using a lipid extract of the New Zealand green-lipped mussel both showed an increase in PEF, which occurred simultaneously with a decrease in FeNO concentrations in one study [56] and a decrease in exhaled H_2O_2 in the other study [54]. FeNO and exhaled H_2O_2 are both markers for airway inflammation and can be analyzed in exhaled breath, and correlate positively with eosinophils in induced sputum [72,73]. Furthermore, FeNO can provide information on the asthmatic state that is consistent with other biomarkers for inflammation in asthma [74] and also decreases after treatment with inhaled corticosteroids [75,76]. The results found in this cluster suggest that the effects of interventions with omega-3 LCPUFAs on asthma-related outcomes are mediated by a decrease in airway immune cell infiltration and local inflammation. These anti-inflammatory effects of omega-3 LCPUFAs and their mediators, such as resolvins and protectins, are generally acknowledged and are in line with earlier findings [77]. Several findings in mouse models confirm the results of the studies described in this review. For example, a study in mice suggested that administration of resolvin E1 to an experimental asthma model resulted in an increased IFN-γ production and a decrease in the proinflammatory lipid mediator leukotriene B4 [78]. Leukotriene B4, as well as other leukotrienes, may be involved in immune cell recruitment in lung tissue of asthma patients [79,80]. Also, leukotriene B4 production in neutrophils was previously found to be reduced after human subjects were supplemented with omega-3 LCPUFA and omega-6 short-chain fatty acids [81]. Another study in Fat-1 transgenic mice, which can endogenously produce omega-3 from omega-6 fatty acids, showed that Fat-1 mice had decreased concentrations of Th2 cytokines IL-5 and IL-13 in their lung tissue as compared to wildtype mice [82]. In short, these results suggest that mediators of eicosapentaenoic acid (EPA) and docosahexaenoic acid (DHA) stimulate IFN-γ production by Th1 cells and inhibit the production of Th2 cytokines and other proinflammatory markers such as leukotrienes, at least in asthma conditions. This could ultimately lead to an inhibition of immune cell recruitment into the airways and therefore contribute to an improvement in asthma-related outcomes. However, not all omega-3 LCPUFA intervention studies in this review showed improvements in asthma-related outcomes that were mediated by the immune system. Strikingly, the three studies with the lowest daily doses of EPA and DHA were the studies that showed beneficial effects on asthma-related outcomes as well as immunological parameters. These studies used intakes between 120 and 300 mg/day. Additionally, one study using a daily dose of EPA and DHA of 630 mg only reported a decrease in FeNO concentrations, but not in asthma-related outcomes [58]. Studies using higher daily intakes of 780 mg or even 1200 mg did not report changes in asthma-related outcomes or in immunological parameters [55,57]. The Food and Agriculture Organisation/World Health Organization set an acceptable macronutrient distribution range for omega-3 LCPUFA between 250 and 2.000 mg/day [83]. Based on the results of this systematic review, asthma patients may benefit from the immunomodulatory effects of omega-3 LCPUFAs when doses on the lower side of this range are consumed. Regarding the effects of higher doses, Yin et al. (2009) showed that supplementing the diet of mice with high doses of fish oil (2% *w/w* and 4% *w/w*) increased the levels of Th2 cytokines IL-5 and IL-13 in lung tissue [84]. It is possible that this mechanism explains why the studies using higher doses of EPA and DHA described in this review did not find the improvements in asthma-related outcomes as observed with the lower doses. The underlying mechanism of the dose-response effect of omega-3 LCPUFAs in asthma patients should be explored further.

The least promising clusters were the supplement cluster, the vitamin D3 cluster and whole-food approaches. Since many different interventions were part of the supplement and whole-food approach clusters, we cannot conclude that these types of interventions will never affect asthma-related outcomes. For vitamin D3, the evidence remains contradictory. We found no indications that vitamin D3 is beneficial for asthma patients. However, future studies should take into account the vitamin D status at the start of the study, dose, timing of the dose (single dose versus multiple doses) and parameters that could be affected by vitamin D3, e.g., immune cells that express the vitamin D receptor.

The current GINA guidelines for asthma state that a diet high in fruit and vegetable intake, as well as weight loss, could improve asthma-related outcomes. Indeed, all interventions of the weight loss cluster had a positive effect on asthma-related outcomes and, more specifically, asthma control. This agrees with the systematic review of Okoniewski and colleagues, who reported that weight loss improved a variety of asthma-related outcomes [85]. However, these beneficial effects hardly coincided with improvements in the response of the immune system in our current review. An explanation for this could be that obesity-related asthma has lower eosinophilic inflammation compared to other phenotypes, and therefore the asthma-related changes after weight-loss were mediated by other mechanisms [86]. It has been suggested that adipokines such as leptin and adiponectin could be involved, which can directly affect airway reactivity [87]. Furthermore, two of the whole-food approaches targeted fruit and vegetable intake of asthma patients [62,63]. Only one of these studies, which used a high antioxidant diet, reported changes in asthma-related outcomes. None of these studies, unfortunately, reported changes in immunological parameters. The effect of fruit and vegetable intake on asthma has been described previously and indeed improved asthma-related outcomes, which has been attributed to their high anti-oxidant and fiber contents [18]. The high antioxidant capacity of fruit and vegetables, as well as the short-chain fatty acids formed from fiber by the microbiota have been suggested to reduce airway inflammation [18]. These suggestions are, unfortunately, not in accordance with the results of this review. However, the number of studies included in this review evaluating fruit and vegetable intake was limited, and these studies mainly addressed the short-term intake of fruits and vegetables. It remains unclear if fruit and vegetables may influence asthma-related outcomes via other routes than the immune system.

Finally, as shown in this review, studies using the same nutritional intervention do not always find similar effects on asthma-related outcomes and immunological parameters. This could be explained by several factors that influence the success of nutritional interventions in asthma patients in general. These factors that were unintendedly part of the study populations may certainly have influenced the interpretation of the results described. An example of such a factor is asthma severity at baseline. Scott and co-workers found that a 10-week weight loss intervention was more successful in participants with more severe asthma at baseline. They suggested that asthma severity could have been a motivator for this group of patients since the burden of the severity of asthma was a motivation for weight loss [88]. Moreover, nutritional status at the start of the intervention may influence the success of the nutritional intervention in asthma patients. Poor diet quality, which may lead to deficiencies of several micronutrients, has been associated with severe asthma [89]. Therefore, dietary interventions might be more successful in asthma patients that have deficiencies at baseline [16]. In addition, study duration could have influenced study outcomes. The studies in this review had durations varying from three days to one year but were, in general, relatively short (3–6 months). Therefore, we cannot exclude that longer-term nutritional interventions could result in more beneficial effects for asthma patients. Furthermore, pathophysiologic mechanisms differ between asthma endotypes [90], suggesting that characteristics of the study population (e.g., age, obesity) influence the success of nutritional interventions. We here show the data for the studies presented in this review did not suggest that the success of nutritional interventions was depended on age. However, other characteristics of the study population could have been of influence. Other examples are indications that vitamin C may be relevant in the prevention of viral-induced exacerbations [91], whereas weight loss interventions may be most relevant for the obesity-induced asthma phenotype [86]. Information on asthma phenotypes or endotypes was missing in many of the trials included in this review. A recommendation for future research is to provide this information since it is crucial in order to interpret the effect of nutritional interventions in asthma patients.

In summary, this review provides an overview of studies that examined nutritional interventions in asthma patients and reported changes in asthma-related outcomes as well as immunological parameters. Certain components from the herbs, herbal mixtures, and extract cluster, as well as the omega-3 LCPUFAs, are promising interventions in the context of improving asthma-related outcomes via immunomodulation. Only three interventions showed clinically relevant improvements. Future studies should now focus on how to optimize the beneficial effects of nutritional interventions in asthma patients, e.g., by considering the phenotypes and endotypes of asthma in the study population. The potential of these interventions and underlying pathways should be explored further before any of these interventions could be added to lifestyle guidelines for asthma patients.

Author Contributions: L.v.B., J.P. and R.P.M. interpreted the data and wrote the manuscript. L.v.B. and J.P. conducted the literature review. G.W. reviewed and edited the manuscript. All authors have read and approved the manuscript.

References

1. Global Asthma Network. *The Global Asthma Report 2018*; Global Asthma Network: Auckland, New Zealand, 2018.
2. Maslan, J.; Mims, J.W. What is asthma? Pathophysiology, demographics, and health care costs. *Otolaryngol. Clin. N. Am.* **2014**, *47*, 13–22. [CrossRef] [PubMed]
3. Global Initiative for Asthma. *Global Strategy for Asthma Management and Prevention, 2020*. 2020. Available online: www.ginasthma.org (accessed on 24 March 2020).
4. Amin, S.; Soliman, M.; McIvor, A.; Cave, A.; Cabrera, C. Understanding patient perspectives on medication adherence in asthma: A targeted review of qualitative studies. *Patient Prefer. Adherence* **2020**, *14*, 541–551. [CrossRef] [PubMed]
5. Bårnes, C.B.; Ulrik, C.S. Asthma and adherence to inhaled corticosteroids: Current status and future perspectives. *Respir. Care* **2015**, *60*, 455–468. [CrossRef] [PubMed]
6. Dahl, R. Systemic side effects of inhaled corticosteroids in patients with asthma. *Respir. Med.* **2006**, *100*, 1307–1317. [CrossRef]
7. Tattersall, M.C.; Guo, M.; Korcarz, C.E.; Gepner, A.D.; Kaufman, J.D.; Liu, K.J.; Barr, R.G.; Donohue, K.M.; McClelland, R.L.; Delaney, J.A. Asthma predicts cardiovascular disease events: The multi-ethnic study of atherosclerosis. *Arterioscler. Thromb. Vasc. Biol.* **2015**, *35*, 1520–1525. [CrossRef]
8. Schulze, M.B.; Martínez-González, M.A.; Fung, T.T.; Lichtenstein, A.H.; Forouhi, N.G. Food based dietary patterns and chronic disease prevention. *BMJ* **2018**, *361*, k2396. [CrossRef]
9. Minihane, A.M.; Vinoy, S.; Russell, W.R.; Baka, A.; Roche, H.M.; Tuohy, K.M.; Teeling, J.L.; Blaak, E.E.; Fenech, M.; Vauzour, D. Low-grade inflammation, diet composition and health: Current research evidence and its translation. *Br. J. Nutr.* **2015**, *114*, 999–1012. [CrossRef]
10. Mozaffarian, D. Dietary and policy priorities for cardiovascular disease, diabetes, and obesity: A comprehensive review. *Circulation* **2016**, *133*, 187–225. [CrossRef]
11. Rosato, V.; Temple, N.J.; La Vecchia, C.; Castellan, G.; Tavani, A.; Guercio, V. Mediterranean diet and cardiovascular disease: A systematic review and meta-analysis of observational studies. *Eur. J. Nutr.* **2019**, *58*, 173–191. [CrossRef]
12. Khan, S.U.; Khan, M.U.; Riaz, H.; Valavoor, S.; Zhao, D.; Vaughan, L.; Okunrintemi, V.; Riaz, I.B.; Khan, M.S.; Kaluski, E. Effects of nutritional supplements and dietary interventions on cardiovascular outcomes: An umbrella review and evidence map. *Ann. Intern. Med.* **2019**, *171*, 190–198. [CrossRef]
13. Aune, D.; Giovannucci, E.; Boffetta, P.; Fadnes, L.T.; Keum, N.; Norat, T.; Greenwood, D.C.; Riboli, E.; Vatten, L.J.; Tonstad, S. Fruit and vegetable intake and the risk of cardiovascular disease, total cancer and all-cause mortality—A systematic review and dose-response meta-analysis of prospective studies. *Int. J. Epidemiol.* **2017**, *46*, 1029–1056. [CrossRef] [PubMed]
14. Garcia-Larsen, V.; Del Giacco, S.R.; Moreira, A.; Bonini, M.; Charles, D.; Reeves, T.; Carlsen, K.H.; Haahtela, T.; Bonini, S.; Fonseca, J. Asthma and dietary intake: An overview of systematic reviews. *Allergy* **2016**, *71*, 433–442. [CrossRef]

15. Allan, K.; Devereux, G. Diet and asthma: Nutrition implications from prevention to treatment. *J. Am. Diet. Assoc.* **2011**, *111*, 258–268. [CrossRef] [PubMed]
16. Wang, M.; Liu, M.; Wang, C.; Xiao, Y.; An, T.; Zou, M.; Cheng, G. Association between vitamin D status and asthma control: A meta-analysis of randomized trials. *Respir. Med.* **2019**, *150*, 85–94. [CrossRef] [PubMed]
17. Miyata, J.; Arita, M. Role of omega-3 fatty acids and their metabolites in asthma and allergic diseases. *Allergol. Int.* **2015**, *64*, 27–34. [CrossRef] [PubMed]
18. Guilleminault, L.; Williams, E.J.; Scott, H.A.; Berthon, B.S.; Jensen, M.; Wood, L.G. Diet and asthma: Is it time to adapt our message? *Nutrients* **2017**, *9*, 1227. [CrossRef]
19. Chaudhuri, R.; Livingston, E.; McMahon, A.D.; Lafferty, J.; Fraser, I.; Spears, M.; McSharry, C.P.; Thomson, N.C. Effects of smoking cessation on lung function and airway inflammation in smokers with asthma. *Am. J. Respir. Crit. Care Med.* **2006**, *174*, 127–133. [CrossRef]
20. Jang, A.S.; Park, S.W.; Kim, D.J.; Uh, S.; Kim, Y.H.; Whang, H.G.; Lim, G.; Park, C.S. Effects of smoking cessation on airflow obstruction and quality of life in asthmatic smokers. *Allergy Asthma Immunol. Res.* **2010**, *2*, 254–259. [CrossRef]
21. Boulet, L.P.; Turcotte, H.; Martin, J.; Poirier, P. Effect of bariatric surgery on airway response and lung function in obese subjects with asthma. *Respir. Med.* **2012**, *106*, 651–660. [CrossRef]
22. Dixon, A.E.; Pratley, R.E.; Forgione, P.M.; Kaminsky, D.A.; Whittaker-Leclair, L.A.; Griffes, L.A.; Garudathri, J.; Raymond, D.; Poynter, M.E.; Bunn, J.Y. Effects of obesity and bariatric surgery on airway hyperresponsiveness, asthma control, and inflammation. *J. Allergy Clin. Immunol.* **2011**, *128*, 508–515.e502. [CrossRef]
23. Scott, H.A.; Gibson, P.G.; Garg, M.L.; Pretto, J.J.; Morgan, P.J.; Callister, R.; Wood, L.G. Dietary restriction and exercise improve airway inflammation and clinical outcomes in overweight and obese asthma: A randomized trial. *Clin. Exp. Allergy* **2013**, *43*, 36–49. [CrossRef] [PubMed]
24. Warburton, D.E.R.; Nicol, C.W.; Bredin, S.S.D. Health benefits of physical activity: The evidence. *CMAJ* **2006**, *174*, 801–809. [CrossRef] [PubMed]
25. Brown, D.R.; Carroll, D.D.; Workman, L.M.; Carlson, S.A.; Brown, D.W. Physical activity and health-related quality of life: US adults with and without limitations. *Qual. Life Res.* **2014**, *23*, 2673–2680. [CrossRef] [PubMed]
26. Lange, N.E.; Litonjua, A.; Hawrylowicz, C.M.; Weiss, S. Vitamin D, the immune system and asthma. *Expert Rev. Clin. Immunol.* **2009**, *5*, 693–702. [CrossRef]
27. Mann, E.H.; Chambers, E.S.; Pfeffer, P.E.; Hawrylowicz, C.M. Immunoregulatory mechanisms of vitamin D relevant to respiratory health and asthma. *Ann. N. Y. Acad. Sci.* **2014**, *1317*, 57–69. [CrossRef]
28. Moher, D.; Liberati, A.; Tetzlaff, J.; Altman, D.G. Preferred reporting items for systematic reviews and meta-analyses: The PRISMA statement. *Ann. Intern. Med.* **2009**, *151*, 264–269. [CrossRef]
29. Online Ruler on Screen Pixel Ruler. Available online: https://www.rapidtables.com/web/tools/pixel-ruler.html (accessed on 24 March 2020).
30. Ras, R.T.; Hiemstra, H.; Lin, Y.; Vermeer, M.A.; Duchateau, G.S.M.J.E.; Trautwein, E.A. Consumption of plant sterol-enriched foods and effects on plasma plant sterol concentrations—A meta-analysis of randomized controlled studies. *Atherosclerosis* **2013**, *230*, 336–346. [CrossRef]
31. Trabuco, E.C.; Moorman, P.G.; Algeciras-Schimnich, A.; Weaver, A.L.; Cliby, W.A. Association of ovary-sparing hysterectomy with ovarian reserve. *Obstet. Gynecol.* **2016**, *127*, 819–827. [CrossRef]
32. Meropol, S.B.; Metlay, J.P. Accuracy of pneumonia hospital admissions in a primary care electronic medical record database. *Pharmacoepidemiol. Drug Saf.* **2012**, *21*, 659–665. [CrossRef]
33. Jadad, A.R.; Moore, R.A.; Carroll, D.; Jenkinson, C.; Reynolds, D.J.M.; Gavaghan, D.J.; McQuay, H.J. Assessing the quality of reports of randomized clinical trials: Is blinding necessary? *Control. Clin. Trials* **1996**, *17*, 1–12. [CrossRef]
34. Barlianto, W.; Rachmawati, M.; Irawan, M.; Wulandari, D. Effects of Nigella sativa oil on Th1/Th2, cytokine balance, and improvement of asthma control in children. *Paediatr. Indones* **2017**, *57*, 223–228. [CrossRef]
35. Barlianto, W.; Wulandari, D.; Chusniyah, M.; Chandra Kusuma, H.M.S.; Prawiro, S.R. Improvement of Th17/Treg balance and asthma control test score by nigella sativa supplementation in asthmatic children: A new approach to managing asthma. *Turk. J. Immunol.* **2018**, *6*, 1–7. [CrossRef]
36. Hosseini, S.A.; Zilaee, M.; Shoushtari, M.H.; Ghasemi dehcheshmeh, M. An evaluation of the effect of saffron supplementation on the antibody titer to heat-shock protein (HSP) 70, hsCRP and spirometry test in patients with mild and moderate persistent allergic asthma: A triple-blind, randomized placebo-controlled trial. *Respir. Med.* **2018**, *145*, 28–34. [CrossRef] [PubMed]

37. Zilaee, M.; Hosseini, S.A.; Jafarirad, S.; Abolnezhadian, F.; Cheraghian, B.; Namjoyan, F.; Ghadiri, A. An evaluation of the effects of saffron supplementation on the asthma clinical symptoms and asthma severity in patients with mild and moderate persistent allergic asthma: A double-blind, randomized placebo-controlled trial. *Respir. Res.* **2019**, *20*, 39–49. [CrossRef] [PubMed]
38. Khayyal, M.T.; El-Ghazaly, M.A.; El-Khatib, A.S.; Hatem, A.M.; De Vries, P.J.F.; El-Shafei, S.; Khattab, M.M. A clinical pharmacological study of the potential beneficial effects of a propolis food product as an adjuvant in asthmatic patients. *Fundam. Clin. Pharmacol.* **2003**, *17*, 93–102. [CrossRef] [PubMed]
39. Koshak, A.; Wei, L.; Koshak, E.; Wali, S.; Alamoudi, O.; Demerdash, A.; Qutub, M.; Pushparaj, P.N.; Heinrich, M. Nigella Sativa supplementation improves asthma control and biomarkers: A randomized, double-blind, placebo-controlled trial. *Phytother. Res.* **2017**, *31*, 403–409. [CrossRef]
40. Salem, A.M.; Bamosa, A.O.; Qutub, H.O.; Gupta, R.K.; Badar, A.; Elnour, A.; Afzal, M.N. Effect of Nigella sativa supplementation on lung function and inflammatory mediatorsin partly controlled asthma: A randomized controlled trial. *Ann. Saudi Med.* **2017**, *37*, 64–71. [CrossRef]
41. Yugandhar, P.; Rao, K.M.; Sengupta, K. A novel herbal composition containing extracts of Boswellia serrata gum resin and Aegle marmelos fruit alleviates symptoms of asthma in a placebo controlled double-blind clinical study. *Phytother. Res.* **2017**, *32*, 140–150. [CrossRef]
42. Ghaffari, J.; Hossaini, R.F.; Khalilian, A.; Nahanmoghadam, N.; Salehifar, E.; Rafatpanah, H. Vitamin E supplementation, lung functions and clinical manifestations in children with moderate asthma: A randomized double blind placebo- Controlled trial. *Iran. J. Allergy Asthma Immunol.* **2014**, *13*, 98–103.
43. Pearson, P.J.; Lewis, S.A.; Britton, J.; Fogarty, A. Vitamin E supplements in asthma: A parallel group randomised placebo controlled trial. *Thorax* **2004**, *59*, 652–656. [CrossRef]
44. Smith, L.J.; Kalhan, R.; Wise, R.A.; Sugar, E.A.; Lima, J.J.; Irvin, C.G.; Dozor, A.J.; Holbrook, J.T.; Hanania, N.; Sockrider, M.; et al. Effect of a soy isoflavone supplement on lung function and clinical outcomes in patients with poorly controlled asthma: A randomized clinical trial. *JAMA* **2015**, *313*, 2033–2043. [CrossRef] [PubMed]
45. Wood, L.G.; Garg, M.L.; Powell, H.; Gibson, P.G. Lycopene-rich treatments modify noneosinophilic airway inflammation in asthma: Proof of concept. *Free Radic. Res.* **2008**, *42*, 94–102. [CrossRef] [PubMed]
46. Dias-Junior, S.A.; Reis, M.; de Carvalho-Pinto, R.M.; Stelmach, R.; Halpern, A.; Cukier, A. Effects of weight loss on asthma control in obese patients with severe asthma. *Eur. Respir. J.* **2014**, *43*, 1368–1377. [CrossRef] [PubMed]
47. Jensen, M.E.; Gibson, P.G.; Collins, C.E.; Hilton, J.M.; Wood, L.G. Diet-induced weight loss in obese children with asthma: A randomized controlled trial. *Clin. Exp. Allergy* **2013**, *43*, 775–784. [CrossRef]
48. Toennesen, L.L.; Meteran, H.; Hostrup, M.; Wium Geiker, N.R.; Jensen, C.B.; Porsbjerg, C.; Astrup, A.; Bangsbo, J.; Parker, D.; Backer, V. Effects of exercise and diet in nonobese asthma patients—A randomized controlled trial. *J. Allergy Clin. Immunol. Pract.* **2018**, *6*, 803–811. [CrossRef]
49. Bar Yoseph, R.; Livnat, G.; Schnapp, Z.; Hakim, F.; Dabbah, H.; Goldbart, A.; Bentur, L. The effect of vitamin D on airway reactivity and inflammation in asthmatic children: A double-blind placebo-controlled trial. *Pediatr. Pulmonol.* **2015**, *50*, 747–753. [CrossRef]
50. Castro, M.; King, T.S.; Kunselman, S.J.; Cabana, M.D.; Denlinger, L.; Holguin, F.; Kazani, S.D.; Moore, W.C.; Moy, J.; Sorkness, C.A. Effect of vitamin D3 on asthma treatment failures in adults with symptomatic asthma and lower vitamin D levels: The VIDA randomized clinical trial. *JAMA* **2014**, *311*, 2083–2091. [CrossRef]
51. De Groot, J.C.; Van Roon, E.N.H.; Storm, H.; Veeger, N.J.G.M.; Zwinderman, A.H.; Hiemstra, P.S.; Bel, E.H.D.; Ten Brinke, A. Vitamin D reduces eosinophilic airway inflammation in nonatopic asthma. *J. Allergy Clin. Immunol.* **2015**, *135*, 670–675.e673. [CrossRef]
52. Kerley, C.P.; Hutchinson, K.; Cormican, L.; Faul, J.; Greally, P.; Coghlan, D.; Elnazir, B. Vitamin D3 for uncontrolled childhood asthma: A pilot study. *Pediatr. Allergy Immunol.* **2016**, *27*, 404–412. [CrossRef]
53. Martineau, A.R.; MacLaughlin, B.D.; Hooper, R.L.; Barnes, N.C.; Jolliffe, D.A.; Greiller, C.L.; Kilpin, K.; McLaughlin, D.; Fletcher, G.; Mein, C.A.; et al. Double-blind randomised placebo-controlled trial of bolus-dose vitamin D3 supplementation in adults with asthma (ViDiAs). *Thorax* **2015**, *70*, 451–457. [CrossRef]
54. Emelyanov, A.; Fedoseev, G.; Krasnoschekova, O.; Abulimity, A.; Trendeleva, T.; Barnes, P.J. Treatment of asthma with lipid extract of New Zealand green-lipped mussel: A randomised clinical trial. *Eur. Respir. J.* **2002**, *20*, 596–600. [CrossRef] [PubMed]
55. Hodge, L.; Salome, C.M.; Hughes, J.M.; Liu-Brennan, D.; Rimmer, J.; Allman, M.; Pang, D.; Armour, C.; Woolcock, A.J. Effect of dietary intake of omega-3 and omega-6 fatty acids on severity of asthma in children. *Eur. Respir. J.* **1998**, *11*, 361–365. [CrossRef] [PubMed]

56. Mickleborough, T.D.; Vaughn, C.L.; Shei, R.J.; Davis, E.M.; Wilhite, D.P. Marine lipid fraction PCSO-524TM (lyprinol/omega XL) of the New Zealand green lipped mussel attenuates hyperpnea-induced bronchoconstriction in asthma. *Respir. Med.* **2013**, *107*, 1152–1163. [CrossRef] [PubMed]
57. Moreira, A.; Moreira, P.; Delgado, L.; Fonseca, J.; Teixeira, V.; Padrao, P.; Castel-Branco, G. Pilot study of the effects of n-3 polyunsaturated fatty acids on exhaled nitric oxide in patients with stable asthma. *J. Investig. Allergol. Clin. Immunol.* **2007**, *17*, 309–313. [PubMed]
58. Schubert, R.; Kitz, R.; Beermann, C.; Rose, M.A.; Lieb, A.; Sommerer, P.C.; Moskovits, J.; Alberternst, H.; Bohles, H.J.; Schulze, J.; et al. Effect of n-3 polyunsaturated fatty acids in asthma after low-dose allergen challenge. *Int. Arch. Allergy Immunol.* **2009**, *148*, 321–329. [CrossRef] [PubMed]
59. Bseikri, M.; McCann, J.C.; Lal, A.; Fong, E.; Graves, K.; Goldrich, A.; Block, D.; Gildengoren, G.L.; Mietus-Snyder, M.; Shigenaga, M.; et al. A novel nutritional intervention improves lung function in overweight/obese adolescents with poorly controlled asthma: The Supplemental Nutrition in Asthma Control (SNAC) pilot study. *FASEB J.* **2018**, *32*, 6643–6654. [CrossRef]
60. Papamichael, M.M.; Katsardis, C.; Lambert, K.; Tsoukalas, D.; Koutsilieris, M.; Erbas, B.; Itsiopoulos, C. Efficacy of a Mediterranean diet supplemented with fatty fish in ameliorating inflammation in paediatric asthma: A randomised controlled trial. *J. Hum. Nutr. Diet.* **2019**, *32*, 185–197. [CrossRef]
61. Sexton, P.; Black, P.; Metcalf, P.; Wall, C.R.; Ley, S.; Wu, L.; Sommerville, F.; Brodie, S.; Kolbe, J. Influence of mediterranean diet on asthma symptoms, lung function, and systemic inflammation: A randomized controlled trial. *J. Asthma* **2013**, *50*, 75–81. [CrossRef]
62. Sudini, K.; Diette, G.B.; Breysse, P.N.; McCormack, M.C.; Bull, D.; Biswal, S.; Zhai, S.; Brereton, N.; Peng, R.D.; Matsui, E.C. A randomized controlled trial of the effect of broccoli sprouts on antioxidant gene expression and airway inflammation in asthmatics. *J. Allergy Clin. Immunol. Pract.* **2016**, *4*, 932–940. [CrossRef]
63. Wood, L.G.; Garg, M.L.; Smart, J.M.; Scott, H.A.; Barker, D.; Gibson, P.G. Manipulating antioxidant intake in asthma: A randomized controlled trial. *Am. J. Clin. Nutr.* **2012**, *96*, 534–543. [CrossRef]
64. Balaha, M.F.; Tanaka, H.; Yamashita, H.; Rahman, M.N.A.; Inagaki, N. Oral Nigella sativa oil ameliorates ovalbumin-induced bronchial asthma in mice. *Int. Immunopharmacol.* **2012**, *14*, 224–231. [CrossRef] [PubMed]
65. Iwamoto, I.; Nakajima, H.; Endo, H.; Yoshida, S. Interferon gamma regulates antigen-induced eosinophil recruitment into the mouse airways by inhibiting the infiltration of CD4+ T cells. *J. Exp. Med.* **1993**, *177*, 573–576. [CrossRef] [PubMed]
66. Mehta, A.A.; Mahajan, S. Role of cytokines in pathophysiology of asthma. *Iran. J. Pharmacol. Ther.* **2006**, *5*, 1–14.
67. Keyhanmanesh, R.; Boskabady, M.H.; Khamneh, S.; Doostar, Y. Effect of thymoquinone on the lung pathology and cytokine levels of ovalbumin-sensitized guinea pigs. *Pharmacol. Rep.* **2010**, *62*, 910–916. [CrossRef]
68. Rana Keyhanmanesh, L.P.; Omrani, H.; Mirzamohammadi, Z.; Shahbazfar, A.A. The effect of single dose of thymoquinone, the main constituents of Nigella sativa, in guinea pig model of asthma. *BioImpacts* **2014**, *4*, 75–81.
69. Xiong, Y.; Wang, J.; Yu, H.; Zhang, X.; Miao, C. Anti-asthma potential of crocin and its effect on MAPK signaling pathway in a murine model of allergic airway disease. *Immunopharmacol. Immunotoxicol.* **2015**, *37*, 236–243. [CrossRef]
70. Noorbakhsh, M.F.; Shaterzadeh-Yazdi, H.; Hayati, F.; Samarghandian, S.; Farkhondeh, T. Protective effects of thymoquinon on pulmonary disorders in experimental studies. *Tanaffos* **2018**, *17*, 211–222.
71. Pashirzad, M.; Shafiee, M.; Avan, A.; Ryzhikov, M.; Fiuji, H.; Bahreyni, A.; Khazaei, M.; Soleimanpour, S.; Hassanian, S.M. Therapeutic potency of crocin in the treatment of inflammatory diseases: Current status and perspective. *J. Cell. Physiol.* **2019**, *234*, 14601–14611. [CrossRef]
72. Berry, M.A.; Shaw, D.E.; Green, R.H.; Brightling, C.E.; Wardlaw, A.J.; Pavord, I.D. The use of exhaled nitric oxide concentration to identify eosinophilic airway inflammation: An observational study in adults with asthma. *Clin. Exp. Allergy* **2005**, *35*, 1175–1179. [CrossRef]
73. Fireman, E.; Shtark, M.; Priel, I.E.; Shiner, R.; Mor, R.; Kivity, S.; Fireman, Z. Hydrogen peroxide in exhaled breath condensate (EBC) vs eosinophil count in induced sputum (IS) in parenchymal vs. airways lung diseases. *Inflammation* **2007**, *30*, 44–51. [CrossRef]
74. Strunk, R.C.; Szefler, S.J.; Phillips, B.R.; Zeiger, R.S.; Chinchilli, V.M.; Larsen, G.; Hodgdon, K.; Morgan, W.; Sorkness, C.A.; Lemanske, R.F., Jr. Relationship of exhaled nitric oxide to clinical and inflammatory markers of persistent asthma in children. *J. Allergy Clin. Immunol.* **2003**, *112*, 883–892. [CrossRef] [PubMed]
75. Kharitonov, S.A.; Yates, D.H.; Barnes, P.J. Inhaled glucocorticoids decrease nitric oxide in exhaled air of asthmatic patients. *Am. J. Respir. Crit. Care Med.* **1996**, *153*, 454–457. [CrossRef] [PubMed]

76. Silkoff, P.E.; McClean, P.; Spino, M.; Erlich, L.A.; Slutsky, A.S.; Zamel, N. Dose-response relationship and reproducibility of the fall in exhaled nitric oxide after inhaled beclomethasone dipropionate therapy in asthma patients. *Chest* **2001**, *119*, 1322–1328. [CrossRef]
77. Calder, P.C. Marine omega-3 fatty acids and inflammatory processes: Effects, mechanisms and clinical relevance. *Biochim. Biophys. Acta Mol. Cell. Biol. Lipids* **2015**, *1851*, 469–484. [CrossRef]
78. Haworth, O.; Cernadas, M.; Yang, R.; Serhan, C.N.; Levy, B.D. Resolvin E1 regulates interleukin 23, interferon-γ and lipoxin A 4 to promote the resolution of allergic airway inflammation. *Nat. Immunol.* **2008**, *9*, 873–879. [CrossRef] [PubMed]
79. Ohnishi, H.; Miyahara, N.; Gelfand, E.W. The role of leukotriene B4 in allergic diseases. *Allergol. Int.* **2008**, *57*, 291–298. [CrossRef]
80. Yates, C.M.; Calder, P.C.; Rainger, G.E. Pharmacology and therapeutics of omega-3 polyunsaturated fatty acids in chronic inflammatory disease. *Pharmacol. Ther.* **2014**, *141*, 272–282. [CrossRef]
81. Weaver, K.L.; Ivester, P.; Seeds, M.; Case, L.D.; Arm, J.P.; Chilton, F.H. Effect of dietary fatty acids on inflammatory gene expression in healthy humans. *J. Biol. Chem.* **2009**, *284*, 15400–15407. [CrossRef]
82. Bilal, S.; Haworth, O.; Wu, L.; Weylandt, K.H.; Levy, B.D.; Kang, J.X. Fat-1 transgenic mice with elevated omega-3 fatty acids are protected from allergic airway responses. *Biochim. Biophys. Acta Mol. Basis Dis.* **2011**, *1812*, 1164–1169. [CrossRef]
83. FAO/WHO. *Expert Consultation on Fats and Fatty Acids in Human Nutrition: Fats and Fatty Acids in Human Nutrition: Report of an Expert Consultation, 10–14 November 2008, Geneva*; Food and Agriculture Organization of the United Nations: Rome, Italy, 2010.
84. Yin, H.; Liu, W.; Goleniewska, K.; Porter, N.A.; Morrow, J.D.; Peebles, R.S., Jr. Dietary supplementation of ω-3 fatty acid-containing fish oil suppresses F2-isoprostanes but enhances inflammatory cytokine response in a mouse model of ovalbumin-induced allergic lung inflammation. *Free Radic. Biol. Med.* **2009**, *47*, 622–628. [CrossRef]
85. Okoniewski, W.; Lu, K.D.; Forno, E. Weight loss for children and adults with obesity and asthma. A systematic review of randomized controlled trials. *Ann. Am. Thorc. Soc.* **2019**, *16*, 613–625. [CrossRef] [PubMed]
86. Farzan, S. The asthma phenotype in the obese: Distinct or otherwise? *J. Allergy* **2013**, *2013*. [CrossRef]
87. Sideleva, O.; Suratt, B.T.; Black, K.E.; Tharp, W.G.; Pratley, R.E.; Forgione, P.; Dienz, O.; Irvin, C.G.; Dixon, A.E. Obesity and asthma: An inflammatory disease of adipose tissue not the airway. *Am. J. Respir. Crit. Care Med.* **2012**, *186*, 598–605. [CrossRef] [PubMed]
88. Scott, H.A.; Gibson, P.G.; Garg, M.L.; Pretto, J.J.; Morgan, P.J.; Callister, R.; Wood, L.G. Determinants of weight loss success utilizing a meal replacement plan and/or exercise, in overweight and obese adults with asthma. *Respirology* **2015**, *20*, 243–250. [CrossRef] [PubMed]
89. Berthon, B.S.; Macdonald-Wicks, L.K.; Gibson, P.G.; Wood, L.G. Investigation of the association between dietary intake, disease severity and airway inflammation in asthma. *Respirology* **2013**, *18*, 447–454. [CrossRef]
90. Kuruvilla, M.E.; Lee, F.E.H.; Lee, G.B. Understanding asthma phenotypes, endotypes, and mechanisms of disease. *Clin. Rev. Allergy Immunol.* **2019**, *56*, 219–233. [CrossRef]
91. Han, Y.Y.; Forno, E.; Holguin, F.; Celedón, J.C. Diet and asthma: An update. *Curr. Opin. Allergy Clin. Immunol.* **2015**, *15*, 369–374. [CrossRef]

2

Vitamin C—An Adjunctive Therapy for Respiratory Infection, Sepsis and COVID-19

Patrick Holford [1,*], Anitra C. Carr [2], Thomas H. Jovic [3,4], Stephen R. Ali [3,4], Iain S. Whitaker [3,4], Paul E. Marik [5] and A. David Smith [6]

1 Institute for Optimum Nutrition, Ambassador House, Richmond TW9 1SQ, UK
2 Nutrition in Medicine Research Group, Department of Pathology & Biomedical Science, University of Otago, Christchurch 8140, New Zealand; anitra.carr@otago.ac.nz
3 Reconstructive Surgery & Regenerative Medicine Research Group, Institute of Life Sciences, Swansea University Medical School, Swansea University, Swansea SA2 8PY, UK; Thomas.Jovic@wales.nhs.uk (T.H.J.); Stephen.Ali@wales.nhs.uk (S.R.A.); Iain.Whitaker@wales.nhs.uk (I.S.W.)
4 Welsh Centre for Burns & Plastic Surgery, Morriston Hospital, Swansea SA6 6NL, UK
5 Division of Pulmonary and Critical Care Medicine, Eastern Virginia Medical School, Norfolk, VA 23507, USA; marikpe@evms.edu
6 Department of Pharmacology, University of Oxford, Oxford OX1 3QT, UK; david.smith@pharm.ox.ac.uk
* Correspondence: pat@patrickholford.com

Abstract: There are limited proven therapies for COVID-19. Vitamin C's antioxidant, anti-inflammatory and immunomodulating effects make it a potential therapeutic candidate, both for the prevention and amelioration of COVID-19 infection, and as an adjunctive therapy in the critical care of COVID-19. This literature review focuses on vitamin C deficiency in respiratory infections, including COVID-19, and the mechanisms of action in infectious disease, including support of the stress response, its role in preventing and treating colds and pneumonia, and its role in treating sepsis and COVID-19. The evidence to date indicates that oral vitamin C (2–8 g/day) may reduce the incidence and duration of respiratory infections and intravenous vitamin C (6–24 g/day) has been shown to reduce mortality, intensive care unit (ICU) and hospital stays, and time on mechanical ventilation for severe respiratory infections. Further trials are urgently warranted. Given the favourable safety profile and low cost of vitamin C, and the frequency of vitamin C deficiency in respiratory infections, it may be worthwhile testing patients' vitamin C status and treating them accordingly with intravenous administration within ICUs and oral administration in hospitalised persons with COVID-19.

Keywords: COVID-19; SARS-CoV-2; coronavirus; vitamin C; ascorbate; colds; pneumonia; sepsis; immunonutrition; supplementation

1. Introduction

Vitamin C, ascorbic acid, is an essential water-soluble nutrient. It is synthesised in plants from fructose and in almost all animals from glucose. It is not synthesised by primates, most bats, guinea pigs, and a small number of birds and fish since the final enzyme, gulonolactone oxidase (GULO), required for ascorbic acid synthesis is missing due to gene mutations that occurred prior to the evolution of Homo sapiens [1]. All these species are therefore dependent on vitamin C in their food. Primates are dependent on an adequate supply provided by fruits and vegetation intake ranging from 4.5 g/day for gorillas [2] to 600 mg/day for smaller monkeys (7.5 kg—a tenth of human size) [3].

The EU Average Requirement of 90 mg/day for men and 80 mg/day for women is to maintain a normal plasma level of 50 μmol/L [4], which is the mean plasma level in UK adults [5]. This is sufficient to prevent scurvy but may be inadequate when a person is under viral exposure and physiological stress. An expert panel in cooperation with the Swiss Society of Nutrition recommended that everyone supplement with 200 mg "to fill the nutrient gap for the general population and especially for the adults age 65 and older. This supplement is targeted to strengthen the immune system" [6]. The Linus Pauling Institute recommends 400 mg for older adults (>50 years old) [7].

Pharmacokinetic studies in healthy volunteers support a 200 mg daily dose to produce a plasma level of circa 70 to 90 μmol/L [8,9]. Complete plasma saturation occurs between 1 g daily and 3 g every four hours, being the highest tolerated oral dose, giving a predicted peak plasma concentration of circa 220 μmol/L [10]. The same dose given intravenously raises plasma vitamin C levels approximately ten-fold. Higher intakes of vitamin C are likely to be needed during viral infections with 2–3 g/day required to maintain normal plasma levels between 60 and 80 μmol/L [11,12]. Whether higher plasma levels have additional benefit is yet to be determined, but would be consistent with the results of the clinical trials discussed in this review.

2. Vitamin C Deficiency in Pneumonia, Sepsis and COVID-19

Human plasma vitamin C levels decline rapidly under conditions of physiological stress including infection, trauma, and surgery, not uncommonly resulting in overt vitamin C deficiency in hospitalised patients, defined as a plasma level of vitamin C ≤ 11 μmol/L [13–18]. Two studies in hospitals in Paris reported that 17 to 44% of patients had vitamin C plasma levels less than ≤ 11 μmol/L [14,15]. In a Canadian university hospital, it was found that 19% of patients had vitamin C plasma levels ≤ 11 μmol/L [16]. In a study of surgical patients in Australia, it was found that 21% had vitamin C plasma levels ≤ 11 μmol/L [17]. A survey of elderly Scottish patients hospitalised as a consequence of acute respiratory infections reported that 35% of patients had vitamin C plasma levels ≤ 11 μmol/L [18]. The UK's National Diet and Nutrition Survey, based on a cross section of the UK population, reports that 4% of 65+ year olds and 40% of those institutionalised in care homes have vitamin C levels ≤ 11 μmol/L [5,19], indicating the way in which older people with low vitamin C status may be especially susceptible to critical infection.

The vitamin C-deficiency disease scurvy has long been associated with pneumonia which led to the view that vitamin C may influence susceptibility to respiratory infections [20]. In other words, people deficient in vitamin C may be more susceptible to severe respiratory infections such as pneumonia. A prospective study of 19,357 men and women followed over 20 years found that people in the top quartiles of baseline plasma vitamin C concentrations had a 30% lower risk of pneumonia [21]. Furthermore, meta-analysis has indicated a reduction in the risk of pneumonia with oral vitamin C supplementation, particularly in individuals with low dietary intakes [22].

Post-mortem investigations of severe COVID-19 have demonstrated a secondary organising pneumonia phenomenon [23]; therefore, studies investigating vitamin C in relation to pneumonia may be relevant [18,24–27] (Table 1). The most recent study, from New Zealand, reported that patients with pneumonia had depleted vitamin C levels compared with healthy controls (23 μmol/L vs. 56 μmol/L, $p < 0.001$). The pneumonia cohort comprised 62% with hypovitaminosis C and 22% with vitamin C ≤ 11 μmol/L, compared with 8% hypovitaminosis C and no cases with ≤11μmol/L in the healthy controls [24]. The more severely ill patients in the ICU had mean vitamin C levels of 11 μmol/L. Similar findings have been reported in other studies of critically ill septic patients [28–33] (Table 1). A New Zealand study of patients with sepsis found that 40% had vitamin C ≤ 11 μmol/L and the majority of the patients had hypovitaminosis C (serum level < 23 μmol/L), despite receiving recommended enteral and parenteral intakes of the vitamin [29].

Table 1. Vitamin C status of patients with pneumonia, sepsis and severe COVID-19.

Study Type	Cohort	Vitamin C (μmol/L) (% Deficient, % Hypovitaminosis C)	Refs.
Pneumonia			
Case control	Healthy volunteers (n = 50)	56 ± 2 [a] (0% [b], 8% [c])	[24]
	Community-acquired pneumonia (n = 50)	23 ± 3 (22%, 62%)	
Case control	Healthy volunteers (n = 20)	66 ± 3	[25]
	Pneumonia cases (n = 11)	31 ± 9	
Case control	Healthy participants (n = 28)	49 ± 1	[26]
	Lobular pneumonia (n = 35):		
	Acute—did not survive (n = 7)	17 ± 1	
	Acute—survived (n = 15)	24 ± 1	
	Convalescent cases (n = 13)	34 ± 1	
Intervention (placebo group)	Pneumonia/bronchitis (n = 29):		[18]
	Week 0	24 ± 5 (40%) [b]	
	Week 2	19 ± 3 (37%)	
	Week 4	24 ± 6 (25%)	
Intervention (control group)	Pneumonia cases (n = 70):		[27]
	Day 0	41	
	Day 5–10	23–24	
	Day 15–20	32–35	
	Day 30	39	
Sepsis			
Intervention (baseline)	Sepsis with ARDS (n = 83):		[28]
	Day 0	22 (11–37) [d]	
	Day 2	23 (9–37)	
	Day 4	26 (9–41)	
	Day 7	29 (12–39)	
Observational	Septic shock patients (n = 24)	15 ± 2 (38% [b], 88% [c])	[29]
Intervention (baseline)	Severe sepsis patients (n = 24)	18 ± 2	[30]
Case control	Healthy controls (n = 6)	48 ± 6	[31]
	Severe sepsis (n = 19)	14 ± 3	
	Septic shock (n = 37)	14 ± 3	
Case control	Healthy controls (n = 14)	76 ± 6	[32]
	Septic encephalopathy (n = 11)	19 ± 11	
Case control	Healthy controls (n = 34)	62 (55–72) [d]	[33]
	ICU (injury, surgery, sepsis) (n = 62)	11 (8–22)	
Severe COVID-19			
Observational	Critically ill COVID-19 (n = 21)	22 ± 4 (45% [b], 70% [c]) [e]	[34]
	Survivors (n = 11)	29 ± 7 (40%, 50%)	
	Non-survivors (n = 10)	15 ± 2 (50%, 90%)	
Observational	COVID-associated ARDS (n = 18)	17 with <9 μmol/L	[35]
		1 with 14 μmol/L	

[a]—Data represent mean and SEM; [d]—median (and interquartile range); [b]—Percentage of patients with vitamin C deficiency (<11 μmol/L); [c]—Percentage of patients with hypovitaminosis C (<23 μmol/L); [e]—Personal communication (Cristian Arvinte, North Suburban Medical Center, Thornton, CO, USA). COVID—coronavirus disease; ICU—intensive care unit; ARDS—acute respiratory distress syndrome. A part of this table has been reproduced from [36].

As yet, there have been few studies reporting the vitamin C status of patients with COVID-19 (Table 1). A study of 21 critically ill COVID-19 patients admitted to ICU in the US found a mean level of 22 μmol/L, thus a majority had hypovitaminosis C. The mean level for 11 survivors was 29 μmol/L compared to 15 μmol/L for the 10 non-survivors; of these five (50%) had ≤11 μmol/L [34]. A study in an ICU in Barcelona of 18 COVID-19 patients meeting acute respiratory distress syndrome (ARDS) criteria found that 17 had undetectable levels of vitamin C (i.e., <9 μmol/L) and one patient had a low vitamin C (14 μmol/L) [35]. Thus, low vitamin C levels are common in critically ill hospitalised patients with respiratory infections, pneumonia, sepsis and COVID-19, the most likely explanation being increased metabolic consumption [37].

3. Mechanisms of Action of Vitamin C in Infections, Sepsis and COVID-19

Vitamin C has important anti-inflammatory, immunomodulating, antioxidant, antithrombotic and antiviral properties [38–40]. The vitamin demonstrates direct virucidal activity and has effector mechanisms in both the innate and adaptive immune systems [41–44]. The effects of vitamin C on immunity during infection are many and include the development and maturation of T-lymphocytes and the functions of phagocytosis and chemotaxis of leucocytes [45]. It also has a vital role as an antioxidant whereby phagocytes import oxidised vitamin C (dehydroascorbic acid) and regenerate it to reduced vitamin C (ascorbic acid) [46,47].

Importantly, and with specific reference to the critical phase of COVID-19, vitamin C contributes to the downregulation of cytokines, protecting the endothelium from oxidant injury and has an essential role in tissue repair [48,49]. The interaction between oxidative stress and the induction of genes integral to the inflammatory response, including TNFα, IL-1, IL-8, and ICAM-1 has been shown to be mediated through activation of NF-κB [50]. Vitamin C lessens reactive oxidative species (ROS) and inflammation via attenuation of NF-κB activation [51]. Vitamin C significantly increases superoxide dismutase, catalase and glutathione and decreases serum TNFα and IL-1β levels in a rat ARDS model [52]. These effects of vitamin C may be due to its epigenetic regulation of various genes, i.e., upregulation of antioxidant proteins and downregulation of proinflammatory cytokines, rather than its direct scavenging of oxidants.

While SARS-CoV-2 downregulates the expression of type-1 interferons (the host's primary anti-viral defence mechanism) [53], vitamin C upregulates these key host defence proteins [40]. In GULO knockout mice, vitamin C shows in vivo anti-viral immune responses and a reduction in viral titres in the lung in the early stage of infection, especially against influenza virus, through increased production of interferon [54]. Animal studies show that vitamin C reduces the incidence and severity of bacterial and viral infections [55], including increased resistance of chick embryo tracheal organ cultures to coronavirus infection and protection of broiler chicks against avian coronavirus [56,57].

Based on the identification of ACE2 as the receptor for SARS-CoV-2 entry, there is a hypothesis that the increased risk of severe COVID-19 is a function of upregulated ACE2, as is found in the co-morbidities of diabetes, cardiovascular disease and hypertension [58]. The SARS-CoV-2 spike glycoprotein is able to bind to ACE2 [59]. It is noteworthy that, in human arterial endothelial cells, vitamin C abolished ACE2 upregulation induced by IL-7 [60].

Although there are many potential targets for vitamin C in the process of infection, viral replication and pathology in COVID-19, it is noteworthy that a key protease in the virus, Mpro, whose function is to activate several viral non-structural proteins, has been proposed as a target. In a modelling study using the crystal structure of Mpro, the active site of this enzyme was found to bind magnesium ascorbate, which had the strongest binding out of 106 nutraceuticals. The authors suggested that ascorbate might, therefore, be a powerful inhibitor of the enzyme [61].

The critical and often fatal phase of COVID-19, primarily triggered by the host's reaction to dead virus particles, occurs with increased production of potent proinflammatory cytokines and chemokines, resulting in the development of multi-organ failure [62]. This may result in neutrophil migration and accumulation in the lung interstitium and bronchoalveolar space and is considered a key determinant of progression of ARDS [63]. Neutrophil extracellular trap formation (NETosis) is a cell death pathway different from apoptosis and necrosis that traps and inactivates pathogens [64]. This is a maladaptive response that may contribute to tissue and organ damage leading to organ failure. Vitamin C deficiency in GULO-knockout mice showed enhanced NETosis in the lungs of septic animals and increased circulating cell-free DNA suggesting that vitamin C is a novel regulator of NETosis [65]. Furthermore, vitamin C enhances lung epithelial barrier function in an animal model of sepsis by promoting epigenetic and transcriptional expression of protein-channels at the alveolar capillary membrane that regulate alveolar fluid clearance which include cystic fibrosis transmembrane conductance regulator, aquaporin-5, the Na^+/K^+-ATPase pump and epithelial sodium channel [66].

There is also increasing evidence that vitamin C, which is a pleiotropic stress hormone, may be playing a critical role in mediating the adrenocortical stress response, particularly in sepsis [38]. Vitamin C concentrations are three to ten times higher in the adrenal glands than in any other organ [67]. It is released from the adrenal cortex under conditions of physiological stress (ACTH stimulation), including viral exposure, raising plasma levels fivefold [68]. Vitamin C enhances cortisol production and potentiates the anti-inflammatory and endothelial cytoprotective effects of glucocorticoids [69,70]. Exogenous glucocorticoid steroids are the only proven disease-modifying treatment for COVID-19 [71]. The postulated mechanisms for vitamin C's amelioration of COVID-19 pathology are shown in Figure 1.

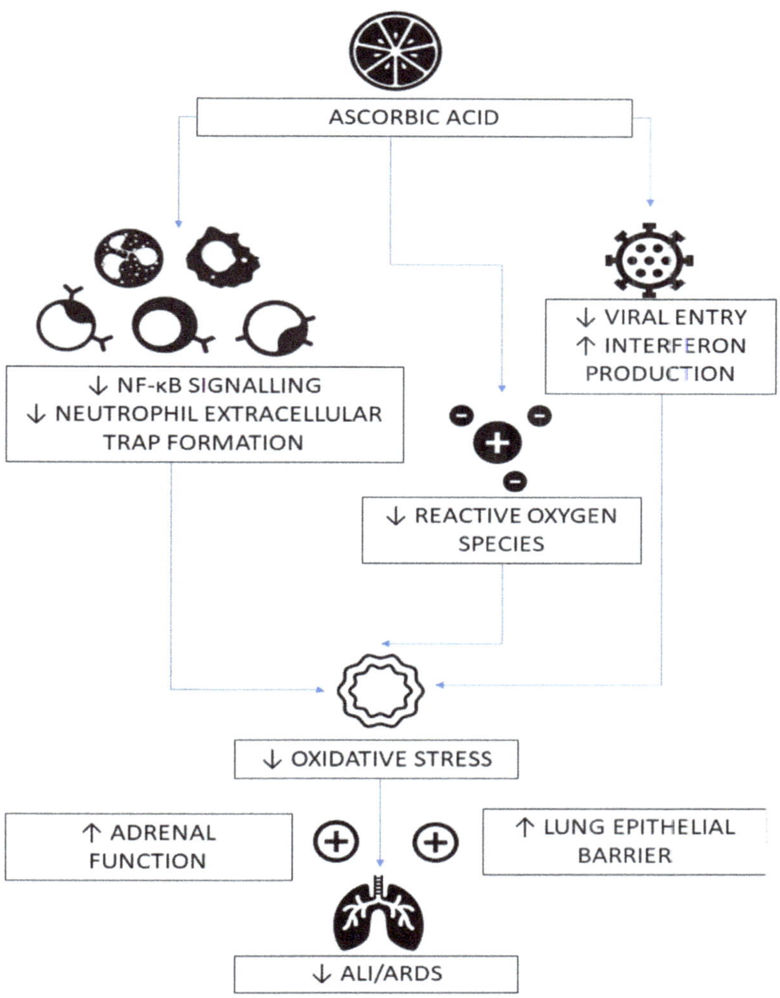

Figure 1. Postulated mechanisms for vitamin C's amelioration of COVID-19 pathology. ↓—decreased; ↑—increased; ALI—acute lung injury; ARDS—acute respiratory distress syndrome; NF-κB—nuclear factor kappa B.

4. Clinical Evidence for the Role of Vitamin C in Colds

Nobel laureate Linus Pauling concluded from randomised controlled trials (RCTs) that vitamin C prevented and alleviated colds thus popularising its use in the 1970s [72,73]. A Cochrane Review of placebo-controlled trials giving oral vitamin C for preventing and treating colds found that supplementation above 200 mg did not reduce the incidence in the general population [74]. However, in five trials involving a total of 598 marathon runners, skiers and soldiers on subarctic exercises vitamin C reduced the incidence of colds by 52% ($p < 0.0001$) [74]. Based on these findings, vitamin C appears to influence resistance to viral infections in special conditions, such as during brief periods of severe physical exercise.

Whereas trials where vitamin C has been administered only after the onset of symptoms have not shown consistent benefits, trials which regularly administered vitamin C reduced the duration of infections in adults by 8% and in children by 14%, with an apparent dose-dependency up to 6–8 g/day [55,74]. In children, 1 to 2 g/day vitamin C reduced cold duration by 18%, with the severity of colds being reduced by regular administration [74].

The latest UK placebo-controlled trial illustrates the meaningful clinical difference between the number of colds, cold duration and severity [75]. This trial comprised 168 volunteers who were randomised to receive a placebo or vitamin C (2 × 500 mg daily) over a 60-day winter period. The vitamin C group had fewer colds (37 vs. 50, $p = 0.05$), and even fewer virally challenged 'cold' days (85 vs. 178, $p = 0.03$) and a shorter duration of severe symptom days (1.8 vs. 3.1 days, $p = 0.03$). The number of participants who had two colds during the trial was significantly reduced (2/84 on vitamin C vs. 16/84 in the placebo group; $p = 0.04$) [75].

In summary, cold symptoms have been shown to be less severe and resolve more quickly with oral vitamin C with a dose-dependent effect. Colds, caused by over 100 different virus strains, some of which are coronaviruses, are defined by a group of symptoms similar to the majority of those who get SARS-CoV-2 infection and do not convert into the acute illness phase. This similarity of symptoms and the disease-modifying effect of vitamin C across a wide range of cold-related viruses is further rationale for considering that vitamin C's effects in reducing severity and duration of infection is not virus-specific and could thus also potentially alleviate SARS-CoV-2 related symptoms. Each of these effects—reduced duration, severity and number of colds—could reasonably be hypothesised, in the context of SARS-CoV-2, to reduce conversion from mild infection to the critical phase of COVID-19. Given the consistent effect of regular vitamin C intake on the duration and severity of colds, and the low cost and safety, it would be appropriate for patients with respiratory virus infections to have the benefits of therapeutic vitamin C assessed.

Since the disease caused by the novel coronavirus can be more severe than ordinary viral infections, the above estimates may justify a regular increased daily intake of vitamin C for the period when the prevalence of the virus is high, when a patient suffers from a virus infection with active cold symptoms, in those testing PCR positive to SARS-CoV-2 and in COVID-19 hospitalised patients; an oral dose of up to 6–8 g/day might be considered. Pauling's recommendation of 1 g every hour of oral ascorbic acid during active infection has yet to be studied in an RCT, therefore, the most effective dose has yet to be determined.

5. Clinical Evidence for the Role of Vitamin C in Pneumonia

In 1951, Klenner investigated the effects of high doses of vitamin C, given intravenously, against viral diseases including pneumonia [76]. A Cochrane review on pneumonia and vitamin C identified three prophylactic RCTs reporting the number of pneumonia cases in participants who were administered oral vitamin C [22]. Each of these found a ≥80% lower incidence of pneumonia for the vitamin C group [77–79]. One was an RCT giving 2 g/day versus placebo to US Marine recruits during a two-month recruit training period and reported 1/331 cases of pneumonia in the vitamin C group versus 7/343 cases in the placebo group ($p = 0.044$) [77].

Two therapeutic trials were identified (Table 2). One was an RCT with elderly people in the UK (mean age 81 years), hospitalised with acute bronchitis or pneumonia. The study found that the plasma vitamin C level at baseline was 23 µmol/L (hypovitaminosis C) and one third of the patients had a vitamin C level of ≤11 µmol/L [18]. Vitamin C (0.2 g/day) reduced the respiratory symptom score in the more ill patients but not the less ill. There were six deaths during the study, all among the more ill patients: five in the placebo group, but only one in the vitamin C group. The other RCT, in the former Soviet Union, administered two different doses, a variable high or low dose relating to the dosage of antibiotics given [27]. The duration of hospital stay in the control group was 23.7 days. In the low dose vitamin C group (0.25–0.8 g/day) hospital stay was 19% shorter and in the high-dose group (0.5–1.6 g/day) it was 36% shorter. A benefit was also reported in relation to erythrocyte sedimentation rate and the normalisation of chest X-ray and temperature.

Table 2. Vitamin C trials in patients with pneumonia, sepsis and severe COVID-19.

Patients	Intervention Dose (Duration)	Patient Outcomes	Refs.
Pneumonia			
Pneumonia/bronchitis (n = 57):	Oral vitamin C (28 day):	↓ respiratory symptom score in most severely ill	[18]
• Placebo (n = 29)	0 g/day	17% mortality in placebo group	
• Treatment (n = 28)	0.2 g/day	4% mortality in treatment group	
Pneumonia (n = 140):	Oral vitamin C (10 day):	↓ hospital length of stay:	[27]
• Control (n = 70)	0 g/day	24 days in control group	
• Low dose (n = 39)	0.25–0.8 g/day	19 days in low dose group	
• High dose (n = 31)	0.5–1.6 g/day	15 days in high dose group	
Sepsis			
Sepsis and ARDS (n = 167):	IV vitamin C (4 day):	X systemic organ failure score X C-reactive protein, thrombomodulin X ventilator-free days ↓ 28 day mortality ↑ ICU-free days ↑ hospital-free days	[28]
• Placebo (n = 83)	0 mg/kg bw/day		
• Treatment (n = 84)	200 mg/kg/day		
Septic shock (n = 100):	IV vitamin C (until ICU discharge)	↓ vasopressor duration ↓ ICU length of stay X length of mechanical ventilation X renal replacement therapy X ICU mortality	[80]
• Placebo (n = 50)	0 g/day		
• Treatment (n = 50)	6 g/day		
Septic shock (n = 28):	IV vitamin C (3 day):	↓ norepinephrine dose and duration ↓ 28 day mortality X ICU length of stay	[81]
• Placebo (n = 14)	0 mg/kg bw/day		
• Treatment (n = 14)	100 mg/kg bw/day		
Severe sepsis (n = 24)	IV vitamin C (4 day):	↓ systemic organ failure score ↓ C-reactive protein, procalcitonin, thrombomodulin	[30]
• Placebo (n = 8)	0 mg/kg bw/day		
• Low dose (n = 8)	50 mg/kg bw/day		
• High dose (n = 8)	200 mg/kg bw/day		
Severe COVID-19			
Critical COVID-19 (n = 54)	IV vitamin C (7 day):	X ventilation-free days ↑ PaO_2/FiO_2 ↓ Interleukin-6 ↓ 28 day mortality in patients with SOFA scores ≥ 3	[82]
• Placebo (n = 28)	0 g/day		
• Treatment (n = 26)	24 g/day		

ARDS—acute respiratory distress syndrome; COVID—coronavirus disease; FiO_2—fraction of inspired oxygen; IV—intravenous; PaO_2—partial pressure of oxygen; SOFA—sequential organ failure assessment; ↓—decrease; X—no change. A part of this table has been reproduced from [36].

6. Clinical Evidence for the Role of Vitamin C in Critically Ill Septic Patients

The major cause for concern regarding COVID-19 is the high frequency of ICU treatment that is needed. Meta-analyses of intravenous vitamin C supplementation in critically ill (burns, sepsis and septic shock) patients indicated that it can lead to vasopressor sparing effects, reduced duration of ICU stay and a reduced need for mechanical ventilation [83]. In six trials, orally administered vitamin C in doses of 1–3 g/day reduced the length of ICU stay by 8.6% ($p = 0.003$) [84]. In five trials including 471 patients requiring ventilation for over 10 h, a dosage of 1–6 g/day of vitamin C reduced ventilation time by 25% ($p < 0.0001$) [85].

There is clear evidence that vitamin C levels decline precipitously in critically ill patients and in those with sepsis (Table 1) [36]. Although 0.1 g/day of vitamin C can maintain a normal plasma level in a healthy person, much higher doses (2–3 g/day) are needed to keep plasma vitamin C levels of critically ill patients within the normal range [11,86]. Being water-soluble, and thus excreted within hours, frequency of dose is important to maintain sufficient blood levels during active infection. Limitations in bioavailability in conditions of rapid vitamin C depletion in critically unwell patients have generated the hypothesis that the required therapeutic plasma levels to optimally reduce oxidative stress and exert an anti-inflammatory effect are more effectively achieved with intravenous administration than with oral administration alone [29,87].

Clinicians using intravenous vitamin C in severely ill COVID-19 patients have reported clinical effects upon administration of 3 g every 6 h together with steroids and anti-coagulants [88]. However, clear evidence for the most effective dose and frequency has not yet been determined. A four-group randomised pharmacokinetic trial testing 2 or 10 g/day, either delivered as a twice-daily bolus infusion or continuous infusion, found that the 2 g/day dose was associated with normal plasma concentrations, and the 10 g/day dose was associated with supranormal plasma concentrations, increased oxalate excretion, and metabolic alkalosis. The study's authors also concluded that sustained therapy is needed to prevent hypovitaminosis C [11].

Vitamin C has been reported to reduce mortality in septic patients requiring vasopressor treatment randomly assigned to be given 25 mg/kg body weight/day intravenous vitamin C every 6 h versus placebo (Table 2). Mortality at 28 days was significantly lower in the ascorbic acid than the placebo group (14% vs. 64%, respectively; $p = 0.009$) [81].

In the largest trial of intravenous vitamin C in sepsis-associated ARDS, the CITRIS-ALI trial, patients were given placebo or vitamin C at a dose of 50 mg/kg every 6 h for 4 days, thus providing 15 g/day for a 75 kg person (Table 2). Patients in the vitamin C group did not have significantly improved markers of inflammation, vascular injury or organ dysfunction which were the primary outcomes [28]. However, there were statistically significant benefits in three of the four clinically relevant outcomes, i.e., mortality ($p = 0.03$), duration of ICU-free days ($p = 0.03$) and hospital-free days ($p = 0.04$). Reanalysis of the data indicated that, during the 4-day vitamin C administration, mortality was 81% lower, but after the cessation of vitamin C administration, there was no difference between the two trial groups [89]. By the end of the 4-day vitamin C administration, the mortality rate was 23% (19/83) in the placebo group and 5% (4/84) in the vitamin C group ($p = 0.0007$). This difference of 18% corresponds to the number needed to treat of 5.5. Furthermore, the study authors, in recognition of the exclusion of sequential organ failure assessment (SOFA) scores in deceased patients, reported in a post hoc analysis assigning deceased patients a SOFA score of 20 and discharged patients a SOFA score of zero, that there was a 60% probability that any random patient from the placebo group had a higher SOFA score than any random patient from the vitamin C group ($p = 0.03$) at 96 h [90].

Another trial randomised 216 patients to low-dose intravenous vitamin C (1.5 g every 6 h thus providing 7.5 g/day), thiamine, and hydrocortisone for up to 10 days or until septic shock resolved, with a mean of 3.4 days, versus hydroxycortisone alone, and found no effect on the primary outcome of vasopressor-free time to 7 days or on 90-day mortality [91]. Two limitations of this study are the delay in giving vitamin C [92], and the absence of a vitamin C only arm [93]; hence, this study only shows that the addition of vitamin C, possibly too late in the disease process and for too short a time, to hydroxycortisone treatment added no treatment advantage.

7. Clinical Evidence for the Role of Vitamin C in COVID-19

Given the potential benefit of vitamin C, in oral and intravenous doses of 2–8 g/day, to reduce duration and severity of the common cold, pneumonia, sepsis and ARDS, this warrants investigation in relation to whether early oral supplementation could be beneficial in preventing conversion from mild infection to more critical COVID-19 infection and, if given intravenously to those with critical COVID-19 symptoms, in reducing mortality and ICU stay, thus speeding up recovery.

Interestingly, many of the risk factors for COVID-19 overlap with those for vitamin C deficiency [94]. Certain sub-groups (male, African American, older, those suffering with co-morbidities of diabetes, hypertension, COPD), all at higher risk of severe COVID-19, have also been shown to have lower serum vitamin C levels [95]. Average plasma vitamin C levels are generally lower in men than women, even with comparative intakes of vitamin C, which has been attributed to their higher body weight [94]. A hypothesis of altered sodium-dependent vitamin C transporter (SVCT1 and 2) expression in these sub-groups has also been proposed [95]. In old versus young rat hepatocytes, the vitamin C level declines by 66%, which is largely attributed to reduced absorption due to a 45% decline in SVCT1 with age [96]. It is noteworthy that inflammatory cytokines, also present in co-morbidities, downregulate SVCT2, resulting in the depletion of intracellular vitamin C [97,98].

There are currently 45 trials registered on Clinicaltrials.gov investigating vitamin C with or without other treatments for COVID-19. In the first RCT to test the value of vitamin C in critically ill COVID-19 patients, 54 ventilated patients in Wuhan, China, were treated with a placebo (sterile water) or intravenous vitamin C at a dose of 24 g/day for 7 days [82] (Table 2). After 7 days of treatment, the ratio of PaO_2/FiO_2 in the vitamin C group was 229 mmHg versus 151 mmHg in the control group ($p = 0.01$), and this also improved over time in the vitamin C group, but fell in the control group. On day 7, the IL-6 level was lower in the vitamin C group than in the placebo group: 19 pg/mL versus 158 pg/mL ($p = 0.04$). The more severely ill patients with SOFA scores ≥ 3 in the vitamin C group exhibited a reduction in 28-day mortality: 18% versus 50% ($p = 0.05$) in univariate survival analysis (Figure 2). No study-related adverse events were reported. The effects of treatment on the ratio PaO_2/FiO_2 and on IL-6 are clinically important, but further studies are needed to determine if the trend in lower mortality can be confirmed. The trial was originally designed for 140 subjects and was thus underpowered, with only 54 patients due to a lack of new admissions.

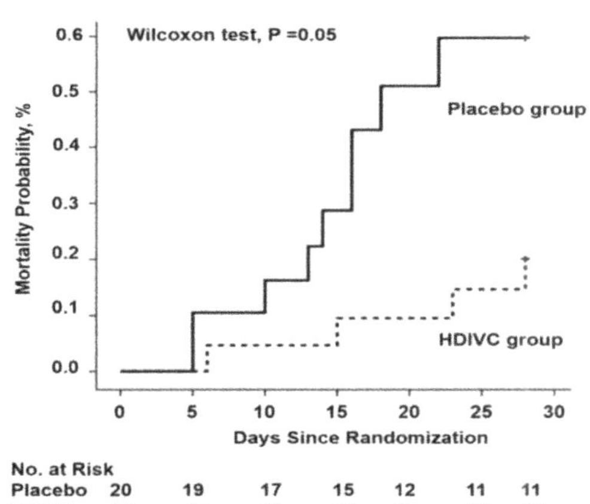

Figure 2. The 28-day mortality from randomization (day 1) to day 28 in a trial of high-dose intravenous vitamin C (HDIVC) in patients with COVID-19. Kaplan–Meier analysis was used to estimate the 28-day mortality and survival curves were compared with the Wilcoxon test ($p = 0.05$) among severe COVID-19 patients (baseline SOFA score ≥ 3). Cox regression was used as multiple comparisons (HR, 0.32 (95%CI, 0.10–1.06); $p = 0.06$). HDIVC—high-dose intravenous vitamin C. Reproduced with permission from Zhang J. et al. [82].

The largest registered trial is the Lessening Organ Dysfunction with Vitamin C-COVID (LOVIT-COVID) trial in Canada, which is recruiting 800 patients who are randomly assigned to vitamin C (intravenous, 50 mg/kg every 6 h) or a placebo for 96 h, i.e., equivalent to 15 g/day for a 75 kg person (NCT04401150). This protocol has also been added as a vitamin C arm in the Randomized, Embedded, Multifactorial Adaptive Platform Trial for Community-Acquired Pneumonia (REMAP-CAP; NCT02735707). The study design provides further rationale for the use of vitamin C in COVID-19 patients [99]. There is also a high-dose (10 g/day) vitamin C intervention study in 500 adults is in progress in Palermo, Italy (NCT04323514).

There is concern, however, that these study designs limit the use of vitamin C to a maximum of four days, which may be inadvisable in acutely ill patients due to the potential return of symptoms if the inflammation is not resolved. This issue was illustrated by the CITRIS-ALI trial, which showed a maximum reduction in mortality compared to placebo on day 4, the final day of vitamin C administration, but a decreased difference between the groups after 28 days [87,89].

In the UK, the Chelsea and Westminster hospital ICU, where adult ICU patients were administered 1 g of intravenous vitamin C every 12 h together with anticoagulants [100], has reported 29% mortality [101], compared to the average 41% reported by the Intensive Care National Audit and Research Centre (ICNARC) for all UK ICUs [102]. While the authors have stated that the addition of an antioxidant in the form of vitamin C could have contributed to the lower mortality rate, it should be noted that other clinical factors and procedures could also account for the improved mortality and that the Chelsea and Westminster ICU serves a more affluent sector of the population with less deprivation on the basis of the Index of Multiple Deprivation (IMD). Deprivation, while a risk factor for COVID-19 mortality, is also a predictor of low vitamin C status. In the UK, an estimated 25% of men and 16% of women in the low-income/materially deprived population are deficient in vitamin C > 11 μmol/L [103].

The Frontline COVID-19 Critical Care Expert Group (FLCCC), a group of emergency medicine experts, have reported that, with the combined use of 6 g/day intravenous vitamin C (1.5 g every 6 h), plus steroids and anticoagulants, mortality was 5% in two ICUs in the US (United Memorial Hospital in Houston, Texas, and Norfolk General Hospital in Norfolk, Virginia), the lowest mortality rates in their respective counties [88].

A case report of 17 COVID-19 patients who were given 1 g of intravenous vitamin C every 8 h for 3 days reported a mortality rate of 12% with 18% rates of intubation and mechanical ventilation and a significant decrease in inflammatory markers, including ferritin and D-dimer, and a trend towards decreasing FiO_2 requirements [104]. Another case of unexpected recovery following high-dose intravenous vitamin C has also been reported [105]. While these case reports are subject to confounding and are not prima facie evidence of effects, they do illustrate the feasibility of using vitamin C for COVID-19 with no adverse effects reported.

8. Safety of Oral and Intravenous Vitamin C

The US DRI, having thoroughly considered the wide literature on vitamin C and many kinds of speculated harms, stated that the safe range is up to 2 g/day [106]. The European Food Safety Authority stated that the lowest observable adverse effect level is 3–4 g/day (in relation to gastrointestinal effects) [107]. Injectable vitamin C phials state "there are no contraindications to the administration of ascorbic acid. As much as 6 g has been administered parenterally to normal adults without evidence of toxicity" [108].

Three concerns have been raised regarding high doses of vitamin C: diarrhoea from high oral ingestion, kidney stones, particularly due to kidney dysfunction in the case of intravenous vitamin C (i.e., if high doses cannot be cleared), and unsuitability for those with specific genetically inherited metabolic issues that affect vitamin C utilisation. The latter relates to those with glucose-6-phosphate deficiency (G6PD) and also haemochromatosis and thalassaemia due to enhanced iron absorption with vitamin C. G6PD deficiency is not considered an exclusion criterion in the use of up to 6 g/day oral or intravenous vitamin C [109]. The FLCCC report that 3 g every 6 h appears to be safe in patients with

G6PD. It may be wise for those with haemochromatosis or thalassaemia to avoid high-dose vitamin C taken with iron-rich foods or supplements and short-term high-dose vitamin C to be medically monitored [110].

Looser bowel movements and diarrhoea rarely occur below 3 g/day and tolerance is increased considerably when fighting a viral infection [111]. Diarrhoea has not been reported as a complication in hospital-based oral treatment and does not occur with intravenous vitamin C administration. A survey of 9328 patients given an average intravenous dose of 24 g of vitamin C every 4 days, primarily for cancer, infection or fatigue, reported that 101 (1%) had side effects, mostly minor, including lethargy/fatigue, a change in mental status and vein irritation/phlebitis [112].

Regarding kidney stone formation, the Kidney Stone Research Laboratory of the University of Cape Town conducted a controlled trial in which ten volunteer subjects were required to ingest 4 g of vitamin C per day for five days. Unlike the earlier studies, they put a preservative in the urine collection bottles to prevent the conversion of ascorbate to oxalic acid. The samples were analysed for numerous physicochemical risk factors of kidney stone formation. These risk factors were not significantly altered and the authors concluded that ingestion of large doses of vitamin C does not increase the risk of forming kidney stones and earlier trials had faulty study designs involving unpreserved urine samples [113]. A prospective cohort study of 85,557 women with no history of kidney stones, with 1078 incidences of kidney stones over 14 years of follow-up, reported that vitamin C was not associated with a risk of kidney stone development [114]. A systematic review of studies giving vitamin C found a correlation between ascorbic acid supplementation and the incidence of kidney stones in men, but not women [115]. A study administering intravenous ascorbic acid in doses ranging from 0.2 to 1.5 g/kg body weight measured urinary oxalic excretion during and over 6 h post infusion. The authors conclude that less than 0.5% of a very large intravenous dose of ascorbic acid was recovered as urinary oxalic acid in people with normal renal function [116]. A cautious position would be to exclude those with a history of kidney stones or kidney dysfunction from high-dose oral or intravenous vitamin C unless medically supervised. Short-term high-dose vitamin C in the region of 2–8 g/day is unlikely to be of significant concern in people with normal kidney function.

9. Conclusions

Vitamin C's potential benefits, low cost, safety profile and multiple disease-modifying actions, including antioxidant, anti-inflammatory and immunomodulating effects, make it an attractive therapeutic candidate in reducing viral load with oral supplementation in the range of 2–8 g/day to help attenuate the conversion to the critical phase of COVID-19. Likewise, vitamin C has potential benefits in treating acute respiratory infections and mitigating inflammation in critical COVID-19 patients with intravenous vitamin C infusion in the range of 6–24 g/day, for correcting disease-induced deficiency, reducing inflammation, enhancing interferon production and supporting the anti-inflammatory actions of glucocorticosteroids, especially given the high level of fatality for patients with severe COVID-19.

Given the remarkable safety of vitamin C, frequent deficiency among patients with COVID-19 and extensive evidence of potential benefits, the current treatment is justified on compassionate grounds pending more COVID-19 clinical trial data becoming available, not only for intravenous use within ICUs, but also orally with doses between 2 and 8 g/day in hospitalised patients due to increased need when fighting a viral infection, as concluded in recent reviews [36,117,118]. The clinical choice of oral versus intravenous vitamin C may be guided by similar criteria for administering oral versus intravenous antibiotics, considering both the severity of the illness and whether the patient is able to swallow oral medication at least four times a day.

People in high-risk groups for COVID-19 mortality, and at risk of vitamin C deficiency, should be encouraged to supplement with vitamin C daily to ensure vitamin C adequacy at all times, and to increase the dose when virally infected to up to 6–8 g/day [119]. Whether or not this will prevent conversion to the critical phase of COVID-19 has yet to be determined.

Author Contributions: Conceptualisation, P.H.; writing—original draft preparation, P.H., T.H.J., S.R.A, I.S.W., A.C.C.; writing—review and editing, P.E.M., A.D.S.; visualisation, T.H.J., S.R.A. All authors have read and agreed to the published version of the manuscript.

Acknowledgments: The authors would like to thank Harri Hemila from the Department of Public Health, University of Helsinki, for his helpful feedback, as well as Gordon Brydon and Sheri Friedman for their help with referencing and secretarial support when preparing the paper for publication. A.C.C. is supported by a Health Research Council of New Zealand Sir Charles Hercus Health Research Fellowship.

References

1. Drouin, G.; Godin, J.R.; Page, B. The genetics of vitamin C loss in vertebrates. *Curr. Genomics* **2011**, *12*, 371–378. [CrossRef]
2. Milton, K. Micronutrient intakes of wild primates: Are humans different? *Comp. Biochem. Physiol. A Mol. Integr. Physiol.* **2003**, *136*, 47–59. [CrossRef]
3. Milton, K. Nutritional characteristics of wild primate foods: Do the diets of our closest living relatives have lessons for us? *Nutrition* **1999**, *15*, 488–498. [CrossRef]
4. European Food Safety Authority Panel on Dietetic Products, Nutrition and Allergies. Scientific opinion on dietary reference values for vitamin C. *EFSA J.* **2013**, *11*, 3418. [CrossRef]
5. Bates, B.; Collins, D.; Cox, L.; Nicholson, S.; Page, P.; Roberts, C.; Steer, T.; Swan, G. *National Diet and Nutrition Survey Years 1 to 9 of the Rolling Programme (2008/2009–2016/2017): Time Trend and Income Analyses*; Public Health England: London, UK, 2019.
6. Berger, M.M.; Bischoff-Ferrari, H.A.; Zimmermann, M.; Herter, I.; Spieldenner, J.; Eggersdorfer, M. *White Paper on Nutritional Status in Supporting a Well-Functioning Immune System for Optimal Health with a Recommendation for Switzerland*; SGE: Bern, Switzerland, 2020.
7. Linus Pauling Institute; Micronutrient Information Center. *Micronutrients for Older Adults Oregon State University*. 2020. Available online: https://lpi.oregonstate.edu/mic/life-stages/older-adults (accessed on 20 October 2020).
8. Levine, M.; Conry-Cantilena, C.; Wang, Y.; Welch, R.W.; Washko, P.W.; Dhariwal, K.R.; Park, J.B.; Lazarev, A.; Graumlich, J.F.; King, J.; et al. Vitamin C pharmacokinetics in healthy volunteers: Evidence for a recommended dietary allowance. *Proc. Natl. Acad. Sci. USA* **1996**, *93*, 3704–3709. [CrossRef] [PubMed]
9. Levine, M.; Wang, Y.; Padayatty, S.J.; Morrow, J. A new recommended dietary allowance of vitamin C for healthy young women. *Proc. Natl. Acad. Sci. USA* **2001**, *98*, 9842–9846. [CrossRef]
10. Padayatty, S.J.; Sun, H.; Wang, Y.; Riordan, H.D.; Hewitt, S.M.; Katz, A.; Wesley, R.A.; Levine, M. Vitamin C pharmacokinetics: Implications for oral and intravenous use. *Ann. Intern. Med.* **2004**, *140*, 533–537. [CrossRef]
11. De Grooth, H.J.; Manubulu-Choo, W.P.; Zandvliet, A.S.; Spoelstra-de Man, A.M.E.; Girbes, A.R.; Swart, E.L.; Oudemans-van Straaten, H.M. Vitamin-C pharmacokinetics in critically ill patients: A randomized trial of four intravenous regimens. *Chest* **2018**, *153*, 1368–1377. [CrossRef]
12. Hume, R.; Weyers, E. Changes in leucocyte ascorbic acid during the common cold. *Scott. Med. J.* **1973**, *18*, 3–7. [CrossRef]
13. Evans-Olders, R.; Eintracht, S.; Hoffer, L.J. Metabolic origin of hypovitaminosis C in acutely hospitalized patients. *Nutrition* **2010**, *26*, 1070–1074. [CrossRef]
14. Teixeira, A.; Carrie, A.S.; Genereau, T.; Herson, S.; Cherin, P. Vitamin C deficiency in elderly hospitalized patients. *Am. J. Med.* **2001**, *111*, 502. [CrossRef]
15. Fain, O.; Paries, J.; Jacquart, B.; Le Moel, G.; Kettaneh, A.; Stirnemann, J.; Heron, C.; Sitbon, M.; Taleb, C.; Letellier, E.; et al. Hypovitaminosis C in hospitalized patients. *Eur. J. Intern. Med.* **2003**, *14*, 419–425. [CrossRef] [PubMed]
16. Gan, R.; Eintracht, S.; Hoffer, L.J. Vitamin C deficiency in a university teaching hospital. *J. Am. Coll. Nutr.* **2008**, *27*, 428–433. [CrossRef] [PubMed]
17. Ravindran, P.; Wiltshire, S.; Das, K.; Wilson, R.B. Vitamin C deficiency in an Australian cohort of metropolitan surgical patients. *Pathology* **2018**, *50*, 654–658. [CrossRef]

18. Hunt, C.; Chakravorty, N.K.; Annan, G.; Habibzadeh, N.; Schorah, C.J. The clinical effects of vitamin C supplementation in elderly hospitalised patients with acute respiratory infections. *Int. J. Vitam. Nutr. Res.* **1994**, *64*, 212–219. [PubMed]
19. Bates, C.J.; Prentice, A.; Cole, T.J.; van der Pols, J.C.; Doyle, W.; Finch, S.; Smithers, G.; Clarke, P.C. Micronutrients: Highlights and research challenges from the 1994-5 National Diet and Nutrition Survey of people aged 65 years and over. *Br. J. Nutr.* **1999**, *82*, 7–15. [CrossRef] [PubMed]
20. Hemilä, H.; Louhiala, P. Vitamin C may affect lung infections. *J. R. Soc. Med.* **2007**, *100*, 495–498. [CrossRef] [PubMed]
21. Myint, P.K.; Wilson, A.M.; Clark, A.B.; Luben, R.N.; Wareham, N.J.; Khaw, K.T. Plasma vitamin C concentrations and risk of incident respiratory diseases and mortality in the European Prospective Investigation into Cancer-Norfolk population-based cohort study. *Eur. J. Clin. Nutr.* **2019**, *73*, 1492–1500. [CrossRef] [PubMed]
22. Hemilä, H.; Louhiala, P. Vitamin C for preventing and treating pneumonia. *Cochrane Database Syst. Rev.* **2013**. [CrossRef]
23. Kory, P.; Kanne, J.P. SARS-CoV-2 organising pneumonia: 'Has there been a widespread failure to identify and treat this prevalent condition in COVID-19?'. *BMJ Open Respir. Res.* **2020**, *7*, e000724. [CrossRef]
24. Carr, A.C.; Spencer, E.; Dixon, L.; Chambers, S.T. Patients with community acquired pneumonia exhibit depleted vitamin C status and elevated oxidative stress. *Nutrients* **2020**, *12*, 1318. [CrossRef]
25. Bakaev, V.V.; Duntau, A.P. Ascorbic acid in blood serum of patients with pulmonary tuberculosis and pneumonia. *Int. J. Tuberc. Lung. Dis.* **2004**, *8*, 263–266.
26. Chakrabarti, B.; Banerjee, S. Dehydroascorbic acid level in blood of patients suffering from various infectious diseases. *Proc. Soc. Exp. Biol. Med.* **1955**, *88*, 581–583. [CrossRef] [PubMed]
27. Mochalkin, N.I. Ascorbic acid in the complex therapy of acute pneumonia. *Voen. Med. Zhurnal* **1970**, *9*, 17–21.
28. Fowler, A.A., III; Truwit, J.D.; Hite, R.D.; Morris, P.E.; DeWilde, C.; Priday, A.; Fisher, B.; Thacker, L.R., II; Natarajan, R.; Brophy, D.F.; et al. Effect of vitamin C infusion on organ failure and biomarkers of inflammation and vascular injury in patients with sepsis and severe acute respiratory failure: The CITRIS-ALI randomized clinical trial. *JAMA* **2019**, *322*, 1261–1270. [CrossRef]
29. Carr, A.C.; Rosengrave, P.C.; Bayer, S.; Chambers, S.; Mehrtens, J.; Shaw, G.M. Hypovitaminosis C and vitamin C deficiency in critically ill patients despite recommended enteral and parenteral intakes. *Crit. Care* **2017**, *21*, 300. [CrossRef] [PubMed]
30. Fowler, A.A.; Syed, A.A.; Knowlson, S.; Sculthorpe, R.; Farthing, D.; DeWilde, C.; Farthing, C.A.; Larus, T.L.; Martin, E.; Brophy, D.F.; et al. Phase I safety trial of intravenous ascorbic acid in patients with severe sepsis. *J. Transl. Med.* **2014**, *12*, 32. [CrossRef] [PubMed]
31. Doise, J.M.; Aho, L.S.; Quenot, J.P.; Guilland, J.C.; Zeller, M.; Vergely, C.; Aube, H.; Blettery, B.; Rochette, L. Plasma antioxidant status in septic critically ill patients: A decrease over time. *Fundam. Clin. Pharmacol.* **2008**, *22*, 203–209. [CrossRef] [PubMed]
32. Voigt, K.; Kontush, A.; Stuerenburg, H.-J.; Muench-Harrach, D.; Hansen, H.C.; Kunze, K. Decreased plasma and cerebrospinal fluid ascorbate levels in patients with septic encephalopathy. *Free Radic. Res.* **2002**, *36*, 735–739. [CrossRef] [PubMed]
33. Schorah, C.J.; Downing, C.; Piripitsi, A.; Gallivan, L.; Al-Hazaa, A.H.; Sanderson, M.J.; Bodenham, A. Total vitamin C, ascorbic acid, and dehydroascorbic acid concentrations in plasma of critically ill patients. *Am. J. Clin. Nutr.* **1996**, *63*, 760–765. [CrossRef]
34. Arvinte, C.; Singh, M.; Marik, P.E. Serum levels of vitamin C and vitamin D in a cohort of critically ill COVID-19 patients of a north American community hospital intensive care unit in May 2020: A pilot study. *Med. Drug Discov.* **2020**. [CrossRef] [PubMed]
35. Chiscano-Camón, L.; Ruiz-Rodriguez, J.C.; Ruiz-Sanmartin, A.; Roca, O.; Ferrer, R. Vitamin C levels in patients with SARS-CoV-2-associated acute respiratory distress syndrome. *Crit. Care* **2020**, *24*, 522. [CrossRef] [PubMed]
36. Carr, A.C. Vitamin C in pneumonia and sepsis. In *Vitamin C: New Biochemical and Functional Insights*; Chen, Q., Vissers, M., Eds.; CRC Press/Taylor & Francis: Boca Raton, FL, USA, 2020; pp. 115–135.
37. Marik, P.E.; Hooper, M.H. Doctor-your septic patients have scurvy! *Crit. Care* **2018**, *22*, 23. [CrossRef] [PubMed]

38. Marik, P.E. Vitamin C: An essential "stress hormone" during sepsis. *J. Thorac. Dis.* **2020**, *12*, S84–S88. [CrossRef]
39. Marik, P.E. Vitamin C for the treatment of sepsis: The scientific rationale. *Pharmacol. Ther.* **2018**, *189*, 63–70. [CrossRef]
40. Colunga Biancatelli, R.M.L.; Berrill, M.; Marik, P.E. The antiviral properties of vitamin C. *Expert Rev. Anti Infect. Ther.* **2020**, *18*, 99–101. [CrossRef]
41. Thomas, W.R.; Holt, P.G. Vitamin C and immunity: An assessment of the evidence. *Clin. Exp. Immunol.* **1978**, *32*, 370–379.
42. Dahl, H.; Degre, M. The effect of ascorbic acid on production of human interferon and the antiviral activity in vitro. *Acta Pathol. Microbiol. Scand. B* **1976**, *84*, 280–284. [CrossRef]
43. Webb, A.L.; Villamor, E. Update: Effects of antioxidant and non-antioxidant vitamin supplementation on immune function. *Nutr. Rev.* **2007**, *65*, 181–217. [CrossRef]
44. Hemila, H. Vitamin C and infectious diseases. In *Vitamin C*; Paoletti, R., Sies, H., Bug, J., Grossi, E., Poli, A., Eds.; Springer: Milan, Italy, 1998; pp. 73–85.
45. Carr, A.C.; Maggini, S. Vitamin C and immune function. *Nutrients* **2017**, *9*, 1211. [CrossRef]
46. Wang, Y.; Russo, T.A.; Kwon, O.; Chanock, S.; Rumsey, S.C.; Levine, M. Ascorbate recycling in human neutrophils: Induction by bacteria. *Proc. Natl. Acad. Sci. USA* **1997**, *94*, 13816–13819. [CrossRef] [PubMed]
47. Nualart, F.J.; Rivas, C.I.; Montecinos, V.P.; Godoy, A.S.; Guaiquil, V.H.; Golde, D.W.; Vera, J.C. Recycling of vitamin C by a bystander effect. *J. Biol. Chem.* **2003**, *278*, 10128–10133. [CrossRef] [PubMed]
48. May, J.M.; Qu, Z.C. Ascorbic acid prevents oxidant-induced increases in endothelial permeability. *Biofactors* **2011**, *37*, 46–50. [CrossRef] [PubMed]
49. May, J.M.; Harrison, F.E. Role of vitamin C in the function of the vascular endothelium. *Antioxid. Redox Signal* **2013**, *19*, 2068–2083. [CrossRef]
50. Sen, C.K.; Packer, L. Antioxidant and redox regulation of gene transcription. *FASEB J.* **1996**, *10*, 709–720. [CrossRef]
51. Chen, Y.; Luo, G.; Yuan, J.; Wang, Y.; Yang, X.; Wang, X.; Li, G.; Liu, Z.; Zhong, N. Vitamin C mitigates oxidative stress and tumor necrosis factor-alpha in severe community-acquired pneumonia and LPS-induced macrophages. *Mediators Inflamm.* **2014**, *2014*, 426740. [CrossRef]
52. Erol, N.; Saglam, L.; Saglam, Y.S.; Erol, H.S.; Altun, S.; Aktas, M.S.; Halici, M.B. The protection potential of antioxidant vitamins against acute respiratory distress syndrome: A rat trial. *Inflammation* **2019**, *42*, 1585–1594. [CrossRef]
53. Blanco-Melo, D.; Nilsson-Payant, B.E.; Liu, W.C.; Uhl, S.; Hoagland, D.; Møller, R.; Jordan, T.X.; Oishi, K.; Panis, M.; Sachs, D.; et al. Imbalanced host response to SARS-CoV-2 drives development of COVID-19. *Cell* **2020**, *181*, 1036–1045. [CrossRef] [PubMed]
54. Kim, Y.; Kim, H.; Bae, S.; Choi, J.; Lim, S.Y.; Lee, N.; Kong, J.M.; Hwang, Y.I.; Kang, J.S.; Lee, W.J. Vitamin C is an essential factor on the anti-viral immune responses through the production of interferon-a/b at the initial stage of influenza A virus (H3N2) infection. *Immune Netw.* **2013**, *13*, 70–74. [CrossRef]
55. Hemilä, H. Vitamin C and infections. *Nutrients* **2017**, *9*, 339. [CrossRef]
56. Atherton, J.G.; Kratzing, C.C.; Fisher, A. The effect of ascorbic acid on infection chick-embryo ciliated tracheal organ cultures by coronavirus. *Arch. Virol.* **1978**, *56*, 195–199. [CrossRef] [PubMed]
57. Davelaar, F.G.; Bos, J. Ascorbic acid and infectious bronchitis infections in broilers. *Avian Pathol.* **1992**, *21*, 581–589. [CrossRef] [PubMed]
58. Gan, R.; Rosoman, N.P.; Henshaw, D.J.E.; Noble, E.P.; Georgius, P.; Sommerfeld, N. COVID-19 as a viral functional ACE2 deficiency disorder with ACE2 related multi-organ disease. *Med. Hypotheses* **2020**, *144*, 110024. [CrossRef] [PubMed]
59. Ni, W.; Yang, X.; Yang, D.; Bao, J.; Li, R.; Xiao, Y.; Hou, C.; Wang, H.; Liu, J.; Yang, D.; et al. Role of angiotensin-converting enzyme 2 (ACE2) in COVID-19. *Crit. Care* **2020**, *24*.
60. Ma, S.; Sun, S.; Li, J.; Fan, Y.; Qu, J.; Sun, L.; Wang, S.; Zhang, Y.; Yang, S.; Liu, Z.; et al. Single-cell transcriptomic atlas of primate cardiopulmonary aging. *Cell Res.* **2020**. [CrossRef] [PubMed]
61. Kumar, V.; Jena, M. In silico virtual screening-based study of nutraceuticals predicts the therapeutic potentials of folic acid and its derivatives against COVID-19. *Res. Square* **2020**. [CrossRef]
62. Bosmann, M.; Ward, P.A. The inflammatory response in sepsis. *Trends Immunol.* **2013**, *34*, 129–136. [CrossRef]

63. Grommes, J.; Soehnlein, O. Contribution of neutrophils to acute lung injury. *Mol. Med.* **2011**, *17*, 293–307. [CrossRef]
64. Brinkmann, V.; Reichard, U.; Goosmann, C.; Fauler, B.; Uhlemann, Y.; Weiss, D.S.; Weinrauch, Y.; Zychlinsky, A. Neutrophil extracellular traps kill bacteria. *Science* **2004**, *303*, 1532–1535. [CrossRef]
65. Mohammed, B.M.; Fisher, B.J.; Kraskauskas, D.; Farkas, D.; Brophy, D.F.; Fowler, A.A., III; Natarajan, R. Vitamin C: A novel regulator of neutrophil extracellular trap formation. *Nutrients* **2013**, *5*, 3131–3151. [CrossRef]
66. Fisher, B.J.; Kraskauskas, D.; Martin, E.J.; Farkas, D.; Wegelin, J.A.; Brophy, D.; Ward, K.R.; Voelkel, N.F.; Fowler, A.A., III; Natarajan, R. Mechanisms of attenuation of abdominal sepsis induced acute lung injury by ascorbic acid. *Am. J. Physiol. Lung Cell Mol. Physiol.* **2012**, *303*, L20–L32. [CrossRef] [PubMed]
67. Hornig, D. Distribution of ascorbic acid, metabolites and analogues in man and animals. *Ann. N. Y. Acad. Sci.* **1975**, *258*, 103–118. [CrossRef] [PubMed]
68. Padayatty, S.J.; Doppman, J.L.; Chang, R.; Wang, Y.; Gill, J.; Papanicolaou, D.A.; Levine, M. Human adrenal glands secrete vitamin C in response to adrenocorticotrophic hormone. *Am. J. Clin. Nutr.* **2007**, *86*, 145–149. [CrossRef]
69. Kodama, M.; Kodama, T.; Murakami, M.; Kodama, M. Vitamin C infusion treatment enhances cortisol production of the adrenal via the pituitary ACTH route. *In Vivo* **1994**, *8*, 1079–1085. [PubMed]
70. Barabutis, N.; Khangoora, V.; Marik, P.E.; Catravas, J.D. Hydrocortisone and ascorbic acid synergistically prevent and repair lipopolysaccharide-induced pulmonary endothelial barrier dysfunction. *Chest* **2017**, *152*, 954–962. [CrossRef] [PubMed]
71. Recovery Collaborative Group; Horby, P.; Lim, W.S.; Emberson, J.R.; Mafham, M.; Bell, J.L.; Linsell, L.; Staplin, N.; Brightling, C.; Ustianowski, A.; et al. Dexamethasone in hospitalized patients with Covid-19-preliminary report. *N. Engl. J. Med.* **2020**. [CrossRef] [PubMed]
72. Pauling, L. The significance of the evidence about ascorbic acid and the common cold. *Proc. Natl. Acad. Sci. USA* **1971**, *68*, 2678–2681. [CrossRef]
73. Pauling, L. *Vitamin C the Common Cold and Flu*; Freeman: San Francisco, CA, USA, 1970.
74. Hemilä, H.; Chalker, E. Vitamin C for preventing and treating the common cold. *Cochrane Database Syst. Rev.* **2013**. [CrossRef] [PubMed]
75. Van Straten, M.; Josling, P. Preventing the common cold with a vitamin C supplement: A double-blind, placebo-controlled survey. *Adv. Ther.* **2002**, *19*, 151–159. [CrossRef]
76. Klenner, F.R. Massive doses of vitamin C and the virus diseases. *South Med. Surg.* **1951**, *113*, 101–107.
77. Pitt, H.A.; Costrini, A.M. Vitamin C prophylaxis in marine recruits. *JAMA* **1979**, *241*, 908–911. [CrossRef] [PubMed]
78. Kimbarowski, J.A.; Mokrow, N.J. Colored precipitation reaction of the urine according to Kimbarowski (FARK) as an index of the effect of ascorbic acid during treatment of viral influenza. *Dtsch Gesundheitsw.* **1967**, *22*, 2413–2418. [PubMed]
79. Glazebrook, A.J.; Thomson, S. The administration of vitamin C in a large institution and its effect on general health and resistance to infection. *J. Hyg.* **1942**, *42*, 1–19. [CrossRef]
80. Nabil Habib, T.; Ahmed, I. Early adjuvant intravenous vitamin C treatment in septic shock may resolve the vasopressor dependence. *Int. J. Microbiol. Adv. Immunol.* **2017**, *5*, 77–81.
81. Zabet, M.H.; Mohammadi, M.; Ramezani, M.; Khalili, H. Effect of high-dose ascorbic acid on vasopressor's requirement in septic shock. *J. Res. Pharm. Pract.* **2016**, *5*, 94–100.
82. Zhang, J.; Rao, X.; Li, Y.; Zhu, Y.; Liu, F.; Guo, G.; Luo, G.; Meng, Z.; De Backer, D.; Xiang, H.; et al. High-dose vitamin C infusion for the treatment of critically ill COVID-19. *Res. Square* **2020**. [CrossRef]
83. Zhang, M.; Jativa, D.F. Vitamin C supplementation in the critically ill: A systematic review and meta-analysis. *SAGE Open Med.* **2018**, *6*. [CrossRef]
84. Hemila, H.; Chalker, E. Vitamin C can shorten the length of stay in the ICU: A meta-analysis. *Nutrients* **2019**, *11*, 708. [CrossRef]
85. Hemila, H.; Chalker, E. Vitamin C may reduce the duration of mechanical ventilation in critically ill patients: A meta-regression analysis. *J. Intensive Care* **2020**, *8*, 15. [CrossRef]
86. Long, C.L.; Maull, K.I.; Krishnan, R.S.; Laws, H.L.; Geiger, J.W.; Borghesi, L.; Franks, W.; Lawson, T.C.; Sauberlich, H.E. Ascorbic acid dynamics in the seriously ill and injured. *J. Surg. Res.* **2003**, *109*, 144–148. [CrossRef]

87. Kashiouris, M.G.; L'Heureux, M.; Cable, C.A.; Fisher, B.J.; Leichtle, S.W.; Fowler, A.A. The emerging role of vitamin C as a treatment for sepsis. *Nutrients* **2020**, *12*, 292. [CrossRef] [PubMed]
88. Marik, P.E.; Kory, P.; Varon, J.; Iglesias, J.; Meduri, G.U. MATH+ protocol for the treatment of SARS-CoV-2 infection: The scientific rationale. *Expert Rev. Anti Infect. Ther.* **2020**, 1–7. [CrossRef] [PubMed]
89. Hemilä, H.; Chalker, E. Reanalysis of the effect of vitamin C on mortality in the CITRIS-ALI trial: Important findings dismissed in the trial report. *Front. Med.* **2020**. [CrossRef] [PubMed]
90. Fowler, A.A., III; Fisher, B.J.; Kashiouris, M.G. Vitamin C for sepsis and acute respiratory failure—Reply. *JAMA* **2020**, *323*, 792–793. [CrossRef]
91. Fujii, T.; Luethi, N.; Young, P.J.; Frei, D.R.; Eastwood, G.M.; French, C.J.; Deane, A.M.; Shehabi, Y.; Hajjar, L.A.; Oliveira, G.; et al. Effect of Vitamin C, Hydrocortisone, and Thiamine vs Hydrocortisone Alone on Time Alive and Free of Vasopressor Support Among Patients with Septic Shock: The VITAMINS Randomized Clinical Trial. *JAMA* **2020**, *323*, 423–431. [CrossRef]
92. Long, M.T.; Kory, P.; Marik, P. Vitamin C, hydrocortisone, and thiamine for septic shock. *JAMA* **2020**, *323*, 2203–2204. [CrossRef]
93. Carr, A.C. Is the VITAMINS RCT indicating potential redundancy between corticosteroids and vitamin C? *Crit. Care* **2020**, *24*, 129. [CrossRef]
94. Carr, A.C.; Rowe, S. Factors affecting vitamin C status and prevalence of deficiency: A global health perspective. *Nutrients* **2020**, *12*, 1963. [CrossRef]
95. Patterson, G.; Isales, C.M.; Fulzele, S. Low level of vitamin C and dysregulation of vitamin C transporter might be involved in the severity of COVID-19 Infection. *Aging Dis.* **2020**, *12*.
96. Michels, A.J.; Joisher, N.; Hagen, T.M. Age-related decline of sodium-dependent ascorbic acid transport in isolated rat hepatocytes. *Arch. Biochem. Biophys.* **2003**, *410*, 112–120. [CrossRef]
97. Subramanian, V.S.; Sabui, S.; Subramenium, G.A.; Marchant, J.S.; Said, H.M. Tumor Necrosis Factor alpha (TNF-alpha) reduces intestinal vitamin C uptake: A role for NF-kB-mediated signaling. *Am. J. Physiol. Gastrointest. Liver Physiol.* **2018**, *315*, G241–G248. [CrossRef]
98. Subramanian, V.S.; Sabui, S.; Moradi, H.; Marchant, J.S.; Said, H.M. Inhibition of intestinal ascorbic acid uptake by lipopolysaccharide is mediated via transcriptional mechanisms. *Biochim. Biophys. Acta Biomembr.* **2018**, *1860*, 556–565. [CrossRef] [PubMed]
99. Domain-Specific Appendix: VITAMIN, C. REMAP-CAP: Randomized, Embedded, Multifactorial Adaptive Platform Trial for Community-Acquired Pneumonia 2020. Available online: https://static1.squarespace.com/static/5cde3c7d9a69340001d79ffe/t/5f1bba732cda7f10310643fe/1595652735252/REMAP-CAP+Vitamin+C+Domain+Specific+Appendix+V2+-+08+June+2020_WM.pdf (accessed on 26 September 2020).
100. Vizcaychipi, M.P.; Shovlin, C.L.; McCarthy, A.; Howard, A.; Brown, A.; Hayes, M.; Singh, S.; Christie, L.; Sisson, A.; Davies, R.; et al. Development and implementation of a COVID-19 near real-time traffic light system in an acute hospital setting. *Emerg. Med. J.* **2020**, *37*, 630–636. [CrossRef] [PubMed]
101. ICNARC Report on COVID-19 in Critical Care: Chelsea and Westminster Hospital Intensive Care Unit. London. 2020. Available online: https://www.patrickholford.com/uploads/2020/chelwesticnarcreportjune.pdf (accessed on 12 June 2020).
102. ICNARC Report on COVID-19 in Critical Care. London. 2020. Available online: https://www.patrickholford.com/uploads/2020/nationwideicnarcreportjune.pdf (accessed on 26 June 2020).
103. Mosdol, A.; Erens, B.; Brunner, E.J. Estimated prevalence and predictors of vitamin C deficiency within UK's low-income population. *J. Public Health* **2008**, *30*, 456–460. [CrossRef] [PubMed]
104. Hiedra, R.; Lo, K.B.; Elbashabsheh, M.; Gul, F.; Wright, R.M.; Albano, J.; Azmaiparashvili, Z.; Patarroyo Aponte, G. The use of IV vitamin C for patients with COVID-19: A case series. *Expert Rev. Anti Infect. Ther.* **2020**, *18*, 1259–1261. [CrossRef] [PubMed]
105. Waqas Khan, H.M.; Parikh, N.; Megala, S.M.; Predeteanu, G.S. Unusual early recovery of a critical COVID-19 patient after administration of intravenous vitamin C. *Am. J. Case Rep.* **2020**, *21*, e925521. [PubMed]
106. Vitamin C: Fact Sheet for Health Professionals USA: National Institutes of Health. 2020. Available online: https://ods.od.nih.gov/factsheets/VitaminC-HealthProfessional/ (accessed on 10 October 2020).
107. Scientific Committee on Food Scientific Panel on Dietetic Products Nutrition and Allergies. *Tolerable Upper Intake Levels for Vitamins and Minerals*; EFSA: Parma, Italy, 2006.

108. Phoenix Labs. Ascorbic Acid Injection 500mg/5ml Clonee, Ireland 2014. Available online: https://www.medicines.org.uk/emc/product/1520/smpc#gref (accessed on 23 November 2020).
109. Marik, P.E. Is intravenous vitamin C contraindicated in patients with G6PD deficiency? *Crit. Care* **2019**, *23*, 109. [CrossRef] [PubMed]
110. Gerster, H. High-dose vitamin C: A risk for persons with high iron stores? *Int. J. Vitam. Nutr. Res.* **1999**, *69*, 67–82. [CrossRef] [PubMed]
111. Cathcart, R.F. Vitamin C, titrating to bowel tolerance, anascorbemia, and acute induced scurvy. *Med. Hypotheses* **1981**, *7*, 1359–1376. [CrossRef]
112. Padayatty, S.J.; Sun, A.Y.; Chen, Q.; Espey, M.G.; Drisko, J.; Levine, M. Vitamin C: Intravenous use by complementary and alternative medicine practitioners and adverse effects. *PLoS ONE* **2010**, *5*, e11414. [CrossRef]
113. Auer, B.L.; Auer, D.; Rodgers, A.L. The effect of ascorbic acid ingestion on the biochemical and physicochemical risk factors associated with calcium oxalate kidney stone formation. *Clin. Chem. Lab. Med.* **1998**, *36*, 143–147. [CrossRef] [PubMed]
114. Curhan, G.C.; Willett, W.C.; Speizer, F.E.; Stampfer, M.J. Intake of vitamins B6 and C and the risk of kidney stones in women. *J. Am. Soc. Nephrol.* **1999**, *10*, 840–845.
115. Jiang, K.; Tang, K.; Liu, H.; Xu, H.; Ye, Z.; Chen, Z. Ascorbic acid supplements and kidney stones incidence among men and women: A systematic review and meta-analysis. *Urol. J* **2018**, *16*, 115–120.
116. Robitaille, L.; Mamer, O.A.; Miller, W.H., Jr.; Levine, M.; Assouline, S.; Melnychuk, D.; Rousseau, C.; Hoffer, L.J. Oxalic acid excretion after intravenous ascorbic acid administration. *Metabolism* **2009**, *58*, 263–269. [CrossRef] [PubMed]
117. Calder, P.C. Nutrition, immunity and COVID-19. *BMJ Nutr. Prev. Health* **2020**, *3*, e000085. [CrossRef] [PubMed]
118. Jovic, T.H.; Ali, S.R.; Ibrahim, N.; Jessop, Z.M.; Tarassoli, S.P.; Dobbs, T.D.; Holford, P.; Thornton, C.A.; Whitaker, I.S. Could vitamins help in the fight against COVID-19? *Nutrients* **2020**, *12*, 2550. [CrossRef] [PubMed]
119. Calder, P.C.; Carr, A.C.; Gombart, A.F.; Eggersdorfer, M. Optimal nutritional status for a well-functioning immune system is an important factor to protect against viral infections. *Nutrients* **2020**, *12*, 1181. [CrossRef]

3

The Impact of Food Histamine Intake on Asthma Activity

Emilia Vassilopoulou [1,*], George N. Konstantinou [2], Anastasia Dimitriou [3], Yannis Manios [4], Lemonica Koumbi [1] and Nikolaos G. Papadopoulos [3]

1 Department of Nutritional Sciences and Dietetics, International Hellenic University, 57400 Thessaloniki, Greece; lemonica.koumbi@gmail.com
2 Department of Allergy and Clinical Immunology, 424 General Military Training Hospital, 57400 Thessaloniki, Greece; gnkonstantinou@gmail.com
3 Allergy Department, 2nd Pediatric Clinic, University of Athens, 11528 Athens, Greece; drdimiana@gmail.com (A.D.); ngpallergy@gmail.com (N.G.P.)
4 Department of Nutrition and Dietetics, Harokopio University of Athens, 70 El. Venizelou Avenue, 17671 Kallithea, Greece; manios@hua.gr
* Correspondence: vassilopoulouemilia@gmail.com

Abstract: Asthma is a complex chronic inflammatory disorder. Diet's impact on asthma symptoms is controversial. The objective of this pilot crossover, randomized, two-period study was to examine the effect of dietary histamine intake on asthma symptoms in twenty-one children with mild intermittent asthma. Children were randomly assigned to either a high- or low-histamine diet, based on the Mediterranean pattern, for 4 weeks. After a 2-week washout period, patients crossed to the alternative diet for 4 additional weeks. Asthma symptoms were assessed at baseline and after the completion of each diet period by a clinician. Daily symptoms and peak flow were recorded throughout the intervention. Adherence to the dietary intervention was assessed via analysis of four random 24-h recalls, for each intervention period. Eighteen children completed the study. Significantly higher mean air flow obstruction was recorded and a trend for prolonged and more severe symptoms was observed during the high-histamine period. Diet may have an active and direct impact on asthma symptoms. Food choice is affected and/or may affect symptoms in children with mild asthma. Diet intervention is promising yet challenging, for asthma control.

Keywords: asthma; nutritional intervention; food histamine; Mediterranean diet; Western diet; antioxidants; anti-inflammatory diet

---

1. Introduction

Asthma is a common chronic disorder of the airways, considered nowadays more as an umbrella term to describe a constellation of clinical symptoms, including wheeze, breathlessness, chest tightness, and cough, with various underlying pathophysiologies [1]. Both genetic predisposition and exposure to environmental factors, such as allergens or irritants promoting airway inflammation, are involved [2].

Evidence shows that diet plays a significant role in the development and improvement of asthma control. Mediterranean diet, characterized by high consumption of vegetables, fruits, whole wheat products and fish, has been demonstrated to be beneficial on controlling asthma symptoms [3,4]. In contrast, "Western" diets, containing high amounts of processed food, saturated fat, sugar and salt, have been associated with increased asthma activity [5,6]. Other studies, however, have reached conflicting results on the effect of diet in asthma [7,8].

A number of food ingredients, including histamine, are known to have a pharmacological action and have been suggested to affect the clinical course of asthma, but their exact impact remains unclear [9,10]. Histamine is contained in food mainly in alcoholic beverages such as red wine or highly processed or spoiled food such as cheese and canned fish, while it can also be found in other food sources after the decarboxylation of the amino acid histidine. Histamine's content in food varies considerably even within the same food product and is highly affected by the product's maturity, storage time and processing [11]. It can be metabolized either by oxidative deamination by diamine oxidase (DAO) or by ring methylation by histamine-N-methyltransferase (HNMT). Notably, the last is regarded as the key enzyme for histamine degradation in the bronchial epithelium [10].

The ingestion of histamine-rich foods results in histamine release and blocks the DAO enzyme that is involved in histamine metabolism [11]. A disequelibrium of accumulated histamine and the incapacity of histamine degradation leads to histamine intolerance [11]. The symptoms of this non-allergic adverse reaction involve several organs, such as skin and gastrointestinal system, but also the cardiovascular and respiratory systems, depending on the plasma histamine levels. Specifically, a slight increase in plasma histamine concentrations (i.e., 1–2 ng/mL) has been shown to exert gastrointestinal symptoms or tachycardia, while a 10-fold higher concentration (i.e., 7–12 ng/mL) can lead to a bronchospasm [11]. As recently reported, food histamine intolerance manifests with the appearance of symptoms such as wheeze and asthma [11] and the proposed mechanism for asthma exacerbations is the reduction of HNMT activity [10].

Undisputedly, cellular histamine is involved in asthma pathophysiology. Apart from the mast cells and basophils, there is evidence that cellular histamine is also produced significantly by some gut microbiome phyla in non-obese asthmatic patients [12–14]. Diet has a predominant role in the gut microbiota composition and its metabolic activity, but the precise role of histamine-producing bacteria and of the ingested histamine in the disease course is yet to be discovered.

The present pilot study aims to investigate the potential of controlling dietary histamine intake and whether this can interfere with the development of respiratory symptoms in children with mild asthma.

2. Materials and Methods

2.1. Patients

Twenty-one children (12 boys), diagnosed and followed up in an outpatient allergy unit of a tertiary pediatric hospital in Athens, with mild intermittent asthma (Global Initiative for Asthma (GINA) Stage 1) [15] and documented forced expiratory volume (FEV1) reversibility, were enrolled in the study.

Exclusion criteria included failure to comply with study procedures, presence of other chronic or acute diseases (except rhinitis, allergic conjunctivitis or atopic dermatitis), systematic treatment for diseases other than asthma, and food allergy history. Children and their parents were informed about the study's protocol and procedures and signed consent was obtained. The parents/caregivers gave their signed informed consent for all the children included in the study before their participation. The study was conducted in accordance with the Declaration of Helsinki, and the protocol was approved by the Scientifical Council and Bioethics committee of the Children Hospital Panagiotis & Aglaia Kyriakou Scientific (Project identification code: issue 3; 130406).

2.2. Study Design

A two-period, two-intervention, randomized crossover design was used that, depending on the histamine content, included two types of diet, a low-histamine (LH) and a high-histamine (HH) diet (Table 1). Participants were randomly assigned following simple randomization procedures (computer-generated random numbers) to start with one out of the two proposed diet patterns for eight weeks and continued with the other one for another eight weeks, with a two-week washout period in between. During this time, the volunteers could consume their typical diet without any restriction.

Table 1. Food ranking in low and high histamine content.

Food Group/Type of Diet	Low Histamine	High Histamine
Dairy products	Fresh pasteurised plain milk without additives (cow's or goat's), butter, plain yogurt, ricotta cheese, cottage cheese, cream cheese	All mature cheese, e.g., brie, camembert, cedar, Cheshire, Danish blue, edam, emmental, Gloucester, gouda, mozzarella, parmesan, Roquefort, yogurt with additives such as fruits, cereal, cacao milk, chocolate milk, plain whole fat long life milk
Fruit	Fresh not very mature apple, apricot, peach, pear, melon	Mature dates, kiwi, orange, papaya, tangerine, passion fruit, avocado, banana, fig, grape, lemon, pineapple, plum, berry, strawberry
Vegetables	Asparagus, cabbage, lettuce, green beans, onion, pepper, radish, turnip	Broccoli, cauliflower, eggplant, mushroom, tomato, sauerkraut, spinach, cucumber
Legumes	Peas, lentils, chickpeas	Beans, soybeans
Starchy products/grains	Bread with natural yeast without preservatives, oat cereals, pure corn flakes, potato, sweet potato, rice, spaghetti, any type of pasta excluded pasta stuffed with cheese, mince meat, cold-cuts, (e.g., tortellini) and colored pasta (with spinach, carrot, etc.	Bread with preservatives, long life bread, stuffed pasta with cheese, mince meat, cold cuts, colored pasta, cereals with chocolate, cereals with fruits, cereals with nuts, ready-made meals (frozen)
Nuts	Chestnut, sunflower seeds, pine nuts, pistachios, almonds, coconuts, currants, red currants, cashew nut, macadamia nut	Hazelnuts, brazil nuts, walnuts, pecan, peanuts, peanut butter
Spices	Herbs, spices except for anise, red pepper, curry (ready-made spicy products not allowed)	Malt vinegar, meat products, soy sauce, vinegar, Worcestershire sauce, yeast products
Meat/poultry/fish	Beef, chicken without skin, turkey without skin, fresh fish, lamb, rabbit, veal, cooked eggs, boiled unsalted turkey	Meat, fish and poultry older than two days, any frozen meat, any form of raw or smoked meat or fish, anchovies, beef liver, pies and pasta with meat, fish nuggets, salami, sausages, chicken livers, canned tuna, canned salmon
Fats/oils	All vegetable oils, homemade sauces prepared with permitted ingredients	Ready-made sauces, olives, oils with preservatives and colorants, olives
Beverages	Homemade lemonade	Tea, decaffeinated tea, ready-made juices, chocolate drinks, cacao-drink, soft drinks including cola-type, tomato juice, vegetable juices
Sweets/sweeteners	Sugar, homemade jams, homemade sweets with permitted ingredients	Cocoa, milk chocolate, black chocolate, white chocolate

Foods from all groups (dairy, fruits, vegetables, starch, meat, fat) were ranked according to their histamine content into low or high histamine [9,16–19]. A food list (Table 1), together with eight model diet plans (1800–2000 Kcal; 50% carbohydrates–15% protein–35% fat of which <10 saturated fat) based on the Mediterranean diet prototype, i.e., with a high content of olive oil, whole wheat products, fish, legumes, fruit and vegetables [3], one for each week of the 8-week intervention period, were prepared (example on Table 2). Considering the high variability on histamine content within the same product depending on maturity, storage and processing, a specialized dietitian encouraged patients and their parents to strictly select food products from the LH or HH food list when they were required to make modifications in the respective daily diet plan. Especially for the LH period they were instructed to select fresh not mature of the respective listed fruit and vegetables, to consume fresh meat and fish and to completely avoid frozen and canned products, as well as ready-prepared or packaged food that contain preservatives. Therefore, food recipes for preparing homemade food like juices, jams, burgers, sauces like tomato sauce, lemonade, bread, salads, cake were provided. Hand measures were used to instruct the food portion size measures [20], but each patient decided his portion size ad libitum to avoid weight changes.

Before randomization (t0), participants were evaluated by a clinician to confirm mild intermittent asthma according to GINA [15] and controlled with low inhaled corticosteroids (fluticasone propionate pMDI 100 μg bid). Basic anthropometric measurements (weight and height) were also recorded.

The best out of three morning and evening Peak Expiratory Flow Rate (PEFR) were measured with a flow meter and recorded on diary cards. A reduction of at least 15% reduction in airflow was considered as an asthma episode [21]. Daily symptom scores [22] were documented on diary cards throughout the study. Upper airway symptoms included blocked/stuffy nose, runny nose, sneezing/itchy nose, itchy/sore/watery eyes, hoarse voice, and sore throat. Lower airway symptoms included cough and wheezing/noisy breathing during the day, the night and during exercise. Each symptom was scored from 0 (no symptom) to 3 (severely troublesome). A sum of at least 3 score units for either the upper or the lower respiratory symptomatology was considered as a *"higher score"* day. Symptoms were quantitatively associated and compared between the different dietary intervention periods. The recorded symptom scores (upper, lower or total) were evaluated and analyzed.

After the end of the first (t1) and second (t2) intervention period, asthma symptom records were re-assessed on site, and weights were measured. At t1, guidance for the cross-arm diet plan was provided, for patients to proceed to the second intervention stage after the two weeks washout period. During the intervention periods, eight 24 h recalls were recorded randomly by phone during each diet intervention, in order to assess compliance and provide assistance for better diet implementation. Histidine intake, which is metabolized to histamine, together with the overall energy, macronutrients and micronutrients were further determined via the 24-h diet recalls with the Food-Processor Nutrition Analysis Software [23]. A post-hoc analysis of food choices during the intervention period was performed to evaluate preference changes depending on the provided food lists and symptom fluctuation. Adherence to the Mediterranean diet was explored via the KIDMED questionnaire [24].

Table 2. Model weekly diet plan provided to the patients for the low-histamine (LH) and high-histamine (HH) period of the dietary intervention.

	*Low Histamine **						
Breakfast	1 cup of fresh whole fat plain milk+ 2 slices of whole wheat bread made with fresh yeast+ 1tsp butter+ 1tsp honey	1 cup of fresh whole fat milk+ 1slice of whole wheat bread made with fresh yeast+ 1tsp homemade peach jam	1 cup of fresh whole fat plain milk+ 3 whole wheat bread rusks	1 cup of fresh whole fat plain milk+ 1 whole wheat bread+ 1tsp honey	200gr whole fat Greek yogurt+ 1 pear	1 cup of fresh whole fat plain milk+ 2 slices of whole wheat bread made with fresh yeast+ 1tsp butter+ 1tsp honey	1 cup of fresh whole fat plain milk+ 2 slices of whole wheat bread made with fresh yeast+ 1tsp butter+ 1tsp honey
Snack	1 cup melon	1 cup of fresh apple-pear juice	1 apple	1 pear	1 cup of fresh juice from apple-pear	1 apple	1 cup of fresh apple juice
Lunch	1 portion green fresh beans+ 1 slice of whole wheat bread+ potatoes	1 portion stuffed zucchini or peppers with rice and beef or turkey mince meat+ 1slice of whole-wheat bread	1 portion of boiled fresh fish+ 1 boiled potato+ boiled carrots, zucchini	1 portion ratatouille vegetables (zucchini, carrots, peppers, onion, olive oil, potatoes)+ 1 slice whole wheat bread	1 portion of pasta with turkey/chicken/beef mince meat+ boiled zucchini+ olive oil	4–5 fried meatballs with chicken mince meat+ 15–20 slices of fried potatoes+ lettuce salad	1 portion leek with rice, lemon and olive oil+ 1 slice whole wheat bread+ cottage or cream cheese
Snack	Oven-baked apple with egg and breadcrumbs, sugar and cinnamon	1 milkshake with fresh whole fat plain milk, vanilla flavour, honey	Homemade popcorn with olive oil or butter	1 slice of homemade vanilla cake	1 homemade rice pudding	1 full-fat yogurt+ 1tsp honey	1 apple milk shake: full-fat milk, apple, cinnamon, honey
Dinner	Homemade Caesars Chicken salad with lettuce, boiled corn, cucumber, olive oil	1 homemade chicken burger with whole wheat bread, lettuce	1 homemade sandwich with lettuce, cottage cheese, boiled turkey ham, lettuce	1 homemade souvlaki with chicken meat and whole wheat pita bread, fried potatoes	Egg salad: egg, tomato, lettuce, olive oil	Lettuce salad with baked lamb meat	Baked chicken meat with cucumber-lettuce salad and olive oil

Table 2. *Cont.*

	High Histamine *						
Breakfast	1 cup of whole fat long life milk+ 2whole wheat homemade chocolate biscuits	1 cup of whole fat long life milk+ 1slice of whole wheat bread+ 1tsp Nutella	1 cup of whole fat long life chocolate milk+ 2 homemade vanilla biscuits	1 cup of whole fat long life milk+ 1 whole wheat bread+ 1tsp honey	1 fruit stirred yogurt with strawberries	1 cup of whole fat long life milk+ $\frac{1}{2}$ cup chocolate cereals	1 cup of whole fat long life milk+ 2 slices of toasted bread+ 2tsp strawberry jam
Snack	1 cup of fresh orange juice	1 cup of packed mixed fruit juice	1 banana	1 cup of packed anana juice	1 banana	1 kiwi fruit	1 cup of packed mixed fruit juice
Lunch	1 portion of lentils+ mature yellow cheese (Cretan graviera)+ 1slice of wholewheat bread	1 portion stuffed tomatoes with rice and frozen mince-meat+ 1slice of wholewheat bread+ feta cheese	1 portion of frozen fish sticks+ 1boiled potato+ cauliflower or broccoli	1 portion "tourlou" vegetables (aubergine, carrots, cucumber, tomato, olive oil, potatoes)+ 1 slice whole wheat bread+ feta cheese	1 portion pasta with tomato sauce and mushrooms+ parmesan cheese+ Tomato salad	4-5 fried meatballs from frozen minced-meat+ 15-20 slices of fried potatoes+ broccoli or cauliflower	1 portion spinach with rice and tomato+ feta cheese+ 1 slice of whole wheat bread
Snack	1 yogurt with chocolate slices	Homemade Banana milkshake (banana, whole milk, honey)	Fruit salad: grapes, orange, banana	1 cup strawberries or grapes	chocolate ice cream	50gr milk or back chocolate	Lemon or strawberry Sorbet
Dinner	1 piece of ham and cheese pie	1 burger with pork mince neat_ tomato salad	1 hot dog: whole wheat bread, 1 sausage stuffed with cheese, 1tsp mustard, 1tsp ketchup	1 souvlaki with pork meat and whole wheat pita bread, fried potatoes, tomato	Chef salad: Roquefort cheese, salami, cedar, boiled egg, tomato, lettuce, olive il	1 slice of spinach pie	Baked pork meat with Greek salad

* All meals and salads prepared with fresh olive oil.

Participant's flowchart with a description of the patients' inclusion criteria and study's design is shown in Figure 1.

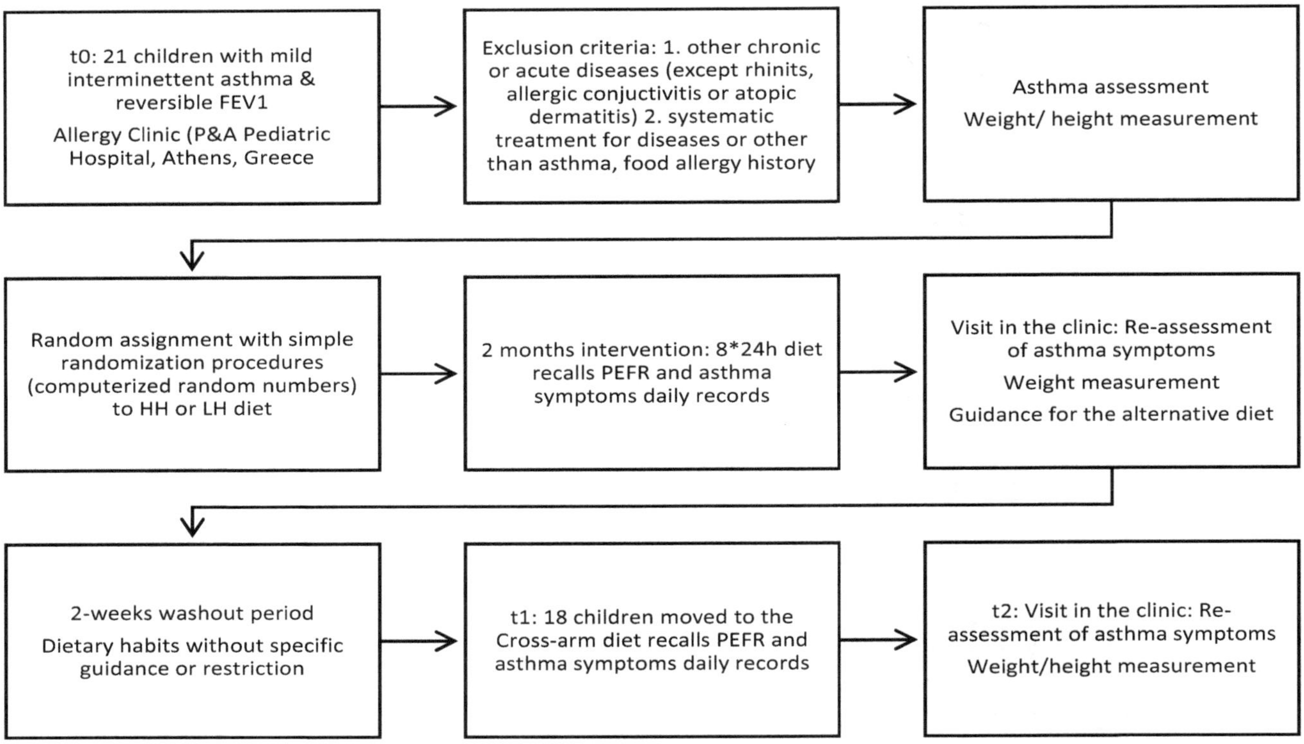

Figure 1. Participant flowchart.

2.3. *Statistical Analysis*

The distributions of all recorded parameters were assessed with the Shapiro–Wilk test. Descriptive statistics are presented as median (inter-quartile range) for non-normally distributed variables and means ± standard deviation for normally distributed parameters. The Wilcoxon rank-sum test and Kruskal–Wallis tests were used to compare continuous variables and the Pearson's X^2 test to compare categorical variables among studied groups. The Wilcoxon matched-pairs rank-sum test was used to compare continuous variables within the same individual between the multiple measurements. All reported *p*-values are based on 2-sided tests and compared with a significance level of 5%. Stata 9.1 for Windows (Stata Corp LP, College Station, TX, USA) was used for all statistical calculations and plots.

3. Results

Eighteen children (10 boys) (mean age 11.5 ± 3.1 years) completed the study successfully. Mean weight at entry point was 47.3 kg (±11.9), mean height was 1.37 m (±9.3) and according to the respective weight to age and height to age growth charts they were within the normal range. No significant weight changes were observed between the different intervention periods ($p = 0.5$).

Mean % predicted FEV1 was 92.6 (±8.6) and no loss of asthma control was recorded during the study period. Nevertheless, the mean PEFR during the LH period was 400 L/min (±55.9) and significantly higher ($p = 0.0006$) than the respective mean PEFR during the HH period 388 L/min (±59).

Both upper and lower respiratory symptom scores were lower during the LH period, but the relevant statistical comparisons were not significant. In addition, the median number of symptom-free days had a two-fold increase during the LH diet period as compared to the HH (5.5 days vs. 9.5), but the differences were non-significant (*p*-value = 0.753) (Table 3).

Table 3. Comparisons between the median number of days with symptoms and median symptom score during the two intervention periods.

		Type of Diet		
		Low Histamine	**High Histamine**	***p*-Values** **
Symptoms duration in days		5.5 (8)	9.5 (4)	0.753
Respiratory Symptoms	Upper *	4.67 (11.5)	12.5 (5.83)	0.780
	Lower *	4.25 (13.1)	14 (12.45)	0.727
	Total *	11.33 (53.5)	30.17 (21.42)	0.889

Data are presented as median (interquartile range). * units in symptom score scale; ** comparisons between different types of diets (Wilcoxon matched-pairs sign test).

Patients' dietary habits during the last year before the intervention were characterized by a high consumption of red meat, processed foods, saturated fat, sodium and sugar and low consumption of fruit, vegetables, legumes and fish. In line with this observation, adhesion to the Mediterranean diet was found low with a need to be improved (mean KIDMED score = 4 ± 2).

Upon intervention, adherence to the diet protocol was assessed via analysis of the 24-h diet recalls, in terms of types of foods consumed (Table 4) as well as macronutrient and micronutrient intake. Histidine intake was found to be higher in the HH diet (Table 5). As anticipated, the food choices varied among the LH and HH periods. During the HH diet, milk, junk food, juices and vegetables intake was higher at symptom-free days than during the LH diet. At higher symptom score days, the intake of oils and butter, fish, chocolate, egg and junk food were higher in the HH diet than in LH. Fish consumption was generally low but increased during days with higher symptom scores independently of the diet assigned, possibly due to caregivers' belief that is a "healthy" choice to relieve symptoms.

Moreover, symptom fluctuation affected food choices within the same intervention period. In the symptom-free days during the HH diet, children consumed more starchy foods, olive oil, chocolate, bacon, ham or sausages and junk food, than in the days with higher symptoms when they consumed more fish and butter. Respectively, in the LH symptom-free days, individuals chose more starchy products, juices from permitted fruit and permitted ham. On the contrary, at higher symptom days during the LH diet, they consumed more olive oil and fresh fish.

In terms of micronutrients, inadequate intake of vitamin D, potassium, and manganese was noted at all stages of intervention. Marginally lower intake of calcium and folate compared to the Dietary Reference Intakes (DRIs) [25] were noted during LH. Furthermore, although zinc's intake was sufficient at all stages, it was double during the HH stage (Table 5).

Table 4. Changes in the frequency of consumption of different foods (food choices) according to symptom fluctuation during and among the two intervention periods.

	LH Period			HH Period			HH vs. LH	
	Remission	Episode		Remission	Episode		Remission	Episode
			p-Value [1]			p-Value [1]	p-Value [2]	p-Value [3]
Milk	1.74 (±1.38)	2.69 (±1.21)	0.064	2.69 (±1.98)	3.77 (±1.35)	0.133	0.004	0.107
Starchy food	3.65 (2.94)	6.04 (2.72)	0.021	4.61 (3.28)	6.27 (±1.85)	0.046	0.972	0.141
Meat	4.01 (±2.91)	5.19 (±2.32)	0.382	3.25 (±2.05)	4.4 (±1.78)	0.133	0.196	0.207
Olive oil	3.24 (±3.12)	0.26 (±0.44)	0.014	0.28 (±0.44)	4.23 (±3.16)	0.002	0.002	0.007
Butter	0.318 (±0.83)	0.05 (±0.14)	0.299	2.56 (±2.62)	0.46 (±0.5)	0.043	0.014	0.007
Fish	0.51 (±0.89)	0.75 (±0.59)	0.184	3.7 (±2.93)	0.29 (±0.47)	0.003	0.059	0.003
Chocolate	0.268 (±0.7)	0.28 (±0.45)	0.657	0.9 (±0.74)	3.33 (±3.06)	0.007	0.002	0.015
Egg	0.05 (±0.15)	0.04 (±0.08)	0.809	0.89 (±1.47)	0.18 (±0.34)	0.053	0.027	0.006
Sweats	0.74 (±0.8)	1.12 (±1.1)	0.328	1.55 (±1.34)	1.46 (±1.08)	0.861	0.463	0.123
Nuts	0.67 (±1.3)	0.4 (±0.42)	0.528	0.61 (±1.39)	0.09 (±0.19)	0.426	0.035	0.514
Bacon or sausages or ham	0.11 (±0.18)	5.08 (±3.21)	0.002	0.31 (±1.11)	0.71 (±0.46)	0.030	0.002	0.242
Junk food	1.01 (±1.27)	0.89 (±1.15)	0.889	0.12 (±0.3)	2.03 (±1.41)	0.002	0.055	0.017
Fried oil	0.79 (±1.25)	0.14 (±0.13)	0.726	1.23 (±1.59)	1.26 (±0.94)	0.917	0.003	0.105
Juices	0	0.8 (0.76)	0.004	0.15 (0.56)	0.12 (0.2)	0.155	0.016	0.317
Fruit	0.29M (±0.37)	0.82 (±0.61)	0.546	1.27 (±2.35)	0.59 (±0.49)	0.726	0.221	0.302
Vegetables	0.66 (±1.02)	0.1 (±0.23)	0.052	0.4 (±0.51)	0.95 (±0.79)	0.028	0.002	0.806

Changes in food choices are presented in mean (±standard deviation). Comparisons (Wilcoxon matched-pairs rank-sum test) of food choices: [1] during episodes vs. remission periods within the same intervention period; [2] during remission between the two intervention periods; [3] during episodes between the two intervention periods.

Table 5. Comparison of micronutrient intake (mean values) with Dietary Reference Intake (DRI).

Type of Diet	High Histamine	Low Histamine	DRI
Sodium (mg) **	3200	1808	1500
Potassium (mg)	2922	2557	4500
Calcium (mg)	1365	807	1300
Iron (mg)	14.5	12	8
Phosphorus (mg)	1603	1208	1250
Magnesium (mg)	280	240	240
Zinc (mg) **	22	8.9	8
Copper (mg)	1.3	1	0.7
Manganese (mg)	1.6	1.7	1.9
Selenium (mg)	0.13	0.1	0.04
Fluoride (μg)	223	300	200
Chromium (mg)	0.03	0.04	0.025
Molybdenum (μg)	43	49	34
Histidine (mg) **	2400	1800	NA
Vitamin A (RE)	637	627	600
Beta-carotene (ug) **	217	494	NA
Vitamin C (mg)	54	46	45
Vitamin D (ug)	4.5	4.46	15
Vitamin E (IU)	11.6	10.4	11
Thiamin (mg)	2	1.26	0.9
Riboflavin (mg)	2.4	1.67	0.9
Niacin (mg)	21.5	20.4	12
Vit B6 (mg)	1.65	1.5	1
Vit B6 (mg)	1.65	1.5	1
Folate (μg)	336	253	300
Vit B12 (μg)	4.98	3.8	1.8
Biotin (μg)	21.5	20.6	20
Pantothenic Acid (mg)	4.4	4	4
Vitamin K (μg)	30	40	60

Deficient intake in specific nutrients is marked in bold letters. ** statistically significant difference ($p = 0.05$) for specific nutrient's intake among the two types of diet. NA: non- applicable.

4. Discussion

Childhood asthma is a complex disease and evidence indicate that diet plays a role on its clinical outcome. This randomized crossover dietary intervention aimed to evaluate the effects of dietary histamine in children with mild asthma. Our results clearly show a significantly higher airflow obstruction during the high-histamine period, whereas a trend towards less symptoms and more symptom-free days during the low histamine intake diet periods was observed.

Histamine is a potent inflammatory mediator and is associated with deleterious inflammation in asthmatic patients, triggering airway hyper-responsiveness and remodelling. The microbial community in the intestine is shaped by the diet and supplies the host with a number of metabolites, including short-chain fatty acids and histamine. Histamine-secreting bacteria are found at a higher frequency in faecal samples from asthmatic patients. The possible contribution to their atopic phenotype is a matter of further investigation, through larger-scale studies on the microbial diversity of asthmatics, especially because it is impossible to distinguish the microbial-derived histamine from the human-produced form [14].

Moreover, food histamine has been demonstrated to be a trigger for worsening asthma symptoms [10]. In line with this, we found higher intake of histamine in the form of histidine in the HH period to be associated with higher airflow obstruction and symptom exacerbation. Histamine intolerance in asthmatics could lead to dyspnea or dysphonia provoked after high histamine ingestion [10]. Notably, histidine is not the only source of histamine from food but is also an autochthonous ingredient in some foods produced by different cooking preparations [17]. Therefore, this finding can be partly accepted as a measure of compliance and as a separate notion.

As the role of diet on asthma symptoms is complex, dietary plans implemented herein were designed under Mediterranean-style eating pattern. This was decided in order to control at most the overall nutrient intake and for the benefit of the patients of the study since it is generally accepted that the specific diet pattern reduces inflammation [7]. Indeed, the analysis of the diet-recalls revealed a desirable high consumption of olive oil (MUFA), as the main source of fat at all stages of the intervention.

The anti-inflammatory n-3 PUFA [26–29] intake though, originating from fish oil, was generally low. Interestingly, when children in both intervention phases developed symptoms, they increased fish consumption. It can be assumed that caregivers considered fish as a "healthy" choice to relieve symptoms. Similarly, our cases presented a deficient vitamin D intake at all times, which has been previously correlated to pulmonary dysfunction in childhood [30], but consumed more butter during the symptomatic periods, which is an external source of vitamin D. Adequate vitamin D intake has been suggested to reduce the number of exacerbations, the requirement of steroids and emergency visits in asthmatic school-aged children. Although no safe conclusions can be produced for the role of vitamin D in this intervention, further evaluations are needed about its beneficial role in asthma, as results so far are unclear [31,32].

Saturated fat intake, originating from milk, egg, fried food, and meat products, was generally high at all intervention stages. Past habits of our participants were closer to the Western diet, with a high intake of SF, refined grains and sugar. Patients were advised at the beginning of the intervention to follow the provided model diets but had the liberty to make changes with foods from the respective provided food list, according to their personal preferences and established dietary habits. As such, they often chose processed foods with higher saturated fat and sugar content. Nevertheless, and although saturated fat is associated with the induction of proinflammatory mediators [33], SF intake was equal in both intervention stages, so no further estimation of its influence can be made.

On the other hand, during the LH period, beta-carotene intake was superior. Beta-carotene is an important antioxidant that has been directly involved in asthma pathogenesis [34]. This positive effect could have added to the shorter and milder periods of symptoms encountered during the low-histamine diet. During the same intervention period, zinc intake was recorded within the recommended DRI's but lower in comparison to the HH period. Zinc has been previously suggested to increase antioxidant function and reduce asthma exacerbations [35]. Nevertheless, these data cannot be better evaluated in the current study's context.

As elucidated from our results, a diet intervention aiming to control a single nutrient's intake is really challenging unless, as elsewhere shown, this is based on a food supplement [36] or ready-prepared meals to control overall intake [37,38]. Both these strategies, though, do not reflect the ability of patients to adapt to the proposed changes of eating habits, nor provide the long-term effect of dietary changes [39]. Irrespective of this, such change is generally difficult to adopt and maintain unless proper therapeutic techniques from medical nutrition and behavioral therapy are incorporated [40].

The present study suggests that food histamine has a significant impact on asthma outcome in children who show a trend for a more "healthy diet" during symptom deterioration periods. Our findings show a significance in mean airflow obstruction and a trend for more symptoms with higher duration during the high-histamine period. As the last did not reach significance, probably due to the small sample of participants, the short intervention period and the mild symptomatology of the selected patients, we could aim for future studies with longer intervention periods, a bigger number of participants or participants with more persistent or severe asthma to confirm this effect.

5. Conclusions

Eating behaviors change in asthmatics during days with symptoms, as also shown here. Histamine intake, along with other dietary factors, influences asthma. In order for the actual effect on the clinical outcomes to emerge, further exploration with long-term dietary interventions are needed, keeping in mind that a diet intervention is promising yet seriously challenging.

Author Contributions: Conceptualization E.V. and N.G.P.; Methodology E.V., G.N.K. and A.D.; Formal Analysis: E.V., G.N.K., Y.M. and L.K.; Writing—Original Draft Preparation: E.V.; Review and Editing: G.N.K., N.G.P., A.D., Y.M. and L.K.; Supervision: N.G.P. All authors have approved the submitted version and agree to be personally accountable for the author's own contributions and for ensuring that questions related to the accuracy or integrity of any part of the work, even ones in which the authors were not personally involved, are appropriately investigated, resolved, and documented in the literature. All authors have read and agreed to the published version of the manuscript.

Acknowledgments: We would like to express our gratitude to the parents of the children included in the study, for their cooperation during the study and the nurses of the Allergy Clinic for their continues support.

References

1. Pavord, I.D.; Beasley, R.; Agusti, A.; Anderson, G.P.; Bel, E.; Brusselle, G.; Cullinan, P.; Custovic, A.; Ducharme, F.M.; Fahy, J.V.; et al. After asthma: Redefining airways diseases. *Lancet* **2018**, *391*, 350–400. [CrossRef]
2. Papadopoulos, N.G.; Arakawa, H.; Lodrup-Carlsen, K.; Custovic, A.; Gern, J.; Lemanske, R.; Le Souef, P.; Mäkelä, M.; Roberts, G.; Wong, G.; et al. International consensus on (ICON) pediatric asthma. *Allergy Eur. J. Allergy Clin. Immunol.* **2012**, *67*, 976–997. [CrossRef] [PubMed]
3. Willett, W.C.; Sacks, F.; Trichopoulou, A.; Drescher, G.; Ferro-Luzzi, A.; Helsing, E.; Trichopoulos, D. Mediterranean diet pyramid: A cultural model for healthy eating. *Am. J. Clin. Nutr.* **1995**, *61* (Suppl. S6). [CrossRef] [PubMed]
4. Calatayud-Sáez, F.M.; Calatayud Moscoso del Prado, B.; Gallego Fernández-Pacheco, J.G.; González-Martín, C.; Alguacil Merino, L.F. Mediterranean diet and childhood asthma. *Allergol. Immunopathol. (Madr)* **2016**, *44*, 99–105. [CrossRef] [PubMed]
5. Berentzen, N.E.; Van Stokkom, V.L.; Gehring, U.; Koppelman, G.H.; Schaap, L.A.; Smit, H.A.; Wijga, A.H. Associations of sugar-containing beverages with asthma prevalence in 11-year-old children: The PIAMA birth cohort. *Eur. J. Clin. Nutr.* **2015**, *69*, 303–308. [CrossRef] [PubMed]
6. Han, Y.-Y.; Forno, E.; Alvarez, M.; Colón-Semidey, A.; Acosta-Perez, E.; Canino, G.; Celedón, J.C. Diet, Lung Function, and Asthma Exacerbations in Puerto Rican Children. *Pediatr. Allergy Immunol. Pulmonol.* **2017**, *30*, 202–209. [CrossRef]
7. Guilleminault, L.; Williams, E.J.; Scott, H.A.; Berthon, B.S.; Jensen, M.; Wood, L.G. Diet and Asthma: Is It Time to Adapt Our Message? *Nutrients* **2017**, *9*, 1227. [CrossRef]
8. Seaton, A.; Godden, D.J.; Brown, K. Increase in asthma: A more toxic environment or a more susceptible population? *Thorax* **1994**, *49*, 171–174. [CrossRef]
9. Wantke, F.; Gotz, M.; Jarisch, R. Histamine-free diet: Treatment of choice for histamine-induced food intolerance and supporting treatment for chronical headaches. *Clin. Exp. Allergy* **1993**, *23*, 982–985. [CrossRef]
10. Maintz, L.; Novak, N. Histamine and Histamine Intolerance. *Am. J. Clin. Nutr.* **2007**, *85*, 1185–1196. [CrossRef]

11. Reese, I.; Ballmer-Weber, B.; Beyer, K.; Fuchs, T.; Kleine-Tebbe, J.; Klimek, L.; Lepp, U.; Niggemann, B.; Saloga, J.; Schäfer, C.; et al. German guideline for the management of adverse reactions to ingested histamine: Guideline of the German Society for Allergology and Clinical Immunology (DGAKI), the German Society for Pediatric Allergology and Environmental Medicine (GPA), the German Association of Allergologists (AeDA), and the Swiss Society for Allergology and Immunology (SGAI). *Allergo J. Int.* **2017**, *26*, 72–79. [CrossRef] [PubMed]
12. Dunford, P.J.; Holgate, S.T. The Role of Histamine in Asthma. In *Histamine in Inflammation*; Advances in Experimental Medicine and Biology; Thurmond, R.L., Ed.; Springer: Boston, MA, USA, 2010; Volume 709. [CrossRef]
13. Yamauchi, K.; Ogasawara, M. The Role of Histamine in the Pathophysiology of Asthma and the Clinical Efficacy of Antihistamines in Asthma Therapy. *Int. J. Mol. Sci.* **2019**, *20*, 1733. [CrossRef] [PubMed]
14. Barcik, W.; Pugin, B.; Westermann, P.; Perez, N.R.; Ferstl, R.; Wawrzyniak, M.; Smolinska, S.; Jutel, M.; Hessel, E.M.; Michalovich, D.; et al. Histamine-secreting microbes are increased in the gut of adult asthma patients. *J. Allergy Clin. Immunol.* **2016**, *138*, 1491–1494.e7. [CrossRef] [PubMed]
15. Pocket Guide for Asthma Management and Prevention (for Adults and Children Older than 5 Years. Available online: https://ginasthma.org/wp-content/uploads/2019/04/GINA-2019-main-Pocket-Guide-wms.pdf (accessed on 2 July 2020).
16. Histamine Intolerance Awareness. The Food List. Available online: https://www.histamineintolerance.org.uk/about/the-food-diary/the-food-list/ (accessed on 9 September 2020).
17. Chung, B.Y.; Park, S.Y.; Byun, Y.S.; Son, J.H.; Choi, Y.W.; Cho, Y.S.; Park, C.W.; Park, C.W. Effect of Different Cooking Methods on Histamine Levels in Selected Foods. *Ann. Dermatol.* **2017**, *29*, 706–714. [CrossRef]
18. Sánchez-Pérez, S.; Comas-Basté, O.; Rabell-González, J.; Eveciana-Nogués, M.; Latorre-Moratalla, M.L.; Vidal-Carou, M. Biogenic Amines in Plant-Origin Foods: Are They Frequently Underestimated in Low-Histamine Diets? *Foods* **2018**, *7*, 205. [CrossRef]
19. San Mauro Martin, I.; Brachero, S.; Garicano Vilar, E. Histamine intolerance and dietary management: A complete review. *Allergol. Immunopathol. (Madr.)* **2016**, *44*, 475–483. [CrossRef]
20. Gibson, A.A.; Hsu, M.S.H.; Rangan, A.M.; Seimon, R.V.; Lee, C.M.Y.; Das, A.; Finch, C.H.; Sainsbury, A. Accuracy of hands v. household measures as portion size estimation aids. *J. Nutr. Sci.* **2016**, *5*, e29. [CrossRef]
21. Adeniyi, A.; Erhabor, G.E.; The peak flow meter and its use in clinical practice. *Afr. J. Respir. Med.* 2011. Available online: https://www.africanjournalofrespiratorymedicine.com/articles/Peak%20flow%20meter.pdf (accessed on 15 October 2020).
22. Konstantinou, G.N.; Xepapadaki, P.; Manousakis, E.; Makrinioti, H.; Kouloufakou-Gratsia, K.; Saxoni-Papageorgiou, P.; Papadopoulos, N.G. Assessment of airflow limitation, airway inflammation, and symptoms during virus-induced wheezing episodes in 4- to 6-year-old children. *J. Allergy Clin. Immunol.* **2013**, *131*. [CrossRef]
23. Esha Research. Food Processor Nutrition Analysis Software. Available online: https://esha.com/products/food-processor/ (accessed on 2 July 2020).
24. Mariscal-Arcas, M.; Rivas, A.; Velasco, J.; Ortega, M.; Caballero, A.M.; Olea-Serrano, F. Evaluation of the Mediterranean Diet Quality Index (KIDMED) in children and adolescents in Southern Spain. *Public Health Nutr.* **2009**, *12*, 1408–1412. [CrossRef]
25. DRI Dietary Reference Intakes. Available online: https://www.ncbi.nlm.nih.gov/books/NBK222890/ (accessed on 2 July 2020).
26. D'Vaz, N.; Meldrum, S.; Dunstan, J.A.; Martino, D.; McCarthy, S.; Metcalfe, J.; Tulic, M.K.; Mori, T.A.; Prescott, S.L. Postnatal fish oil supplementation in high-risk infants to prevent allergy: Randomized controlled trial. *Pediatrics* **2012**, *130*, 674–682. [CrossRef]
27. Schindler, T.; Sinn, J.K.; Osborn, D.A. Polyunsaturated fatty acid supplementation in infancy for the prevention of allergy. *Cochrane Database Syst. Rev.* **2016**, *2016*. [CrossRef] [PubMed]
28. Nagel, G.; Linseisen, J. Dietary intake of fatty acids, antioxidants and selected food groups and asthma in adults'. *Eur. J. Clin. Nutr.* **2005**, *59*, 8–15. [CrossRef] [PubMed]
29. Li, J.; Xun, P.; Zamora, D.; Sood, A.; Liu, K.; Daviglus, M.; Iribarren, C.; Jacobs, D.; Shikany, J.M.; He, K. Intakes of long-chain omega-3 (n-3) PUFAs and fish in relation to incidence of asthma among American young adults: The CARDIA study. *Am. J. Clin. Nutr.* **2013**, *97*, 173–178. [CrossRef] [PubMed]

30. Han, Y.-Y.; Forno, E.; Celedón, J.C. Vitamin D Insufficiency and Asthma in a US Nationwide Study. *J. Allergy Clin. Immunol. Pract.* **2017**, *5*, 790–796. [CrossRef]
31. Yadav, M.; Mittal, K. Effect of vitamin D supplementation on moderate to severe bronchial asthma. *Indian J. Pediatr.* **2014**, *81*, 650–654. [CrossRef]
32. Kerley, C.P.; Hutchinson, K.; Cormican, L.; Faul, J.; Greally, P.; Coghlan, D.; Elnazir, B. Vitamin D3 for uncontrolled childhood asthma: A pilot study. *Pediatr. Allergy Immunol.* **2016**, *27*, 404–412. [CrossRef]
33. Wendell, S.G.; Baffi, C.; Holguin, F. Fatty acids, inflammation, and asthma. *J. Allergy Clin. Immunol.* **2014**, *133*, 1255–1264. [CrossRef]
34. Allen, S.; Britton, J.R.; Leonardi-Bee, J.A. Association between antioxidant vitamins and asthma outcome measures: Systematic review and meta-analysis. *Thorax* **2009**, *64*, 610–619 [CrossRef]
35. Ghaffari, J.; Khalilian, A.; Salehifar, E.; Khorasani, E.; Rezaii, M. Effect of zinc supplementation in children with asthma: A randomized, placebo-controlled trial in northern Islamic Republic of Iran. *East. Mediterr. Health J.* **2014**, *20*, 391–396. [CrossRef]
36. Rago, D.; Rasmussen, M.A.; Lee-Sarwar, K.A.; Weiss, S.T.; Lasky-Su, J.; Stokholm, J.; Bønnelykke, K.; Chawes, B.L.; Bisgaard, H. Fish-oil supplementation in pregnancy, child metabolomics and asthma risk. *EBioMedicine* **2019**, *46*, 399–410. [CrossRef]
37. Brigham, E.P.; Matsui, E.C.; Appel, L.J.; Bull, D.A.; Curtin-Brosnan, J.; Zhai, S.; White, K.; Charleston, J.B.; Hansel, N.N.; Diette, G.B.; et al. A pilot feeding study for adults with asthma: The healthy eating better breathing trial. *PLoS ONE* **2017**, *12*. [CrossRef] [PubMed]
38. Ma, J.; Strub, P.; Lavori, P.W.; Buist, A.S.; Camargo, C.A.; Nadeau, K.C.; Wilson, S.R.; Xiao, L. DASH for asthma: A pilot study of the DASH diet in not-well-controlled adult asthma. *Contemp. Clin. Trials.* **2013**, *35*, 55–67. [CrossRef] [PubMed]
39. Stoodley, I.; Williams, L.; Thompson, C.; Scott, H.; Wood, L. Evidence for lifestyle interventions in asthma. *Breathe* **2019**, *15*, e50–e61. [CrossRef] [PubMed]
40. Vassilopoulou, E.; Efthymiou, D.; Elissavet, V.; Agorastos, A. Case Report Integrative Food, Nutrition and Metabolism. *Integr. Food Nutr. Metab.* **2019**. [CrossRef]

4

The Role of Omega-3 Fatty Acids in the Setting of Coronary Artery Disease and COPD

Alex Pizzini [1,†], Lukas Lunger [2,†], Thomas Sonnweber [1], Guenter Weiss [1] and Ivan Tancevski [1,*]

1 Department of Internal Medicine II, Infectious Diseases, Pneumology, Rheumatology, Medical University of Innsbruck, 6020 Innsbruck, Austria; alex.pizzini@i-med.ac.at (A.P.); Thomas.Sonnweber@i-med.ac.at (T.S.); Guenter.Weiss@i-med.ac.at (G.W.)

2 Department of Urology, Klinikum rechts der Isar, Technische Universität München, 81675 Munich, Germany; lukas.lunger@tum.de

* Correspondence: Ivan.Tancevski@i-med.ac.at;

† Authors with equal contribution.

Abstract: Chronic obstructive pulmonary disease (COPD) is a growing healthcare concern and will represent the third leading cause of death worldwide within the next decade. COPD is the result of a complex interaction between environmental factors, especially cigarette smoking, air pollution, and genetic preconditions, which result in persistent inflammation of the airways. There is growing evidence that the chronic inflammatory state, measurable by increased levels of circulating cytokines, chemokines, and acute phase proteins, may not be confined to the lungs. Cardiovascular disease (CVD) and especially coronary artery disease (CAD) are common comorbidities of COPD, and low-grade systemic inflammation plays a decisive role in its pathogenesis. Omega-3 polyunsaturated fatty acids (*n*-3 PUFAs) exert multiple functions in humans and are crucially involved in limiting and resolving inflammatory processes. *n*-3 PUFAs have been intensively studied for their ability to improve morbidity and mortality in patients with CVD and CAD. This review aims to summarize the current knowledge on the effects of *n*-3 PUFA on inflammation and its impact on CAD in COPD from a clinical perspective.

Keywords: omega 3; PUFA; *n*-3 PUFA; COPD; inflammation; coronary artery disease; ischemic heart disease; CAD; CHD

1. Introduction

Chronic obstructive pulmonary disease (COPD) is one of the leading causes of morbidity and mortality worldwide [1]. Data from the Global Burden of Disease Study estimate that, to date, approximately 328 million people suffer from COPD globally, and suggest that this number may be even higher because of a substantial number of undiagnosed cases and increasing exposure to environmental factors, which promote COPD development and progression. It is estimated that, by the year 2030, COPD will represent the third leading cause of death worldwide [1–5].

COPD is the result of a complex interaction between lifestyle factors, especially cigarette smoking and air pollution, and genetic preconditions, resulting in persistent inflammation of the airways even after smoking cessation, causing sustained peripheral airflow limitation [1,6]. The latter is defined as the ratio between forced expiratory volume in one second (FEV1) versus forced vital capacity (FVC) being less than 0.7, determined via spirometry after bronchodilator therapy [1]. The exact mechanisms behind these processes are not yet understood, but the challenge to oxidative stress and the resulting imbalance of proteases and anti-proteases seem to be causative [6]. Moreover, there is growing evidence that the chronic inflammatory state reflected by increased levels of circulating cytokines, chemokines, and acute phase proteins may not be confined to the lungs [7]. Cardiovascular disease (CVD) and coronary artery disease (CAD) are the typical and most common comorbidities of COPD, and significantly impact on patients' prognosis and quality of life (Figure 1) [8–11].

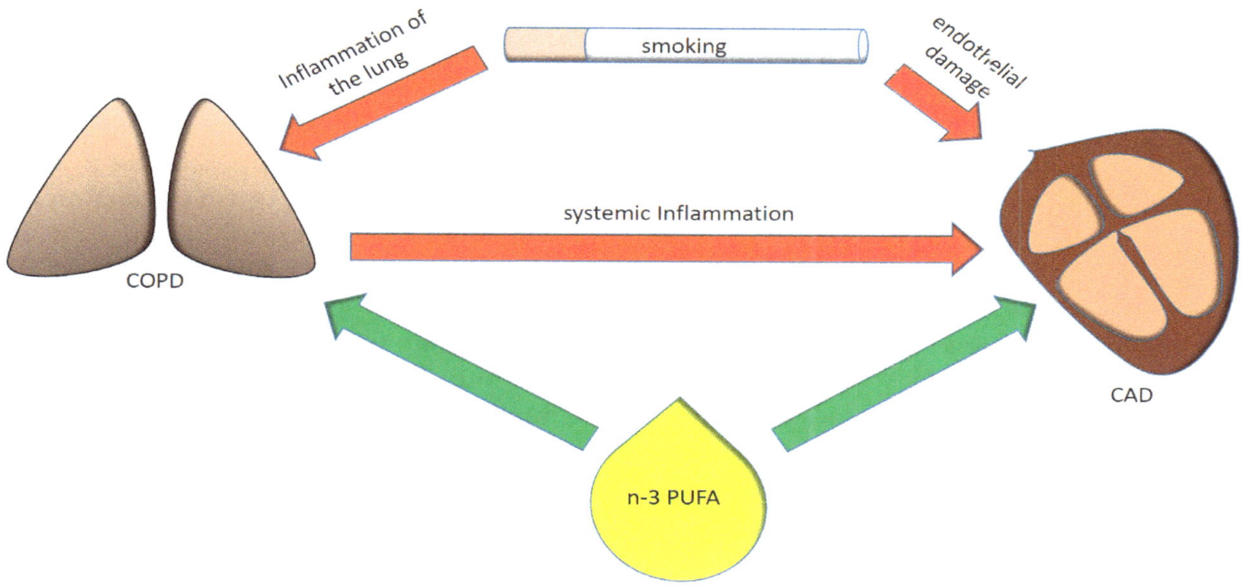

Figure 1. Interplay between smoking, pulmonary and systemic inflammation, coronary artery disease and omega-3 polyunsaturated fatty acids (*n*-3 PUFAs). COPD = chronic obstructive pulmonary disease, CAD = coronary artery disease.

Omega-3 polyunsaturated fatty acids (*n*-3 PUFAs) exert multiple functions in humans and are crucially involved in limiting and resolving inflammatory processes [12,13]. Eicosapentaenoic (EPA) and docosahexaenoic (DHA) acid are the main long-chain PUFA of the *n*-3 PUFA family, and seafood is the richest dietary source of these essential fatty acids, whereas their metabolic precursor, α-linolenic acid (ALA), is contained in substantial amounts only in vegetables [14].

2. Systemic Inflammation in COPD

The principal pathological features of COPD are obstructive bronchiolitis and emphysema, as well as increased mucus secretion. These conditions are the result of a rather complex and chronic inflammatory process, which is initiated mostly by chronic inhalation of irritants, predominantly cigarette smoking, air pollutants, and biomass fuel [6]. In this context, it ought to be mentioned that each puff of a cigarette contains more than 2000 xenobiotic compounds and 1014 free radicals, which injure lung epithelial cells with dose-dependent cytotoxicity [15,16]. These irritants subsequently activate pattern recognition receptors, such as Toll-like receptors (TLR), either directly, or indirectly by causing injury to epithelial cells, which release damage-associated molecular patterns. Interleukin (IL)-1ß has been demonstrated to be crucially involved in this first step, and IL-1 receptor knockout mice exposed to cigarette smoke showed reduced pulmonary inflammation and were significantly protected from development of emphysema compared with littermate controls [17]. On activation, innate immune cells release pro-inflammatory cytokines and chemokines, such as tumor necrosis factor α (TNFα) and IL-8, which leads to further recruitment of neutrophils and inflammatory monocytes to the lung [18]. Activated neutrophils and macrophages, in turn, foster lung destruction through the release of reactive oxygen species and proteolytic enzymes such as neutrophil elastase and matrix metalloproteinases [19,20].

Activation of the adaptive immune system is a second step in the pathogenesis of COPD, and cigarette smoke is crucially involved in activation of dendritic cells in the lower respiratory tract, leading to T cell activation [21]. CD8 cytotoxic T cells are the predominant T cells in the airways of COPD patients [15], however, CD4+ T helper-1 cells and CD4+ T helper-17 cells are also found in high quantities [6,22,23]. Furthermore, B cells organized into lymphoid follicles are frequently detected in the airways of patients with COPD, as shown in central bronchial biopsy specimens [24].

Several inflammatory cytokines, including TNFα; IL-6; IL-8; IL-18; and acute phase proteins such as C-reactive protein (CRP), serum amyloid A, and fibrinogen, as well as white blood cells (WBC), are detected at increased concentrations in the circulation of patients affected by COPD [25,26]. Similarly, these cytokines are also increased in the sputum and bronchoalveolar lavage fluid of COPD patients [8], suggesting a close relationship between airway and systemic inflammation. The latter has been described as an overspill of inflammatory mediators from the peripheral lung to systemic circulation contributing to the development of comorbidities of COPD [7]. Agusti et al. analyzed six inflammatory biomarkers (WBC, CRP, IL-6, IL-8, fibrinogen, and TNFα) in one of the largest available COPD cohorts, the ECLIPSE cohort [26]. The study included COPD patients, smokers without airflow limitation, and non-smokers. Thirty percent of COPD patients had no signs of systemic inflammation, whereas 16% had persistent systemic inflammation. The study group with persistent inflammation had significantly increased all-cause mortality, as compared with individuals without chronic inflammation (13% vs. 2%). The authors concluded that systemic inflammation is not a constant feature in all COPD patients, because approximately one-third of those analyzed did not have any abnormal biomarker neither at baseline nor at one year after follow-up. In a logistic regression analysis, body mass index (BMI), age, current smoking, and airflow limitation were identified as risk factors for persistent inflammation in COPD patients. Similarly, Garcia-Aymerich et al. were able to identify a COPD phenotype characterized by high proportion of obesity, cardiovascular disease, diabetes, and systemic inflammation in approximately one-third of patients recruited at the first hospital admission because of acute exacerbated COPD (AECOPD) [27]. Yet, the mechanisms linking COPD to the development or progression of COPD associated comorbidities are not fully understood, as these studies only show associations and do not prove causality.

3. Coronary Artery Disease in COPD

CAD prevalence rates in COPD patients range from 7% to 34% [28–30]. COPD and CAD have a close relationship, as they share common risk factors such as advanced age, cigarette smoking, and environmental pollution. There are evident epidemiologic data connecting COPD with CAD. In a cross-sectional study of patients with suspected CAD, patients with COPD had a significantly higher frequency of obstructive coronary lesions as compared with CAD patients without airflow limitation [31]. Additionally, the severity of airflow limitation correlated with coronary lesion size and quantity. No difference was found between COPD and non-COPD CAD patients regarding risk factors, and a univariate analysis revealed COPD as an independent predictor of CAD. Multiple other studies have shown similar results and identified COPD as a powerful and independent risk factor for CVD and CAD. Spirometry tests, especially FEV1, and airflow obstruction defined as FEV1/FVC less than 0.70, for instance, have strong predictive potential for CAD. For every 10% decrease in FEV1, cardiovascular mortality was found to increase by about 28%, and even among individuals with severe airways obstruction, the leading causes of death are predominantly sequels of cardiovascular disease [31–34]. On the other side, studies investigating airflow limitation in patients with CAD are scarce, but the prevalence of obstructive ventilation in CAD patients might be underestimated in the literature [28].

The pathophysiological mechanism linking COPD to its comorbidities is not yet certain, but chronic exposure to low-grade systemic inflammation might play a central role. Inflammation is a key factor in the development and progression of atherosclerotic lesions, and numerous cytokines, mediators, and immune cells have been identified to promote vascular inflammation, cholesterol deposition in the arterial wall, and the formation of atherosclerotic plaques [35,36].

Most large epidemiologic studies identified C-reactive protein (CRP) as a key player and predictor of CAD [35,37], as well as "upstream" inflammatory cytokines like IL-6, IL-18, and TNFα strongly correlated with disease activity and severity in CAD [38,39]. Similar systemic alterations of systemic inflammatory markers are found in those COPD patients that revealed an increased prevalence of cardiovascular disease [26].

However, even though persistent inflammation may constitute the pathophysiological link between COPD and CAD, alternative mechanistic approaches ought to be mentioned.

Pulmonary emphysema, a phenotype of COPD, is a pathologic condition characterized by abnormal and permanent enlargement of the airspaces distal to the terminal bronchioles that leads to destruction of airspace walls and usually to progressive airflow limitation [1]. Studies about the pathogenesis of emphysema revealed an association with endothelial apoptosis [40–42] and endothelial dysfunction [43]. The subsequently altered pulmonary perfusion can lead to impaired left ventricular filling, reduced stroke volume, and lower cardiac output [44]. The endothelial damage, however, is not limited to the lungs and large cross-sectional studies linked the presence of emphysema to subclinical atherosclerosis and peripheral arterial stiffness [45] as a consequence of endothelial and vascular smooth muscle dysfunction [46]. Arterial stiffness is a strong predictor of cardiovascular disease [47,48], and emphysema severity based on quantitative computed tomography scans in turn was revealed as the most powerful predictor of arterial stiffness [49]. Moreover, systemic vascular dysfunction seems to already be present in the earlier stages of COPD, and particularly in patients with emphysema, although presenting with a largely preserved FEV1 [50].

Still, many other potential mechanisms, for instance, physical inactivity secondary to more advanced COPD stages, chronic hypoxia, genetic predisposition, as well as direct endothelial damage caused by cigarette smoking, may help to further explain the frequent association between COPD and CAD [51].

4. Anti-Inflammatory Proprieties of *n*-3 PUFA and the Benefits in Cardiovascular Disease

n-3 PUFA exert multiple functions in humans and are crucially involved in limiting and resolving inflammatory processes. A recent American Heart Association science advisory recommends consuming nonfried seafood, especially species higher in long chain *n*-3 PUFA, one to two times per week for cardiovascular benefits [52]. However, data about the specific *n*-3 PUFA supplementation for influencing the risk of CVD are still ambiguous, underlined by recent findings from randomized controlled trials and meta-analyses, which led to a class III recommendation by the American Heart Association for dietary supplementation with *n*-3 PUFAs in populations at high risk of CVD [53]. This is further supported by a Cochrane Systematic Review providing information that EPA and DHA slightly reduce serum triglycerides and raise high density lipoprotein cholesterol (HDL-C), however, little or no effect on all-cause deaths and cardiovascular events and probably little or no difference in terms of cardiovascular death, coronary deaths or events, stroke, or heart irregularities was described. [54]. The hypothesized protective mechanisms are not solely related to reduced overall inflammation, but also include effects on lipid metabolism and thrombogenesis, as well as anti-arrhythmic proprieties, reducing the rate of sudden cardiac death in secondary prevention [53,55,56].

Increased bioavailability of *n*-3 PUFAs, by means of EPA and DHA, change the balance between *n*-3 and *n*-6 PUFA with arachidonic acid (AA) as the major precursor of the latter, favoring the synthesis of anti-inflammatory eicosanoids [57]. The incorporation of EPA and DHA into human inflammatory cells occurs in a dose-response fashion, and because less substrate is available for synthesis of AA-derived eicosanoids, *n*-3 PUFA supplementation to human diet has been shown to result in decreased production of prostaglandin E2 (PGE2), thromboxane A2, Leukotriene B4 (LTB4), 5-hydroxyeicosatetraenoic acid, and leukotriene E4 by inflammatory cells [57]. Plenty of evidence supporting this hypothesis is available from rheumatoid arthritis disease, a disease primarily characterized by inflammation [58]. There are many studies about patients with rheumatoid arthritis, where fish oil supplements decreased LTB4 production by neutrophils and monocytes, 5-hydroxyeicosatetraenoic acid production by neutrophils, and PGE2 production by mononuclear cells [58]. A recently published prospective trial concluded that the intake of fish oil resulted in a shift of n-6/n-3 PUFA ratio and in a higher incorporation of n-3 PUFA precursors for the anti-inflammatory lipid mediators in plasma phospholipids. This further induced a significant improvement in the clinical status by improving joint inflammation, as well as reducing inflammatory parameters (CRP, erythrocyte sedimentation rate) [59]. However, the altered ratio between n-6/n-3 PUFA occurred solely through an increase of n-3 PUFA, while n-6 PUFA remained unchanged. In the literature, similar concerns with the n-6/n-3 PUFA ratio were identified and discussed. Depending on how the proportion of n-6 PUFA changes, the proportion of n-3 PUFA could decrease, remain unchanged, or increase and still lead to a lower n-6/n-3 PUFA ratio, although the active biochemical effects of a decrease, no change, or an increase in the proportion of n-3 PUFA are distinctly different. Moreover, the single aspect of an n-3/n-6 PUFA ratio neglects the source of n-3 PUFA, and it is well established that the biological effects of α-linolenic acid (ALA), EPA, and DHA are diverse [60]. In terms of cardiovascular diseases, one would hypothesize that higher levels of n-6 PUFA and lower levels of n-3 PUFA could increase cardiovascular risk. This has not been demonstrated, as both n-6 and n-3 fatty acids are associated with reduced cardiovascular risk in several studies [61]. Similarly, two prospective trials concluded that the ratio of n-6/n-3 polyunsaturated fatty acids is of no value in modifying cardiovascular disease risk [62–64].

The anti-inflammatory mechanism of n-3 PUFA also expands on leukocyte recruitment by affecting the expression of adhesion molecules on endothelial cells [65]. This step is crucial, as monocytes in particular migrate into the vessel wall, differentiate into macrophages, and may become foam cells, contributing to the initiation and progression of inflammatory atherosclerotic lesions [66,67]. Moreover, resolution of inflammation is an actively programmed biochemical progress, regulated by specialized pro-resolving mediators (SPM) derived from n-3 and n-6 PUFA (Figure 2) [68]. While n-3 PUFAs are synthesized to resolvins, protectins, and maresins, n-6 PUFAs are synthesized to lipoxins [69]. SPMs are predominantly involved in the regulation of neutrophil activity, as well as cyto- and chemokine release, and induce the resolution of an inflammatory tissue state towards tissue homeostasis [70].

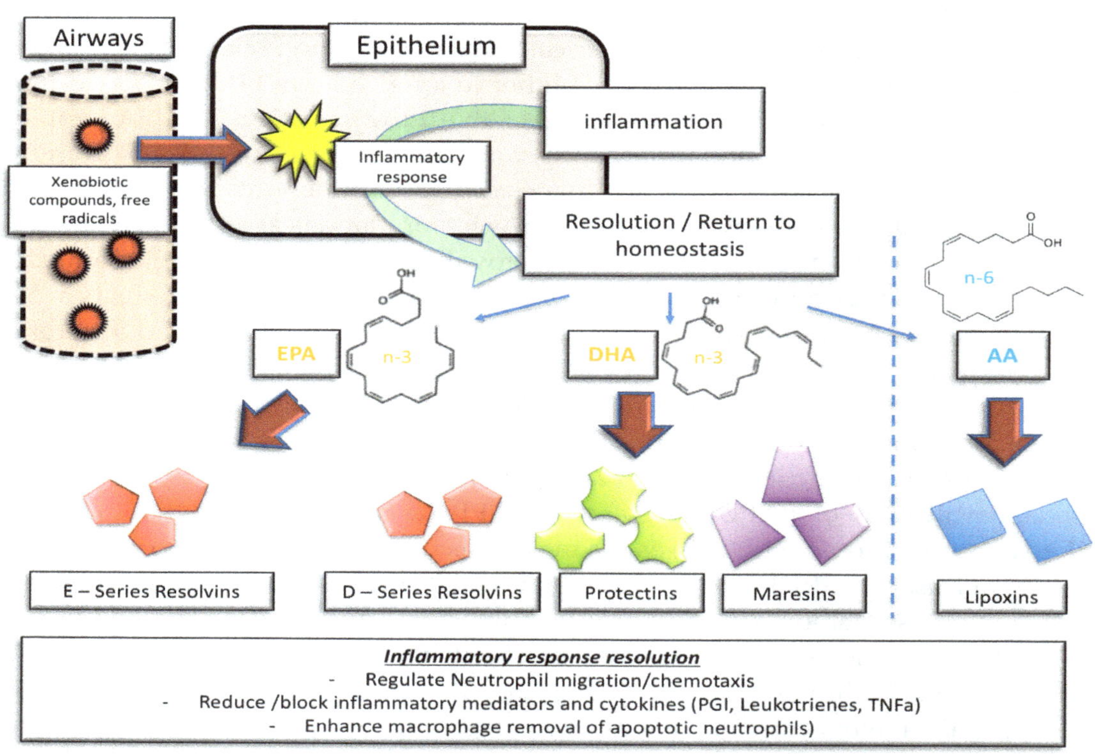

Figure 2. Inflammatory response and inflammatory resolution: the role of molecular mediators derived from n-3 PUFA and n-6 PUFA. EPA = eicosapentaenoic acid, DHA = docosahexaenoic acid, AA = arachidonic acid, PGI = prostaglandins, TNFα = tumor necrosis factor α.

Figure 2 illustrates the complexity of SPM involvement in inflammation resolution. Resolvin E1, derived from EPA, is involved in the limitation of neutrophil migration, the enhancement of neutrophil and eosinophil clearance, and the reduction of IL-23 and 12 release. Also, resolvin E1 inhibits platelet and vascular smooth muscle activation [71].

Similarly, resolvin D1, derived from DHA, limits neutrophil transmigration, and promotes the clearance of apoptotic cells and allergens. Moreover, resolvin D1 stimulates the production of IgM and IgG. Resolvin D2, on top of limiting neutrophil activity and enhancing macrophage activity, reduces the possibility of leukocyte–endothelial interaction by stimulating NO production [71].

Protectin D1 effectively inhibits T cell migration and apoptosis, and reduces the production and release of TNFα and Interferon gamma, besides limiting neutrophil activity and promoting macrophage activation [70].

Maresin 1, on the other hand, predominately affects pulmonary tissue by reducing the overall amount of neutrophils in the lung, limiting edema, tissue hypoxia, and pro-inflammatory cytokines [70]. Also, IL-5 and IL-13 secretion is reduced, thereby affecting innate lymphoid cells. Another beneficial effect of this SPM is the stimulation of regulatory T cells, stimulating innate lymphoid cells type 2 mediated effects [70]. Finally, *n*-3 PUFAs also directly impact arterial stiffness by decreasing the pulse wave velocity and improving arterial compliance [72], as was shown in a meta-analysis by Pase et al. Similarly, the effects were further confirmed by more recent randomized controlled trials in patients with metabolic syndrome and patients at elevated cardiovascular risk [73,74].

5. *n*-3 PUFA in COPD Patients, Smokers, and Subjects at Risk

The beneficial effects of an inflammation-modulating diet using *n*-3 PUFA in patients with acute lung injury or acute respiratory distress syndrome have been reported previously [75,76]. Therefore, it was hypothesized that *n*-3 PUFA might also have beneficial effects in patients with COPD and the effect might extend to linked comorbidities potentially related to systemic inflammation, including CAD.

Investigations on *n*-3 PUFA and the impact on airflow limitation and smoking were published in the past (a schematic overview of the discussed studies is given in Table 1). One of the first available studies was conducted by Sharp et al. in 1994 [77]. A large cross-sectional cohort study (Honolulu Heart Program) revealed a protective function of elevated fish consumption (major source of *n*-3 PUFA) in smokers by decelerating the FEV1 decline. However, the effect was limited to subjects with a maximum inhalation of 30 cigarettes per day, indicating a dose-dependent limitation. Interestingly, an analysis of the same cohort also showed a decrease in the risk of CAD morbidity and mortality in smokers with increased fish intake (defined as >2 times/week), suggesting a relationship between airflow limitation, CAD, and *n*-3 PUFA [78]. No information is available on whether patients matching the current definition of COPD were included in this analysis.

Table 1. Summary of the reviewed studies related to omega-3 polyunsaturated fatty acid (*n*-3 PUFA) in chronic obstructive pulmonary disease (COPD) patients, smokers and subjects at risk. ALA = alpha linoleic acid, CAD = coronary artery diseases, CRP = C-reactive protein, CVD = cardiovascular disease, FFQ = food frequency questionnaire, DHA = docosahexaenoic acid, EPA = eicosapentaenoic acid, FEV1 = forced expiratory volume in one second, FVC = forced vital capacity, HF = heart failure, IL = interleukin, RCT = randomized controlled trial, STA = stearinic acid, TNFα = tumor necrosis factor alpha.

Author/Year/Type	Cohort Size/Description	*n*-3 PUFA Source	Outcome	COPD	Limitations	Association with CAD (Same Study or Same Cohort)
Sharp et al., 1994, observational	*n* = 6346, Honolulu Heart Program—mean age 54 years	Fish consumption/week—FFQ	Slower decline of FEV1 in smokers.	Obstructive lung disease was solely based on FEV1<65%. Symptoms are not reported.	No details provided about COPD patients. PUFA source reported as fish consumption per week.	Decrease in the risk of coronary heart disease morbidity and mortality in smokers with elevated fish intake.
Shahar et al., 1994, observational	*n* = 8960, Atherosclerosis Risk in Communities Study (ARIC); age: 45–64 years	*n*-3 PUFA (EPA and DHA)—FFQ	Strong inverse relation between COPD and intake of *n*-3 PUFA. Besides COPD, better lung function also in smokers and former smokers.	COPD patients included, however, using a different definition.	Outdated definition of COPD.	*n*-3 PUFAs were associated with hypocoagulable hemostasis. Lower levels of plasma PUFA (especially *n*-6 PUFA) among participants who developed coronary heart disease. Increased risk of HF in subjects with higher plasma levels of saturated fatty acids. *n*-3 PUFAs were associated with a decreased risk of HF in women.
Garcia-Larsen et al., 2015, cross-sectional	*n* = 1232, age 22–28 y	*n*-3 PUFA—FFQ	Positive association between *n*-3 PUFA consumption and ventilatory function (FEV1% and FVC%).	-	Results were not significant after adjustment for multiple comparisons.	-
Leng et al., 2017, observational	*n* = 1829, Lovelace Smokers cohort and *n* = 508 the Veterans Smokers cohort, age 40–74 years	*n*-3 PUFA, EPA, DPA, DHA—FFQ	EPA, DPA, and DHA were associated with better FEV1; DPA was associated with a lower age-related FEV1 decline.	25% COPD patients.	Both cohorts showed a mean FEV1/FVC ratio of >0.7. Included COPD patients mild-to-moderate stages.	-
Wood et al., 2010, observational	*n* = 195, Hunter community study, age 55–85 years	*n*-3 PUFA—FFQ	Increased proportion of dietary fat was associated with increased IL-6 levels, which were significant predictors of FEV1% and FVC in men. No association between *n*3-PUFA and %FEV1.	No information given (no absolute limitation of FEV1% and FEV1/FVC > 0.7).	No information is given about the relation between *n*-3 PUFA and IL-6.	IL-6 is an important marker of cardiovascular and coronary artery disease. No data about CAD or CVD reported.
Scaglia et al., 2016, cross-sectional	*n* = 100 (1:1 smokers vs. never-smokers), 18–75 years	Red blood cell membrane determination of ALA, EPA, DPA, and DHA	Significantly lower levels of DHA in smokers compared with non-smokers.	-	Spirometry not included; no information about lung diseases.	-

Table 1. *Cont.*

Author/Year/Type	Cohort Size/Description	*n*-3 PUFA Source	Outcome	COPD	Limitations	Association with CAD (Same Study or Same Cohort)
Matsuyama et al., 2005, prospective interventional, 2 years duration	*n* = 64, mean age 66 years.	Supplementation *n*-3 PUFA vs. *n*-6 PUFA	Decrease of Borg dyspnea scale and a decrease of arterial oxygen saturation after 6 min walking test in *n*-3 PUFA group. Leukotriene B4 levels in serum and sputum and tumor necrosis factor alpha and interleukin-8 levels in sputum decreased significantly in the *n*-3 group. No change in FEV1.	Limited to COPD only with FEV1% < 60% and BMI <25 kg/m^2, no active smokers.	Sample size	Impact on inflammatory parameters related to CAD and CVD, however, no data about CAD and CVD in this population are reported.
De Batlle, 2012, cross-sectional	*n* = 250, PAC-COPD study group, mean age 68 years	*n*-3 PUFA: DHA, EPA, ALA—FFQ	ALA was associated with lower TNFα concentrations in serum. AA (*n*-6 PUFA) was related to higher IL-6 and CRP serum concentrations.	COPD patients recruited during their first hospital admission. Mostly moderate to severe COPD.	No repeated measurements, inflammatory sputum parameters not assessed.	Association between ALA and cardiovascular disease, however, no information about CVD or CAD in this population are reported.
Broekhuizen et al., 2005, prospective interventional double-blind RCT over 8 weeks (PUFA vs. Placebo)	*n* = 80, mean age 63 years	9 g PUFA (STA, ALA, EPA, DHA) or placebo daily	Increase in peak exercise capacity and duration of constant work rate. No changes in terms of CRP, IL-6 and TNFa	Mostly severe to very severe COPD patients with mean FEV1% 35–38%.	Limited observation period of 8 weeks.	Association between the analyzed inflammatory parameters and CAD and CVD, however, no information about CVD or CAD in this population are reported.
Calder et al., 2018, prospective interventional RCT over 12 weeks	*n* = 45, mean age 69 years	2.0 g DHA + EPA, 10 g whey protein concentrate and 10 µg 25-hydroxy-vitamin D3 twice daily for 12 weeks vs. a milk-based comparator	Intervention group gained more fat mass. Reductions in systolic blood pressure, triglycerides and exercise-induced fatigue and dyspnoea, and increases in high-density lipoprotein cholesterol.	Moderate-to-severe COPD and involuntary weight loss or low body mass index (16–18 kg/m^2).	Sample size	Inclusion of metabolic parameters and inflammatory parameters clearly associated with CVD and CAD.

Shahar et al. analyzed the dietary impact of *n*-3 PUFA (assessment of EPA and DHA intake via questionnaire) on 8960 current or former smokers from the "Atherosclerosis Risk in Communities—ARIC" study cohort and studied its relation with COPD [79]. COPD was assessed by a questionnaire on respiratory symptoms and by spirometry. The definition of COPD, however, was slightly different when compared with the current GOLD definition [1]. The authors describe a strong inverse relation between COPD severity and intake of *n*-3 PUFA. Moreover, higher intake of *n*-3 PUFA and fish consumption also predicted better lung function in smokers and former smokers. Many other investigations, including the same cohort, were subsequently published; *n*-3 PUFAs were associated with a modification of hemostatic factors—key components of CAD and acute myocardial infarction—resulting in a hypocoagulable profile [80]. Data from the same cohort also revealed lower levels of plasma PUFA (especially *n*-6 PUFA) among participants who developed CAD [81]. Yamagishi et al. found an increased risk of heart failure in subjects with higher plasma levels of saturated fatty acids, and *n*-3 PUFAs were associated with a decreased risk of heart failure in women in the ARIC cohort [82].

A positive association between *n*-3 PUFA (assessment of *n*-3 PUFA via questionnaire) consumption and ventilatory function (FEV1% and FVC%) was found in 1232 adults aged between 22 and 28 years [83]. The analyzed cohort had no signs of obstructive ventilatory dysfunction, and statistical significance was lost after adjusting for multiple comparisons, suggesting only a weak effect of *n*-3 PUFA. The idea of analyzing a cohort of young adults was related to the fact that reduced maximal attained lung function (as measured by spirometry) may identify individuals who are at increased risk for the subsequent development of COPD [1,84].

Leng et al. conducted a nutritional epidemiological study in two separate cohorts (Hispanic and non-Hispanic white smokers; assessment of EPA, DHA, and docosapentaenoic acid (DPA) intake via questionnaire) to identify nutrients associated with FEV1 and its decline [85]. Of the analyzed *n*-3 PUFAs, EPA, DHA, and DPA intake were positively associated with better FEV1 volumes, and DPA was associated with a reduced age-related FEV1 decline. No increased FEV1 decline of currently smoking participants was observed in one of the two cohorts (Lovelace Smoker's cohort) if high amounts of DPA were consumed. The study only included approximately 25% COPD patients, and both cohorts showed a mean FEV1/FVC ratio of >0.7, limiting the disease to mild-to-moderate stages. No data about CVD prevalence in the two analyzed cohorts are provided.

Conflicting evidence came from another population-based cohort study showing that an increased proportion of dietary fat consumption was associated with increased IL-6 levels, which were significant predictors of FEV1 and FVC [86]. Plasma IL-6 is a clinically relevant marker of inflammation and has been linked to cardiovascular outcomes in some epidemiological studies [87]. *n*-3 PUFA (assessment via questionnaire) intake was not found to be associated with %FEV1 in the linear regression model, and no information is given about the relation between *n*-3 PUFA and IL-6. Overall, the patients included in the study had no absolute limitation of FEV1 (approximately 80% predicted) and obstructive ventilation, a typical feature of COPD, was not found (FEV1/FVC > 0.7.) Moreover, the assessed smoking status revealed non-smokers in 73% of female patients and 39% of male patients and, therefore, the odds of COPD patients being included in the study are low.

In 2016, Scaglia et al. analyzed dietary habits related to PUFA consumption (red blood cell membrane determination of alpha linoleic acid (ALA), EPA, DPA, and DHA) in smokers and lifetime non-smokers [88]. They found significant differences in the dietary consumption of *n*-3 PUFA between the two groups and showed lower levels of DHA and EPA in smokers. They hypothesized that PUFA might interfere with smoking habits, suggesting dietary supplementation as a potential therapeutic option for smoking cessation. Still, this observation was not confirmed in follow up studies thus far and urges further elucidation.

The anti-inflammatory proprieties of *n*-3 PUFA in COPD patients have been studied [89] in sixty-four patients receiving either an *n*-3 PUFA (ALA) or an *n*-6 PUFA (linoleic acid) supplementation diet for two years. Apart from clinical improvements (decrease of dyspnea according to Borg scale and decrease of arterial oxygen saturation after a 6 min walking test), leukotriene B4 levels in serum and sputum, as well as TNFα and IL-8 levels in sputum, decreased significantly in patients consuming an *n*-3 PUFA rich diet, while there was no significant change in individuals receiving dietary supplementation of *n*-6 PUFA.

A cross-sectional study including 250 COPD patients analyzed inflammatory parameters related to dietary intake of *n*-3 (EPA, DHA, ALA) and *n*-6 PUFA [90]. Higher intake of alpha linoleic acid (ALA) was associated with lower TNFα concentrations in serum, while no differences were seen with other assessed inflammatory parameters (IL-6, IL-8, and CRP). A higher ALA intake was related to higher IL-6 and CRP serum concentrations.

The effects of PUFA supplementation (blend of PUFA, 9 g, mainly *n*-3 PUFA, namely ALA, EPA, and DHA) on the outcome of pulmonary rehabilitation were studied in 80 COPD patients randomized to an intervention or a placebo group [91]. The peak exercise capacity increased in both groups. However, a significantly higher increase was observed in the intervention group after eight weeks of training. Also, the duration of the constant work rate increased far more in patients receiving PUFA. However, the measured systemic inflammatory parameters, namely CRP, IL-6, and TNFα, did not change after rehabilitation or after PUFA intervention, contrasting the results of others [89,90], who observed modulation of systemic inflammation after *n*-3 PUFA supplementation. Thus, systemic inflammation is not a common feature of all COPD patients. Therefore, a more detailed analysis of the subgroup of "inflamed COPD" patients would be desirable. Still, it is unanswered as to how the biochemical phenotype of an "inflamed COPD" patient is defined.

The beneficial effects of *n*-3 PUFA in COPD associated cachexia were studied in a randomized controlled trial including 45 patients [92]. Patients in the intervention group received 2.0 g DHA + EPA as well as 10 g whey protein concentrate and 10 μg 25-hydroxy-vitamin D3 twice daily for 12 weeks versus a milk-based comparator. Both groups gained weight, but the intervention group gained more fat mass. Moreover, a significant reduction in systolic blood pressure and increases in high-density lipoprotein cholesterol were observed in the intervention group compared with controls, parameters that can be regarded as risk factors for CAD [93]. No significant changes in the measured inflammatory parameters (CRP, IL-6, IL-8, and TNF) were observed.

In summary, several limitations of the described studies must be discussed. First, the most important limitation is that most of the studies are cross-sectional observational cohort studies. Second, *n*-3 PUFA sources are indirectly measured using food frequency questionnaires. Dietary habits reported from questionnaires are surrogate parameters of the real dietary consumption of *n*-3 PUFA; this may lead to inaccurate *n*-3 PUFA consumption estimations, although studies suggest a plausible correlation between the two factors [94,95]. Third, the causality and the direction of a causal relation cannot be explained when considering a cross-sectional study design. Finally, COPD patients and smokers may have changed their lifestyles and dietary habits, reducing fish consumption. Therefore, further prospective studies are warranted to investigate the impact of *n*-3 PUFA consumption on systemic inflammatory parameters in such patients.

6. *n*-3 PUFA, CAD, and COPD

Evidence on the beneficial effects of *n*-3 PUFA on CAD and CVD in COPD patients is scarce. Many large randomized controlled trials have been conducted to study the benefits of *n*-3 PUFA in CAD and CVD [53,54], however, although most of the included patients were smokers, the prevalence and severity of COPD were rarely reported.

We reviewed all included studies from the Cochrane systematic database review, "Polyunsaturated fatty acids for the primary and secondary prevention of cardiovascular disease", and the American Heart Association Science Advisory, "Omega-3 Polyunsaturated Fatty Acid (Fish Oil) Supplementation and the Prevention of Clinical Cardiovascular Disease", in regard to included COPD patients [53,54]. Of the included 65 studies, only 4 reported on COPD patients in their cohort.

Nodari et al. analyzed the benefits of *n*-3 PUFA (850 to 882 mg of EPA and DHA) in the prevention of atrial fibrillation (AF) recurrence rates after electrical cardioversion in a prospective randomized controlled trial, including 199 patients [96]. After one year of follow-up, the probability of maintained sinus rhythm was significantly higher in the *n*-3 PUFAs-treated patients as compared with the placebo group. A small subgroup of approximately 10% COPD patients ($n = 12$ placebo vs. $n = 13$ intervention) was included in the study, however, no separate details on the subgroup were discussed.

Rauch et al. analyzed the effect of *n*-3 PUFA (460 mg EPA, 380 mg DHA) if given on top of modern guideline-adjusted therapy in survivors of acute myocardial infarction [97]. The study was designed as a randomized, placebo-controlled trial with a duration of one year, and included 3851 patients, of whom approximately 6% were highlighted as COPD patients ($n = 122$ placebo vs. $n = 108$ intervention group). Overall, guideline-adjusted treatment of acute myocardial infarction already resulted in a low rate of sudden cardiac death and other clinical events within one year of follow-up, and the application of *n*-3 PUFA could not further improve the outcome. No details are provided regarding such effects in the COPD subgroup.

The GISSI-HF investigators published a randomized, double-blind, placebo-controlled trial analyzing the effect of *n*-3 PUFA (850–882 mg EPA and DHA) in patients with chronic heart failure [98]. In total, 6975 patients with chronic heart failure of New York Heart Association class II–IV were randomly assigned to *n*-3 PUFA intervention or placebo. A subpopulation of 205 COPD patients was included in the study ($n = 793$ placebo vs. $n = 740$ intervention). Primary endpoints were time to death from any cause or death/admission to hospital for a cardiovascular reason. A slight, yet significant reduction of death from any cause or death/admission to hospital for cardiovascular reasons was found in the PUFA group. No specific details are provided for the COPD subpopulation.

Finally, Mozaffarin et al. analyzed the effect of *n*-3 PUFA (EPA 465 mg and DHA 375 mg) in the prevention of AF in 1516 patients who underwent cardiac surgery [99]. Patients were randomized to receive fish oil or placebo until hospital discharge or postoperative day 10. A small subgroup of approximately 11% of COPD patients (placebo $n = 90$ vs. intervention $n = 80$) was included in the study. The authors concluded that perioperative supplementation with *n*-3 PUFA did not reduce the risk of postoperative AF and, similarly to the aforementioned studies, no details are provided about the COPD subgroup.

In summary, these studies showed a weak benefit of *n*-3 PUFA supplementation in the setting of atrial fibrillation recurrence rate after electrical cardioversion and a slight reduction of death and hospital admission in patients with left heart failure, both diseases closely associated with CAD. No benefits were seen in survivors of acute myocardial infarction or patients with atrial fibrillation after cardiac surgery. The weak benefits seem to also apply to COPD patients, which were included in 5–20% of the discussed studies. However, as already mentioned earlier, the high number of undiagnosed COPD cases and low awareness of investigators towards this chronic disease in patients with cardiac pathologies led to neglect of this important aspect even in large and prospective trials. In our opinion, it seems plausible that other studies also included COPD patients at a rate of at least 5–10%. Thus, the results from the Cochrane systematic database review and the American Heart Association Science Advisory might also apply to COPD patients.

7. Conclusions and Future Perspectives

COPD represents a growing healthcare concern worldwide. Pathophysiological aspects of COPD imply a local inflammatory reaction, initiated by inhalation of noxious substances, which, in some cases, led to the emergence of inflammatory mediators in the systemic circulation. Epidemiologic and mechanistic studies indicate that COPD is frequently associated with CAD, congestive heart failure, and cardiac arrhythmias, independent of shared risk factors. A possible pathway is highlighted as chronic low-grade systemic inflammation, an aspect that likely also contributes to coronary artery disease. *n*-3 PUFAs have been intensively studied for their ability to improve morbidity and mortality in patients with CAD. However, little evidence exists toward the beneficial anti-inflammatory aspects of *n*-3 PUFA in COPD patients, and even less evidence is available in regard to patients with COPD and associated CAD.

Overall, the available literature suggests a weak benefit of n-3 PUFA in COPD patients related to clinical outcomes, and n-3 PUFA mediated borderline amelioration of local and systemic inflammation. To date, the specific interplay between n-3 PUFA, COPD, and CAD has not been investigated in prospective trials.

In-depth keyword guided research on ongoing trials on n-3 PUFA in COPD and CAD revealed a relatively small number of registered trials on http://ClinicalTrials.gov. To date, only one trial investigating the effect of fish oil on endothelial function by FMD (flow-mediated dilation) in COPD has been registered (NCT00835289). Another trial has investigated the effect of both training and nutritional supplementation on body composition, activity, and cardiometabolic risk in COPD (NCT01344135). However, as nutritional supplementation has not occurred in all subjects and as an observational period of eight months may not be enough to reach clinically important cardiovascular and COPD endpoints, prospective, randomized controlled studies are warranted. Future studies ought to measure atherosclerotic disease progression, as well as establish relevant COPD inflammation parameters in order to determine the role of PUFA in inflammation-mediated diseases such as COPD and CAD. Moreover, standardized PUFA administration as well as a sufficient observation period may be crucial to understanding the role of PUFA in these diseases. Successful trials may help introduce a standardized supplementation of PUFA in patients with CAD or COPD or both to reduce disease progression or development.

Author Contributions: Conceptualization, A.P., L.L., and T.S.; writing—original draft preparation, A.P. and L.L.; writing—review and editing, G.W., I.T.; visualization, L.L.; supervision, I.T.

Acknowledgments: Support by the "Verein zur Förderung von Forschung und Weiterbildung in Infektiologie und Immunologie an der Medizinischen Universität Innsbruck" is gratefully acknowledged.

References

1. Vogelmeier, C.F.; Criner, G.J.; Martinez, F.J.; Anzueto, A.; Barnes, P.J.; Bourbeau, J.; Celli, B.R.; Chen, R.; Decramer, M.; Fabbri, L.M.; et al. Global strategy for the diagnosis, management, and prevention of chronic obstructive lung disease 2017 report. GOLD executive summary. *Am. J. Respir. Crit. Care Med.* **2017**, *195*, 557–582. [CrossRef] [PubMed]
2. Lozano, R.; Naghavi, M.; Foreman, K.; Lim, S.; Shibuya, K.; Aboyans, V.; Abraham, J.; Adair, T.; Aggarwal, R.; Ahn, S.Y.; et al. Global and regional mortality from 235 causes of death for 20 age groups in 1990 and 2010: A systematic analysis for the global burden of disease study 2010. *Lancet* **2012**, *380*, 2095–2128. [CrossRef]
3. WHO. Projections of Mortality and Causes of Death, 2015 and 2030. Available online: http://www.who.int/healthinfo/global_burden_disease/projections2015_2030/en/ (accessed on 1 June 2018).
4. WHO. Chronic Obstructive Pulmonary Disease (COPD). Available online: http://www.who.int/respiratory/copd/en/ (accessed on 1 September 2018).
5. Lindberg, A.; Bjerg, A.; Ronmark, E.; Larsson, L.G.; Lundback, B. Prevalence and underdiagnosis of COPD by disease severity and the attributable fraction of smoking report from the obstructive lung disease in Northern Sweden studies. *Respir. Med.* **2006**, *100*, 264–272. [CrossRef] [PubMed]
6. Barnes, P.J.; Burney, P.G.; Silverman, E.K.; Celli, B.R.; Vestbo, J.; Wedzicha, J.A.; Wouters, E.F. Chronic obstructive pulmonary disease. *Nat. Rev. Dis. Primers* **2015**, *1*, 15076. [CrossRef] [PubMed]
7. Barnes, P.J. Chronic obstructive pulmonary disease: Effects beyond the lungs. *PLoS Med.* **2010**, *7*, e1000220. [CrossRef] [PubMed]
8. Barnes, P.J.; Celli, B.R. Systemic manifestations and comorbidities of COPD. *Eur. Respir. J.* **2009**, *33*, 1165–1185. [CrossRef] [PubMed]
9. Soriano, J.B.; Visick, G.T.; Muellerova, H.; Payvandi, N.; Hansell, A.L. Patterns of comorbidities in newly diagnosed COPD and asthma in primary care. *Chest* **2005**, *128*, 2099–2107. [CrossRef] [PubMed]
10. Mannino, D.M.; Thorn, D.; Swensen, A.; Holguin, F. Prevalence and outcomes of diabetes, hypertension and cardiovascular disease in COPD. *Eur. Respir. J.* **2008**, *32*, 962–969. [CrossRef] [PubMed]

11. Miller, J.; Edwards, L.D.; Agusti, A.; Bakke, P.; Calverley, P.M.; Celli, B.; Coxson, H.O.; Crim, C.; Lomas, D.A.; Miller, B.E.; et al. Comorbidity, systemic inflammation and outcomes in the ECLIPSE cohort. *Respir. Med.* **2013**, *107*, 1376–1384. [CrossRef] [PubMed]
12. Serhan, C.N.; Chiang, N.; Van Dyke, T.E. Resolving inflammation: Dual anti-inflammatory and pro-resolution lipid mediators. *Nat. Rev. Immunol.* **2008**, *8*, 349–361. [CrossRef] [PubMed]
13. Calder, P.C. Omega-3 polyunsaturated fatty acids and inflammatory processes: Nutrition or pharmacology? *Br. J. Clin. Pharmacol.* **2013**, *75*, 645–662. [CrossRef] [PubMed]
14. Davis, B.C.; Kris-Etherton, P.M. Achieving optimal essential fatty acid status in vegetarians: Current knowledge and practical implications. *Am. J. Clin. Nutr.* **2003**, *78*, 640S–646S. [CrossRef] [PubMed]
15. Cosio, M.G.; Saetta, M.; Agusti, A. Immunologic aspects of chronic obstructive pulmonary disease. *N. Engl. J. Med.* **2009**, *360*, 2445–2454. [CrossRef] [PubMed]
16. Pryor, W.A.; Prier, D.G.; Church, D.F. Electron-spin resonance study of mainstream and sidestream cigarette smoke: Nature of the free radicals in gas-phase smoke and in cigarette tar. Environ. *Health Perspect.* **1983**, *47*, 345–355. [CrossRef] [PubMed]
17. Churg, A.; Zhou, S.; Wang, X.; Wang, R.; Wright, J.L. The role of interleukin-1beta in murine cigarette smoke-induced emphysema and small airway remodeling. *Am. J. Respir. Cell Mol. Biol.* **2009**, *40*, 482–490. [CrossRef] [PubMed]
18. Brusselle, G.G.; Joos, G.F.; Bracke, K.R. New insights into the immunology of chronic obstructive pulmonary disease. *Lancet* **2011**, *378*, 1015–1026. [CrossRef]
19. Chung, K.F.; Adcock, I.M. Multifaceted mechanisms in COPD: Inflammation, immunity, and tissue repair and destruction. *Eur. Respir. J.* **2008**, *31*, 1334–1356. [CrossRef] [PubMed]
20. Demedts, I.K.; Morel-Montero, A.; Lebecque, S.; Pacheco, Y.; Cataldo, D.; Joos, G.F.; Pauwels, R.A.; Brusselle, G.G. Elevated MMP-12 protein levels in induced sputum from patients with COPD. *Thorax* **2006**, *61*, 196–201. [CrossRef] [PubMed]
21. Freeman, C.M.; Martinez, F.J.; Han, M.K.; Ames, T.M.; Chensue, S.W.; Todt, J.C.; Arenberg, D.A.; Meldrum, C.A.; Getty, C.; McCloskey, L.; et al. Lung dendritic cell expression of maturation molecules increases with worsening chronic obstructive pulmonary disease. *Am. J. Respir. Crit. Care Med.* **2009**, *180*, 1179–1188. [CrossRef] [PubMed]
22. Di Stefano, A.; Caramori, G.; Gnemmi, I.; Contoli, M.; Vicari, C.; Capelli, A.; Magno, F.; D'Anna, S.E.; Zanini, A.; Brun, P.; et al. T helper type 17-related cytokine expression is increased in the bronchial mucosa of stable chronic obstructive pulmonary disease patients. *Clin. Exp. Immunol.* **2009**, *157*, 316–324. [CrossRef] [PubMed]
23. Barnes, P.J. Cellular and molecular mechanisms of chronic obstructive pulmonary disease. *Clin. Chest Med.* **2014**, *35*, 71–86. [CrossRef] [PubMed]
24. Hogg, J.C.; Chu, F.; Utokaparch, S.; Woods, R.; Elliott, W.M.; Buzatu, L.; Cherniack, R.M.; Rogers, R.M.; Sciurba, F.C.; Coxson, H.O.; et al. The nature of small-airway obstruction in chronic obstructive pulmonary disease. *N. Engl. J. Med.* **2004**, *350*, 2645–2653. [CrossRef] [PubMed]
25. Gan, W.Q.; Man, S.F.; Senthilselvan, A.; Sin, D.D. Association between chronic obstructive pulmonary disease and systemic inflammation: A systematic review and a meta-analysis. *Thorax* **2004**, *59*, 574–580. [CrossRef] [PubMed]
26. Agusti, A.; Edwards, L.D.; Rennard, S.I.; MacNee, W.; Tal-Singer, R.; Miller, B.E.; Vestbo, J.; Lomas, D.A.; Calverley, P.M.; Wouters, E.; et al. Persistent systemic inflammation is associated with poor clinical outcomes in COPD: A novel phenotype. *PLoS ONE* **2012**, *7*, e37483. [CrossRef] [PubMed]
27. Garcia-Aymerich, J.; Gomez, F.P.; Benet, M.; Farrero, E.; Basagana, X.; Gayete, A.; Pare, C.; Freixa, X.; Ferrer, J.; Ferrer, A.; et al. Identification and prospective validation of clinically relevant chronic obstructive pulmonary disease (COPD) subtypes. *Thorax* **2011**, *66*, 430–437. [CrossRef] [PubMed]
28. Soriano, J.B.; Rigo, F.; Guerrero, D.; Yanez, A.; Forteza, J.F.; Frontera, G.; Togores, B.; Agusti, A. High prevalence of undiagnosed airflow limitation in patients with cardiovascular disease. *Chest* **2010**, *137*, 333–340. [CrossRef] [PubMed]
29. Behar, S.; Panosh, A.; Reicher-Reiss, H.; Zion, M.; Schlesinger, Z.; Goldbourt, U. Prevalence and prognosis of chronic obstructive pulmonary disease among 5,839 consecutive patients with acute myocardial infarction. SPRINT Study Group. *Am. J. Med.* **1992**, *93*, 637–641. [CrossRef]
30. Cazzola, M.; Calzetta, L.; Bettoncelli, G.; Cricelli, C.; Romeo, F.; Matera, M.G.; Rogliani, P. Cardiovascular disease in asthma and COPD: A population-based retrospective cross-sectional study. *Respir. Med.* **2012**, *106*, 249–256. [CrossRef] [PubMed]

31. Mota, I.L.; Sousa, A.C.S.; Almeida, M.L.D.; de Melo, E.V.; Ferreira, E.J.P.; Neto, J.B.; Matos, C.J.O.; Telino, C.; Souto, M.J.S.; Oliveira, J.L.M. Coronary lesions in patients with COPD (Global Initiative for Obstructive Lung Disease stages I-III) and suspected or confirmed coronary arterial disease. *Int. J. Chronic Obstr. Pulm. Dis.* **2018**, *13*, 1999–2006. [CrossRef] [PubMed]
32. Sin, D.D.; Man, S.F. Chronic obstructive pulmonary disease as a risk factor for cardiovascular morbidity and mortality. *Proc. Am. Thorac. Soc.* **2005**, *2*, 8–11. [CrossRef] [PubMed]
33. Anthonisen, N.R.; Connett, J.E.; Enright, P.L.; Manfreda, J.; Lung Health Study Research, G. Hospitalizations and mortality in the Lung Health Study. *Am. J. Respir. Crit. Care Med.* **2002**, *166*, 333–339. [CrossRef] [PubMed]
34. Curkendall, S.M.; DeLuise, C.; Jones, J.K.; Lanes, S.; Stang, M.R.; Goehring, E., Jr.; She, D. Cardiovascular disease in patients with chronic obstructive pulmonary disease, Saskatchewan Canada cardiovascular disease in COPD patients. *Ann. Epidemiol.* **2006**, *16*, 63–70. [CrossRef] [PubMed]
35. The Emerging Risk Factors Collaboration; Kaptoge, S.; Di Angelantonio, E.; Pennells, L.; Wood, A.M.; White, I.R.; Gao, P.; Walker, M.; Thompson, A.; Sarwar, N.; et al. C-reactive protein, fibrinogen, and cardiovascular disease prediction. *N. Engl. J. Med.* **2012**, *367*, 1310–1320. [CrossRef] [PubMed]
36. Libby, P.; Ridker, P.M.; Hansson, G.K. Progress and challenges in translating the biology of atherosclerosis. *Nature* **2011**, *473*, 317–325. [CrossRef] [PubMed]
37. The Emerging Risk Factors Collaboration; Kaptoge, S.; Di Angelantonio, E.; Lowe, G.; Pepys, M.B.; Thompson, S.G.; Collins, R.; Danesh, J. C-reactive protein concentration and risk of coronary heart disease, stroke, and mortality: An individual participant meta-analysis. *Lancet* **2010**, *375*, 132–140.
38. Kaptoge, S.; Seshasai, S.R.; Gao, P.; Freitag, D.F.; Butterworth, A.S.; Borglykke, A.; Di Angelantonio, E.; Gudnason, V.; Rumley, A.; Lowe, G.D.; et al. Inflammatory cytokines and risk of coronary heart disease: New prospective study and updated meta-analysis. *Eur. Heart J.* **2014**, *35*, 578–589. [CrossRef] [PubMed]
39. Danesh, J.; Kaptoge, S.; Mann, A.G.; Sarwar, N.; Wood, A.; Angleman, S.B.; Wensley, F.; Higgins, J.P.; Lennon, L.; Eiriksdottir, G.; et al. Long-term interleukin-6 levels and subsequent risk of coronary heart disease: Two new prospective studies and a systematic review. *PLoS Med.* **2008**, *5*, e78. [CrossRef] [PubMed]
40. Petrache, I.; Natarajan, V.; Zhen, L.; Medler, T.R.; Richter, A.T.; Cho, C.; Hubbard, W.C.; Berdyshev, E.V.; Tuder, R.M. Ceramide upregulation causes pulmonary cell apoptosis and emphysema-like disease in mice. *Nat. Med.* **2005**, *11*, 491–498. [CrossRef] [PubMed]
41. Demedts, I.K.; Demoor, T.; Bracke, K.R.; Joos, G.F.; Brusselle, G.G. Role of apoptosis in the pathogenesis of COPD and pulmonary emphysema. *Respir. Res.* **2006**, *7*, 53. [CrossRef] [PubMed]
42. Kasahara, Y.; Tuder, R.M.; Cool, C.D.; Lynch, D.A.; Flores, S.C.; Voelkel, N.F. Endothelial cell death and decreased expression of vascular endothelial growth factor and vascular endothelial growth factor receptor 2 in emphysema. *Am. J. Respir. Crit. Care Med.* **2001**, *163*, 737–744. [CrossRef] [PubMed]
43. Barr, R.G.; Mesia-Vela, S.; Austin, J.H.; Basner, R.C.; Keller, B.M.; Reeves, A.P.; Shimbo, D.; Stevenson, L. Impaired flow-mediated dilation is associated with low pulmonary function and emphysema in ex-smokers: The Emphysema and Cancer Action Project (EMCAP) Study. *Am. J. Respir. Crit. Care Med.* **2007**, *176*, 1200–1207. [CrossRef] [PubMed]
44. Barr, R.G.; Bluemke, D.A.; Ahmed, F.S.; Carr, J.J.; Enright, P.L.; Hoffman, E.A.; Jiang, R.; Kawut, S.M.; Kronmal, R.A.; Lima, J.A.; et al. Percent emphysema, airflow obstruction, and impaired left ventricular filling. *N. Engl. J. Med.* **2010**, *362*, 217–227. [CrossRef] [PubMed]
45. Barr, R.G.; Ahmed, F.S.; Carr, J.J.; Hoffman, E.A.; Jiang, R.; Kawut, S.M.; Watson, K. Subclinical atherosclerosis, airflow obstruction and emphysema: The MESA Lung Study. *Eur. Respir. J.* **2012**, *39*, 846–854. [CrossRef] [PubMed]
46. Zieman, S.J.; Melenovsky, V.; Kass, D.A. Mechanisms, pathophysiology, and therapy of arterial stiffness. *Arterioscler. Thromb. Vasc. Biol.* **2005**, *25*, 932–943. [CrossRef] [PubMed]
47. Vlachopoulos, C.; Aznaouridis, K.; Stefanadis, C. Prediction of cardiovascular events and all-cause mortality with arterial stiffness: A systematic review and meta-analysis. *J. Am. Coll. Cardiol.* **2010**, *55*, 1318–1327. [CrossRef] [PubMed]
48. Cooper, L.L.; Palmisano, J.N.; Benjamin, E.J.; Larson, M.G.; Vasan, R.S.; Mitchell, G.F.; Hamburg, N.M. Microvascular function contributes to the relation between aortic stiffness and cardiovascular events: The framingham heart study. *Circ. Cardiovasc. Imaging* **2016**, *9*. [CrossRef] [PubMed]

49. McAllister, D.A.; Maclay, J.D.; Mills, N.L.; Mair, G.; Miller, J.; Anderson, D.; Newby, D.E.; Murchison, J.T.; Macnee, W. Arterial stiffness is independently associated with emphysema severity in patients with chronic obstructive pulmonary disease. *Am. J. Respir. Crit. Care Med.* **2007**, *176*, 1208–1214. [CrossRef] [PubMed]
50. Zelt, J.T.; Jones, J.H.; Hirai, D.M.; King, T.J.; Berton, D.C.; Pyke, K.E.; O'Donnell, D.E.; Neder, J.A. Systemic vascular dysfunction is associated with emphysema burden in mild COPD. *Respir. Med.* **2018**, *136*, 29–36. [CrossRef] [PubMed]
51. Roversi, S.; Fabbri, L.M.; Sin, D.D.; Hawkins, N.M.; Agusti, A. Chronic obstructive pulmonary disease and cardiac diseases. An urgent need for integrated care. *Am. J. Respir. Crit. Care Med.* **2016**, *194*, 1319–1336. [CrossRef] [PubMed]
52. Rimm, E.B.; Appel, L.J.; Chiuve, S.E.; Djousse, L.; Engler, M.B.; Kris-Etherton, P.M.; Mozaffarian, D.; Siscovick, D.S.; Lichtenstein, A.H.; American Heart Association Nutrition Committee of the Council on Lifestyle and Cardiometabolic Health; et al. Seafood long-chain n-3 polyunsaturated fatty acids and cardiovascular disease: A science advisory from the American Heart Association. *Circulation* **2018**, *138*, e35–e47. [CrossRef] [PubMed]
53. Siscovick, D.S.; Barringer, T.A.; Fretts, A.M.; Wu, J.H.; Lichtenstein, A.H.; Costello, R.B.; Kris-Etherton, P.M.; Jacobson, T.A.; Engler, M.B.; Alger, H.M.; et al. Omega-3 polyunsaturated fatty acid (fish oil) supplementation and the prevention of clinical cardiovascular disease: A science advisory from the American Heart Association. *Circulation* **2017**, *135*, e867–e884. [CrossRef] [PubMed]
54. Abdelhamid, A.S.; Martin, N.; Bridges, C.; Brainard, J.S.; Wang, X.; Brown, T.J.; Hanson, S.; Jimoh, O.F.; Ajabnoor, S.M.; Deane, K.H.; et al. Polyunsaturated fatty acids for the primary and secondary prevention of cardiovascular disease. *Cochrane Database Syst. Rev.* **2018**, *7*, CD012345. [CrossRef] [PubMed]
55. Pizzini, A.; Lunger, L.; Demetz, E.; Hilbe, R.; Weiss, G.; Ebenbichler, C.; Tancevski, I. The role of omega-3 fatty acids in reverse cholesterol transport: A review. *Nutrients* **2017**, *9*, 1099. [CrossRef] [PubMed]
56. Back, M. Omega-3 fatty acids in atherosclerosis and coronary artery disease. *Future Sci. OA* **2017**, *3*, FSO236. [CrossRef] [PubMed]
57. Calder, P.C. n-3 polyunsaturated fatty acids, inflammation, and inflammatory diseases. *Am. J. Clin. Nutr.* **2006**, *83*, 1505S–1519S. [CrossRef] [PubMed]
58. Miles, E.A.; Calder, P.C. Influence of marine *n*-3 polyunsaturated fatty acids on immune function and a systematic review of their effects on clinical outcomes in rheumatoid arthritis. *Br. J. Nutr.* **2012**, *107*, S171–S184. [CrossRef] [PubMed]
59. Veselinovic, M.; Vasiljevic, D.; Vucic, V.; Arsic, A.; Petrovic, S.; Tomic-Lucic, A.; Savic, M.; Zivanovic, S.; Stojic, V.; Jakovljevic, V. Clinical benefits of n-3 pufa and -linolenic acid in patients with rheumatoid arthritis. *Nutrients* **2017**, *9*, 325. [CrossRef] [PubMed]
60. Stanley, J.C.; Elsom, R.L.; Calder, P.C.; Griffin, B.A.; Harris, W.S.; Jebb, S.A.; Lovegrove, J.A.; Moore, C.S.; Riemersma, R.A.; Sanders, T.A. UK Food Standards Agency Workshop Report: The effects of the dietary n-6:n-3 fatty acid ratio on cardiovascular health. *Br. J. Nutr.* **2007**, *98*, 1305–1310. [CrossRef] [PubMed]
61. Chowdhury, R.; Warnakula, S.; Kunutsor, S.; Crowe, F.; Ward, H.A.; Johnson, L.; Franco, O.H.; Butterworth, A.S.; Forouhi, N.G.; Thompson, S.G.; et al. Association of dietary, circulating, and supplement fatty acids with coronary risk: A systematic review and meta-analysis. *Ann. Int. Med.* **2014**, *160*, 398–406. [CrossRef] [PubMed]
62. Griffin, B.A. How relevant is the ratio of dietary n-6 to n-3 polyunsaturated fatty acids to cardiovascular disease risk? Evidence from the OPTILIP study. *Curr. Opin. Lipidol.* **2008**, *19*, 57–62. [CrossRef] [PubMed]
63. Sanders, T.A.; Lewis, F.; Slaughter, S.; Griffin, B.A.; Griffin, M.; Davies, I.; Millward, D.J.; Cooper, J.A.; Miller, G.J. Effect of varying the ratio of n-6 to n-3 fatty acids by increasing the dietary intake of alpha-linolenic acid, eicosapentaenoic and docosahexaenoic acid, or both on fibrinogen and clotting factors VII and XII in persons aged 45–70 y: The OPTILIP study. *Am. J. Clin. Nutr.* **2006**, *84*, 513–522. [CrossRef] [PubMed]
64. Goyens, P.L.; Spilker, M.E.; Zock, P.L.; Katan, M.B.; Mensink, R.P. Conversion of alpha-linolenic acid in humans is influenced by the absolute amounts of alpha-linolenic acid and linoleic acid in the diet and not by their ratio. *Am. J. Clin. Nutr.* **2006**, *84*, 44–53. [CrossRef] [PubMed]
65. Baker, E.J.; Yusof, M.H.; Yaqoob, P.; Miles, E.A.; Calder, P.C. Omega-3 fatty acids and leukocyte-endothelium adhesion: Novel anti-atherosclerotic actions. *Mol. Asp. Med.* **2018**, *64*, 169–181. [CrossRef] [PubMed]
66. Rosenfeld, M.E.; Palinski, W.; Yla-Herttuala, S.; Carew, T.E. Macrophages, endothelial cells, and lipoprotein oxidation in the pathogenesis of atherosclerosis. *Toxicol. Pathol.* **1990**, *18*, 560–571. [PubMed]

67. Rosenfeld, M.E.; Tsukada, T.; Chait, A.; Bierman, E.L.; Gown, A.M.; Ross, R. Fatty streak expansion and maturation in Watanabe Heritable Hyperlipemic and comparably hypercholesterolemic fat-fed rabbits. *Arteriosclerosis* **1987**, *7*, 24–34. [CrossRef] [PubMed]
68. Spite, M.; Claria, J.; Serhan, C.N. Resolvins, specialized proresolving lipid mediators, and their potential roles in metabolic diseases. *Cell Metab.* **2014**, *19*, 21–36. [CrossRef] [PubMed]
69. Norling, L.V.; Ly, L.; Dalli, J. Resolving inflammation by using nutrition therapy: Roles for specialized proresolving mediators. *Curr. Opin. Clin. Nutr. Metab. Care* **2017**, *20*, 145–152. [CrossRef] [PubMed]
70. Duvall, M.G.; Levy, B.D. DHA- and EPA-derived resolvins, protectins, and maresins in airway inflammation. *Eur. J. Pharmacol.* **2016**, *785*, 144–155. [CrossRef] [PubMed]
71. Barnig, C.; Frossard, N.; Levy, B.D. Towards targeting resolution pathways of airway inflammation in asthma. *Pharmacol. Ther.* **2018**, *186*, 98–113. [CrossRef] [PubMed]
72. Pase, M.P.; Grima, N.A.; Sarris, J. Do long-chain n-3 fatty acids reduce arterial stiffness? A meta-analysis of randomised controlled trials. *Br. J. Nutr.* **2011**, *106*, 974–980. [CrossRef] [PubMed]
73. Casanova, M.A.; Medeiros, F.; Trindade, M.; Cohen, C.; Oigman, W.; Neves, M.F. Omega-3 fatty acids supplementation improves endothelial function and arterial stiffness in hypertensive patients with hypertriglyceridemia and high cardiovascular risk. *J. Am. Soc. Hypertens.* **2017**, *11*, 10–19. [CrossRef] [PubMed]
74. Tousoulis, D.; Plastiras, A.; Siasos, G.; Oikonomou, E.; Verveniotis, A.; Kokkou, E.; Maniatis, K.; Gouliopoulos, N.; Miliou, A.; Paraskevopoulos, T.; et al. Omega-3 PUFAs improved endothelial function and arterial stiffness with a parallel antiinflammatory effect in adults with metabolic syndrome. *Atherosclerosis* **2014**, *232*, 10–16. [CrossRef] [PubMed]
75. Zhu, D.; Zhang, Y.; Li, S.; Gan, L.; Feng, H.; Nie, W. Enteral omega-3 fatty acid supplementation in adult patients with acute respiratory distress syndrome: A systematic review of randomized controlled trials with meta-analysis and trial sequential analysis. *Intensive Care Med.* **2014**, *40*, 504–512. [CrossRef] [PubMed]
76. Pontes-Arruda, A.; Demichele, S.; Seth, A.; Singer, P. The use of an inflammation-modulating diet in patients with acute lung injury or acute respiratory distress syndrome: A meta-analysis of outcome data. *J. Parenter. Enteral Nutr.* **2008**, *32*, 596–605. [CrossRef] [PubMed]
77. Sharp, D.S.; Rodriguez, B.L.; Shahar, E.; Hwang, L.J.; Burchfiel, C.M. Fish consumption may limit the damage of smoking on the lung. *Am. J. Respir. Crit. Care Med.* **1994**, *150*, 983–987. [CrossRef] [PubMed]
78. Rodriguez, B.L.; Sharp, D.S.; Abbott, R.D.; Burchfiel, C.M.; Masaki, K.; Chyou, P.H.; Huang, B.; Yano, K.; Curb, J.D. Fish intake may limit the increase in risk of coronary heart disease morbidity and mortality among heavy smokers. The Honolulu Heart Program. *Circulation* **1996**, *94*, 952–956. [CrossRef] [PubMed]
79. Shahar, E.; Folsom, A.R.; Melnick, S.L.; Tockman, M.S.; Comstock, G.W.; Gennaro, V.; Higgins, M.W.; Sorlie, P.D.; Ko, W.J.; Szklo, M. Dietary n-3 polyunsaturated fatty acids and smoking-related chronic obstructive pulmonary disease. Atherosclerosis Risk in Communities Study Investigators. *N. Engl. J. Med.* **1994**, *331*, 228–233. [CrossRef] [PubMed]
80. Shahar, E.; Folsom, A.R.; Wu, K.K.; Dennis, B.H.; Shimakawa, T.; Conlan, M.G.; Davis, C.E.; Williams, O.D. Associations of fish intake and dietary n-3 polyunsaturated fatty acids with a hypocoagulable profile. The Atherosclerosis Risk in Communities (ARIC) Study. *Arterioscler. Thromb.* **1993**, *13*, 1205–1212. [CrossRef] [PubMed]
81. Wang, L.; Folsom, A.R.; Eckfeldt, J.H. Plasma fatty acid composition and incidence of coronary heart disease in middle aged adults: The Atherosclerosis Risk in Communities (ARIC) Study. *Nutr. Metab. Cardiovasc. Dis.* **2003**, *13*, 256–266. [CrossRef]
82. Yamagishi, K.; Nettleton, J.A.; Folsom, A.R.; Investigators, A.S. Plasma fatty acid composition and incident heart failure in middle-aged adults: The Atherosclerosis Risk in Communities (ARIC) Study. *Am. Heart J.* **2008**, *156*, 965–974. [CrossRef] [PubMed]
83. Garcia-Larsen, V.; Amigo, H.; Bustos, P.; Bakolis, I.; Rona, R.J. Ventilatory function in young adults and dietary antioxidant intake. *Nutrients* **2015**, *7*, 2879–2896. [CrossRef] [PubMed]
84. Stern, D.A.; Morgan, W.J.; Wright, A.L.; Guerra, S.; Martinez, F.D. Poor airway function in early infancy and lung function by age 22 years: A non-selective longitudinal cohort study. *Lancet* **2007**, *370*, 758–764. [CrossRef]
85. Leng, S.; Picchi, M.A.; Tesfaigzi, Y.; Wu, G.; Gauderman, W.J.; Xu, F.; Gilliland, F.D.; Belinsky, S.A. Dietary nutrients associated with preservation of lung function in Hispanic and non-Hispanic white smokers from New Mexico. *Int. J. Chronic Obstr. Pulm. Dis.* **2017**, *12*, 3171–3181. [CrossRef] [PubMed]

86. Wood, L.G.; Attia, J.; McElduff, P.; McEvoy, M.; Gibson, P.G. Assessment of dietary fat intake and innate immune activation as risk factors for impaired lung function. *Eur. J. Clin. Nutr.* **2010**, *64*, 818–825. [CrossRef] [PubMed]
87. Ridker, P.M.; Rifai, N.; Stampfer, M.J.; Hennekens, C.H. Plasma concentration of interleukin-6 and the risk of future myocardial infarction among apparently healthy men. *Circulation* **2000**, *101*, 1767–1772. [CrossRef] [PubMed]
88. Scaglia, N.; Chatkin, J.; Chapman, K.R.; Ferreira, I.; Wagner, M.; Selby, P.; Allard, J.; Zamel, N. The relationship between omega-3 and smoking habit: A cross-sectional study. *Lipids Health Dis.* **2016**, *15*, 61. [CrossRef] [PubMed]
89. Matsuyama, W.; Mitsuyama, H.; Watanabe, M.; Oonakahara, K.; Higashimoto, I.; Osame, M.; Arimura, K. Effects of omega-3 polyunsaturated fatty acids on inflammatory markers in COPD. *Chest* **2005**, *128*, 3817–3827. [CrossRef] [PubMed]
90. De Batlle, J.; Sauleda, J.; Balcells, E.; Gomez, F.P.; Mendez, M.; Rodriguez, E.; Barreiro, E.; Ferrer, J.J.; Romieu, I.; Gea, J.; et al. Association between Omega3 and Omega6 fatty acid intakes and serum inflammatory markers in COPD. *J. Nutr. Biochem.* **2012**, *23*, 817–821. [CrossRef] [PubMed]
91. Broekhuizen, R.; Wouters, E.F.; Creutzberg, E.C.; Weling-Scheepers, C.A.; Schols, A.M. Polyunsaturated fatty acids improve exercise capacity in chronic obstructive pulmonary disease. *Thorax* **2005**, *60*, 376–382. [CrossRef] [PubMed]
92. Calder, P.C.; Laviano, A.; Lonnqvist, F.; Muscaritoli, M.; Ohlander, M.; Schols, A. Targeted medical nutrition for cachexia in chronic obstructive pulmonary disease: A randomized, controlled trial. *J. Cachexia Sarcopenia Muscle* **2018**, *9*, 28–40. [CrossRef] [PubMed]
93. Piepoli, M.F.; Hoes, A.W.; Agewall, S.; Albus, C.; Brotons, C.; Catapano, A.L.; Cooney, M.T.; Corra, U.; Cosyns, B.; Deaton, C.; et al. 2016 European Guidelines on cardiovascular disease prevention in clinical practice: The Sixth Joint Task Force of the European Society of Cardiology and Other Societies on Cardiovascular Disease Prevention in Clinical Practice (constituted by representatives of 10 societies and by invited experts) Developed with the special contribution of the European Association for Cardiovascular Prevention & Rehabilitation (EACPR). *Eur. Heart J.* **2016**, *37*, 2315–2381. [PubMed]
94. London, S.J.; Sacks, F.M.; Caesar, J.; Stampfer, M.J.; Siguel, E.; Willett, W.C. Fatty acid composition of subcutaneous adipose tissue and diet in postmenopausal US women. *Am. J. Clin. Nutr.* **1991**, *54*, 340–345. [CrossRef] [PubMed]
95. Silverman, D.I.; Reis, G.J.; Sacks, F.M.; Boucher, T.M.; Pasternak, R.C. Usefulness of plasma phospholipid N-3 fatty acid levels in predicting dietary fish intake in patients with coronary artery disease. *Am. J. Cardiol.* **1990**, *66*, 860–862. [CrossRef]
96. Nodari, S.; Triggiani, M.; Campia, U.; Manerba, A.; Milesi, G.; Cesana, B.M.; Gheorghiade, M.; Dei Cas, L. N-3 polyunsaturated fatty acids in the prevention of atrial fibrillation recurrences after electrical cardioversion: A prospective, randomized study. *Circulation* **2011**, *124*, 1100–1106. [CrossRef] [PubMed]
97. Rauch, B.; Schiele, R.; Schneider, S.; Diller, F.; Victor, N.; Gohlke, H.; Gottwik, M.; Steinbeck, G.; Del Castillo, U.; Sack, R.; et al. OMEGA, a randomized, placebo-controlled trial to test the effect of highly purified omega-3 fatty acids on top of modern guideline-adjusted therapy after myocardial infarction. *Circulation* **2010**, *122*, 2152–2159. [CrossRef] [PubMed]
98. Tavazzi, L.; Maggioni, A.P.; Marchioli, R.; Barlera, S.; Franzosi, M.G.; Latini, R.; Lucci, D.; Nicolosi, G.L.; Porcu, M.; Tognoni, G.; et al. Effect of n-3 polyunsaturated fatty acids in patients with chronic heart failure (the GISSI-HF trial): A randomised, double-blind, placebo-controlled trial. *Lancet* **2008**, *372*, 1223–1230. [PubMed]
99. Mozaffarian, D.; Marchioli, R.; Macchia, A.; Silletta, M.G.; Ferrazzi, P.; Gardner, T.J.; Latini, R.; Libby, P.; Lombardi, F.; O'Gara, P.T.; et al. Fish oil and postoperative atrial fibrillation: The Omega-3 Fatty Acids for Prevention of Post-operative Atrial Fibrillation (OPERA) randomized trial. *JAMA* **2012**, *308*, 2001–2011. [CrossRef] [PubMed]

5

Impact of Nutrition on Pulmonary Arterial Hypertension

María Callejo [1,2,3], Joan Albert Barberá [2,4], Juan Duarte [5,6,7,8] and Francisco Perez-Vizcaino [1,2,3,*]

1. Department of Pharmacology and Toxicology, School of Medicine, Universidad Complutense de Madrid, 28040 Madrid, Spain; maria.callejo@ucm.es
2. CIBER Enfermedades Respiratorias, Ciberes, 28029 Madrid, Spain; jbarbera@clinic.cat
3. Instituto de Investigación Sanitaria Gregorio Marañón (IISGM), 28007 Madrid, Spain
4. Department of Pulmonary Medicine, Hospital Clínic-Institut d'Investigacions Biomèdiques August Pi i Sunyer (IDIBAPS), Universitat de Barcelona, 08036 Barcelona, Spain
5. Department of Pharmacology, School of Pharmacy, Universidad de Granada, 18071 Granada, Spain; jmduarte@ugr.es
6. CIBER Enfermedades Cardiovasculares, CiberCV, 28029 Madrid, Spain
7. Instituto de Investigación Biosanitaria (ibs.Granada), 18012 Granada, Spain
8. Centro de Investigaciones Biomédicas (CIBM), 18016 Granada, Spain

* Correspondence: fperez@med.ucm.es

Abstract: Pulmonary arterial hypertension (PAH) is characterized by sustained vasoconstriction, vascular remodeling, inflammation, and in situ thrombosis. Although there have been important advances in the knowledge of the pathophysiology of PAH, it remains a debilitating, limiting, and rapidly progressive disease. Vitamin D and iron deficiency are worldwide health problems of pandemic proportions. Notably, these nutritional alterations are largely more prevalent in PAH patients than in the general population and there are several pieces of evidence suggesting that they may trigger or aggravate disease progression. There are also several case reports associating scurvy, due to severe vitamin C deficiency, with PAH. Flavonoids such as quercetin, isoflavonoids such as genistein, and other dietary polyphenols including resveratrol slow the progression of the disease in animal models of PAH. Finally, the role of the gut microbiota and its interplay with the diet, host immune system, and energy metabolism is emerging in multiple cardiovascular diseases. The alteration of the gut microbiota has also been reported in animal models of PAH. It is thus possible that in the near future interventions targeting the nutritional status and the gut dysbiosis will improve the outcome of these patients.

Keywords: pulmonary hypertension; microbiota; vitamin C; vitamin D; iron; diet

---

1. Pulmonary Hypertension

The pulmonary circulation in healthy individuals is a high flow, low resistance circuit. It accommodates a similar cardiac output as the systemic circulation but with one sixth of its pressure. Normal mean pulmonary arterial pressure (mPAP) at rest is 14.0 ± 3.3 mmHg, with an upper limit of normal of 20 mmHg [1]. Pulmonary hypertension (PH) is due to a rise in pulmonary vascular resistance and mPAP. It is a chronic vascular disorder resulting in progressive right heart failure and eventually death [2,3]. A clinical classification categorizes PH into five groups according to their pathophysiological mechanisms, clinical presentation, hemodynamic characteristics, and treatment strategy [1,3]. Group 1, Pulmonary Arterial Hypertension (PAH) is also subclassified into idiopathic, familial, associated with other disorders or infections, or resulting from drug or toxin exposure [3,4]. The definition of PAH has been revised in the 6th World Symposium on Pulmonary Hypertension. PAH is now defined as a mPAP > 20 mmHg at right heart catheterization, normal left atrial pressure, and pulmonary vascular resistance ≥ 3 Wood units [1]. In Europe, PAH prevalence is in the range of 15–60 subjects per million population and an incidence of 5–10 cases per million per year [5,6]. In addition to poor prognosis, with one- and three-year survival rates around 87% and 67%, respectively, limitations in functional status affect the patient's quality of life, daily life activities, and employment [7,8].

1.1. Etiology

Several genetic and environmental factors for the development and progression of PAH have been identified [3,4,9]. In the West, idiopathic PAH, i.e., without any familial history or known triggering factor, is the most common subtype (30–50% of all cases of PAH), followed by connective tissue disease-associated PAH, congenital heart disease-associated PAH, and heritable PAH [5]. Mutations in *BMPR2* (bone morphogenetic protein receptors type II) can be detected in approximately 70% of cases of heritable PAH and they are also identified in 10–20% of IPAH [10]. In addition, mutations in other genes related to BMPR2 signaling axis have been discovered [9]: *ACVRL1/ALK1* (Activin receptor-like kinase 1), *ENG* (endoglin), and *SMAD9* (decapentaplegic homolog 9) [9,11]. Mutations in the *KCNK3* gene, which encodes the potassium channel TASK-1 [12], and in *KCNA5,* which encodes the voltage-dependent potassium channel Kv1.5, have also been identified in PAH patients [13]. Numerous drugs and substances have been involved in the development of PAH, including anorexigens, selective serotonin reuptake inhibitors, interferons, antiviral therapies, chemotherapeutic agents, and tyrosine kinase inhibitors such as dasatinib [3,14]. Finally, PAH is also associated with other systemic disorders, such as connective tissue diseases and portal hypertension, and infections, such as HIV and schistosomiasis [3]. In summary, with the exception of idiopathic PAH, in all forms of the disease, there is a factor known to be involved in its etiopathogeny, including mutations, systemic diseases, congenital heart defects, infections, drugs, and toxins. However, none of them by itself can trigger the disease and the need for a second hit has been proposed. For instance, *BMPR2* mutations present low penetrance: only 42% of the women and 14% of the men carrying the mutation develop the disease [11,15]. Similarly, about 30% of patients with scleroderma and 0.5% of HIV patients develop it [16,17].

1.2. Pathophysiology

The main pathophysiological mechanisms of PAH are sustained vasoconstriction, endothelial dysfunction, pulmonary vascular remodeling, in situ thrombosis, and inflammation [2,18,19]. Sustained vasoconstriction and endothelial dysfunction are due to an altered production of endothelial vasoactive mediators. These include decreased vasodilator and antiplatelet factors such as nitric oxide (NO) and prostacyclin (PGI_2), and increased vasoconstrictors and/or prothrombotic factors such as endothelin-1 (ET-1), serotonin (5-HT), thromboxane (TXA_2), angiotensin II (Ang II), and diverse growth factors, which also contribute to a hyperproliferative and procoagulant state. Ionic remodeling is also a key feature of PAH. The downregulation of voltage potassium channels, notably Kv1.5 [20,21] and TASK-1 [22,23], results in a more depolarized membrane potential in pulmonary arterial smooth muscle cells (PASMC) in PAH patients, leading to increased intracellular calcium and consequently PASMC vasoconstriction and also PASMC proliferation. Excessive smooth muscle proliferation and resistance to apoptosis due to paracrine growth factors, dysregulation of BMPR2 signaling pathway, dysfunctional potassium channels, and rise of anti-apoptotic proteins, among other factors, lead to smooth muscle hyperplasia. These deranged processes culminate in the obliteration of the pulmonary artery by enlarged intima and media layers [18,24] and the formation of proliferating vascular structures called plexiform lesions [24,25]. Thrombotic events in situ are frequent in PAH and contribute to the narrowing of pulmonary arteries too [19]. Altered immune mechanisms also play a significant role in the pathogenesis of PAH. Pulmonary vascular lesions in PAH patients and animal models reveal a recruitment of inflammatory cells as T- and B-lymphocytes, macrophages, dendritic cells, and mast cells [2,18]. In addition, there is an abnormal circulating level of certain cytokines, such as IL-1β, IL-6,

IL-17, TNF-α, and CCL5. Notably, some of these cytokines correlate with a worse prognosis in PAH patients [26].

1.3. Current Pharmacological Therapies

Over the last decades, intensive research on the cellular and molecular mechanisms and signaling pathways has provided a better understanding of the pathophysiology of PAH and consequently the identification of different pharmacological treatments. Unfortunately, a definitive cure does not exist for PAH. Currently, the five classes of therapies approved for PAH target the Ca^{2+} entry and the three main dysfunctional endothelial pathways: NO, prostacyclin, and endothelin-1 pathways [27,28]. Inhibitors of cyclic nucleotide phosphodiesterase type 5 (PDE-5), sildenafil and tadalafil, potentiate the action of endogenous NO and promote vasodilation [5,27,28]. Soluble guanylate cyclase (sGC) also acts in the NO signaling pathway catalyzing the transformation of GTP to cGMP. The sGC stimulator riociguat promotes the synthesis of cGMP favoring vasodilation and inhibiting cell proliferation. The action of riociguat is independent of the NO availability. Available prostacyclin-related therapies include synthetic (epoprostenol), prostacyclin analogs (treprostinil and iloprost) and the prostacyclin receptor agonist selexipag [27,28]. Endothelin-1 receptor antagonists (ERAs) include bosentan, macitentan, and ambrisentan [5,27,28].

Despite the current approved drugs as monotherapy have shown a favorable impact on clinical, functional, and hemodynamic outcomes, disease progression is frequently observed. At the 5th World Symposium of PH and based on the high level of evidence gathered from numerous randomized, controlled trials, the use of sequential combination therapy was proposed, at least in PAH patients with inadequate response to monotherapy, and possible first-line therapy in patients with advanced disease (New York Heart Association Functional Class III/IV). In addition, to achieve greater therapeutic response, currently, initial combination therapy at the time of diagnosis is recommended. Moreover, triple combination regimens are also considered in severe PAH, when double therapy fails [27,29].

1.4. Non-Pharmacological Therapies

In randomized controlled trials, exercise therapy improves exercise tolerance, functional capacity, and quality of life, with a positive impact on social, emotional, and psychological aspects [3,30]. Therefore, supervised exercise rehabilitation programs are recommended [3]. In addition, it is recommended that patients should avoid excessive physical activity that leads to distressing symptoms such as due to poor gas exchange or improper ventilation. Moreover, exercise programs are not well-stablished and present several limitations based on the gaps in the knowledge of the optimal method, intensity, and duration of the training [31].

Dietary modification is one of the first steps in the treatment of cardiovascular diseases. The routine treatment of systemic arterial hypertension involves dietary interventions for all patients including salt and alcohol restriction; increased consumption of vegetables, fresh fruits, whole grains, soluble fiber, fish, nuts, and olive oil; low consumption of red meat; and consumption of low-fat dairy products [32]. However, the European Society of Cardiology (ESC) and the European Respiratory Society (ERS) Guidelines [3] have not established specific recommendations for dietary habits or nutrient supplementation for PAH.

Interestingly, associations between nutritional factors and PAH have recently been reported in both human epidemiological studies and animal models. Recently, it has been reported that multiple-target nutritional intervention with extra protein, leucine, fish oil, and oligosaccharides can be a new strategy to prevent the pathophysiological alterations such as cardiac and skeletal muscle hypertrophy in PAH [33].

Herein, we focus on the scientific evidence on how the deficit in iron and vitamins C and D as well as other dietary components such as flavonoids may affect the progression of PAH. Finally, the role of the gut microbiota and its interplay with the diet and the host immune system is emerging in multiple cardiovascular and respiratory diseases including PAH. Other dietary factors such as n-3 polyunsaturated fatty acids (PUFAs), vitamin E, melatonin, and coenzyme Q10 may theoretically have an effect in PAH but there is no experimental or clinical evidence to support it and they are not discussed herein.

2. Dietary Components with an Impact on PAH

2.1. Vitamin C

Vitamin C, also known as ascorbic acid, is a water-soluble vitamin found in several fruits and vegetables. It is required for the activity of several enzymes, involved in tissue repair, important for the immune system function, and functions as an antioxidant. Severe deficit of vitamin C leads to scurvy, causing general weakness, anemia, skin hemorrhages, gum disease, and teeth loss [34,35].

Many studies have shown that oxidative stress is involved in cardiovascular disease [36]. Nitric oxide inactivation by reactive oxygen species is a key event in endothelial dysfunction associated to hypertension and atherosclerosis and other vascular pathologies [37]. On the other hand, oxidation of LDL in the endothelial wall makes these particles more atherogenic and allows them to accumulate in the artery walls [36]. This has led to the wide use of antioxidants including vitamin C to slow the progression of atherosclerosis. However, the meta-analysis of pooled data from randomized controlled trials have concluded that antioxidant vitamin supplementation has no effect on the incidence of major cardiovascular events, myocardial infarction, stroke, total death, and cardiac death [38].

Several case reports have shown that pulmonary hypertension is a complication of scurvy [39–42]. Elevated mPAP was reversible after the administration of ascorbate. Two possible mechanisms for the involvement of vitamin C deficiency in PAH have been proposed [41]. First, vitamin C increases the availability of endothelial NO that has vasodilatory and antiproliferative capacity [43]. Second, a deficiency of vitamin C can inactivate prolyl hydroxylases, the cellular oxygen sensors, uncoupling hypoxia-inducible factor (HIF) from oxygen control [44]. Uncontrolled HIF activity may lead to activation of pulmonary hypertensive mechanisms [45].

Whether moderate vitamin C deficiency rather than clinical scurvy, which is rare in Western societies, plays a role in PAH is unknown. Moreover, the effect of vitamin C supplements on PAH patients has not been well-addressed yet and there is only preliminary experimental evidence of its effectiveness. For example, a study in broiler chickens has shown that vitamin C reduced the incidence of PAH and the associated muscularization of pulmonary arterioles [46].

2.2. Vitamin D

Vitamin D is a fat-soluble vitamin that acts as a steroid hormone. It was discovered as an essential nutrient for the prevention of rickets. Although vitamin D may be obtained from diet, the main source is derived from endogenous synthesis in the skin under the influence of solar ultraviolet B radiation [47]. The inactive precursor synthetized in the skin or diet undergoes a two-step activation process to become biologically active. The first step is the 25-hydroxylation in the liver by CYP2R1 resulting in 25-hydroxyvitamin D_3 ($25(OH)D_3$), also named calcidiol, which has partial activity. The second hydroxylated metabolite is the active 1α, 25-dihydroxyvitamin D_3 ($1,25(OH)_2D_3$), also called calcitriol, by the 1α-hydroxylase enzyme or CYP27B1 mainly in the kidney [47,48]. Although calcitriol is the active metabolite of vitamin D, calcidiol is the best circulating biomarker of vitamin D status because the calcitriol half-life is shorter than that of calcidiol [47,48]. Calcitriol exerts its functions through the vitamin D receptor (VDR). Similar to other steroid receptor family members, VDR acts as a transcription factor [49]. VDR binds calcitriol with high affinity and specificity and then heterodimerizes with the retinoid-X receptor (RXR). After that, the VDR–RXR complex interacts with the vitamin D response elements on the promoter DNA region of target genes, resulting in changes in gene expression [48,50]. VDR regulates the expression of mRNAs as well as several miRNAs, indirectly regulating the expression of other genes [51].

There is no clear consensus on the definition of vitamin D deficiency; the optimum levels and the dietary requirements are uncertain [52,53]. However, even using conservative thresholds, nowadays, there is a pandemic of vitamin D deficiency [54]. The principal causes of low 25(OH)D_3 levels are inadequate sun exposure and/or reduced dietary intake [54].

Classically, vitamin D deficiency was related to bone diseases. Currently, because of VDR is found is many tissues, such as immune and cardiovascular cells, vitamin D deficiency has also been related to infection, cancer, and respiratory and cardiovascular diseases [53,55,56]. In fact, vitamin D deficiency has been associated with increased all-cause and cardiovascular mortality [57,58]. The discovery of VDR in many tissues that do not participate in calcium and phosphorous homeostasis led to identify a great variety of functions mediated by VDR, such as cell proliferation and differentiation, immunomodulation, and intracellular metabolism, among others [48].

In the context of PAH, there is some basic and clinical evidence suggesting a role for vitamin D in the pathophysiology of the disease. VDR was identified in vascular cells, including endothelial and smooth muscle cells. It is involved in numerous processes of potential relevance in cardiovascular diseases, such as cell proliferation, differentiation, and apoptosis; cell adhesion; oxidative stress; angiogenesis; and immunomodulatory and anti-inflammatory activity [53]. Therefore, it is assumed that vitamin D levels may affect the development of PAH.

To clarify whether vitamin D levels could be involved in PAH progression, Tanaka et al. treated PAH rats with a diet containing 10;000 UI/kg of cholecalciferol [59]. Notably, in this study, they found that vitamin D supplementation in PAH rats improved survival and attenuated some typical features in PAH such as right ventricle remodeling, assessed by Fulton index (ratio of right ventricle weight to left ventricle plus septum weight), and medial thickness of muscular pulmonary arteries. Despite these benefits of vitamin D, cholecalciferol treatment did not decrease pulmonary artery pressure [59]. Moreover, in an in vitro setup, calcitriol treatment inhibited the hypoxia-induced proliferation and migration in rat pulmonary artery endothelial cells (PAEC) via miR-204/TGFβ/Smad signaling pathway. Specifically, calcitriol suppressed the expression of Tgfbr2, α-SMA, and Smad7 and induced miR-204, p21, and Smad2 expression [60]. In the same study, similar results were found in an in vivo rat model. Remarkably, intraperitoneal calcitriol administration (20 mg/kg) partly reversed the rise in mPAP and Fulton index induced by three weeks of hypoxia [60].

In the clinical arena, Ulrich et al. showed that secondary hyperparathyroidism is highly prevalent in PAH patients [61]. Physiologically, decreased serum 25(OH)D_3 results in increased parathyroid hormone (PTH) levels in order to maintain adequate serum calcium concentrations. Therefore, low vitamin D status in PAH patients could be the reason for the elevated PTH. Later, epidemiological studies demonstrated that vitamin D deficiency is quite prevalent in PAH patients [59,62,63]. In the prospective study carried out by Demir et al., PAH patients presented much lower vitamin D levels (median of 6.79 ng/mL), considered as severe deficit of vitamin D ($<$10 ng/mL of serum 25(OH)D_3), than controls (18.76 ng/mL) [62]. In line with this result, Tanaka et al. found that, in a cohort of PAH patients, 39 out of 41 (95.1%) presented vitamin D insufficient and 25 patients (61%) showed deficient levels [59].

The relationship between vitamin D deficiency and PAH prognosis was evaluated. Serum 25(OH)D_3 levels were negatively correlated with mPAP assessed by right heart catheterization, and a significant positive correlation with cardiac output was found [59]. The potential benefits of vitamin D replacement on clinical outcomes has been also studied [63]. Twenty-two PAH patients were enrolled in a prospective uncontrolled longitudinal study. All PAH patients received cholecalciferol at a dose of 50,000 IU weekly for three months. In addition to the rise of serum 25(OH)D_3 levels from 14 $\pm$ 9 to 69 $\pm$ 31 ng/mL, remarkably, vitamin D supplements improved the 6-min-walk-distance (6MWD) test by around 80 m and right ventricle size. Mean PAP estimated by echocardiography was reduced from 79 $\pm$ 25 to 69 $\pm$ 23 mmHg but this effect did not reach statistical significance. Pro-BNP (pro-Brain Natriuretic Peptide) and functional class were also unchanged after vitamin D therapy [63].

All these data point to beneficial effects of vitamin D in PAH. However, the therapeutic use of vitamin D in this context has not been validated in randomized clinical trials. Nevertheless, given the high prevalence of vitamin D deficiency associated to PAH, it seems reasonable that serum vitamin D levels should be regularly assessed in these patients. Vitamin D supplements should be used to prevent bone diseases in any subject showing moderate or severe deficiency. Whether the symptoms, quality of life, and prognosis of patients with PAH improve after restoring vitamin D levels is unclear. Vitamin D supplementation has been used in other conditions. For instance, vitamin D supplements succeeded in respiratory diseases, decreasing the incidence of asthma [64] and chronic obstructive pulmonary disease (COPD) [65] exacerbations in patients with baseline 25(OH)D_3 levels lower than 25 nmol/L [65]. On the contrary, vitamin D supplementation has failed in other pathologies. In several of these latter studies, baseline vitamin D levels have not been taken into account [66–68].

In view of these results, it is plausible that vitamin D deficiency in combination with others risk factors could aggravate PAH. Vitamin D deficiency per se does not cause PAH. This is consistent with the fact that vitamin D deficiency is very prevalent in the population [54] while PAH is a rare disease. Therefore, further research is necessary to investigate the harmful effects of vitamin D deficiency in the pathogenesis of PAH and the efficacy and safety of vitamin D treatments.

2.3. *Iron*

Iron is essential in several physiological processes, including oxygen delivery and energy metabolism. In fact, about 70% of iron is bound to hemoglobin and around 5–10% is found in myoglobin. Serum ferritin is the most specific indicator used in laboratories for evaluating iron stores. Ferritin levels below 30 ng/mL are considered iron deficiency with or without anemia [69,70]. Circulating soluble transferrin receptor levels is another biomarker of iron deficiency. Iron deficiency is the most common cause of anemia worldwide and it is particularly common in specific chronic diseases such as heart failure or chronic renal diseases [71].

Recent data indicate that iron deficiency is also prevalent in patients with idiopathic PAH (IPAH) and it correlates with disease severity [72–74]. In fact, anemia is also an indicative of poor prognosis [75,76]. For the first time, Ruiter et al. [73] reported that around of 40% IPAH patients present iron deficiency and it is associated with decreased exercise capacity, assessed by the 6MWD test without anemia. Similar results were found by Yu in patients with PAH associated with congenital heart disease [77]. The significantly decreased 6MWD suggests that iron is essential in maintaining exercise performance. The authors speculated that iron deficiency might impair oxygen transport and delivery and finally disturb muscle oxygen homeostasis. Consequently, the clinical manifestation is shorter 6MWD. Interestingly, restoring iron levels in patients with chronic left heart failure significantly improves 6MWD and New York Heart Association (NYHA)-Functional Class [78,79].

Although epidemiological data show iron deficiency in PAH, the physiological contribution of iron in PAH is unknown. Few studies have been carried out in this context [80–83]. Variation in iron availability without anemia can affect pulmonary vascular tone. Intravenous infusion of iron attenuated the increased in mPAP in response to sustained hypoxia in 16 healthy volunteers with normal iron levels [83]. Likewise, acute iron depletion exacerbates PAP and pulmonary vasoconstrictive response to hypoxia condition [83]. In line with these results, in individuals exposed to high altitude, PAH may be attenuated by iron supplementation [84].

After four weeks of iron deficient diet, rats present vascular remodeling in resistance pulmonary arteries and PAH. These vascular changes were accompanied by activation of HIF, STAT3, and mitochondrial dysfunction. In addition, in this study, mPAP and pulmonary vascular muscularization was reversed by intravenous iron therapy [80]. Transferrin-1 receptor (TfR1) knock-out mice show protection against the development of hypoxia-induced PAH. Similarly, downregulation of TfR1 in vitro also inhibits human PASMC proliferation [85]. Moreover, recently, Lakhal-Littleton et al. demonstrated that intracellular iron deficient in PASMC induces PAH in mice via increasing expression of ET-1 [86].

The cause of the increased prevalence of iron deficiency in PAH is not completely clear. Iron deficiency can be related to reduced intake, impaired uptake, or increased loss of iron. Some authors postulated that the predominance of PAH in women vs. men could be due to a higher prevalence of iron deficiency in premenopausal women compared to postmenopausal women and men [77,87,88]. However, ferritin levels and circulating soluble transferrin receptor levels did not differ with gender or age in a large cohort of IPAH patients [72,73]. On the other hand, it is interesting that only a small proportion of IPAH responded to oral iron therapy, suggesting that, at least in these group of patients, a disturbance in iron absorption could be responsible for iron deficiency [73,89]. In line with this theory, elevated hepcidin levels were found in IPAH patients [72]. Hepcidin is a hormonal inhibitor of the intestinal absorption of dietary iron synthesized by the liver, which is elevated in inflammation [90]. However, plasma hepcidin concentration did not correlate with IL-6 levels, suggesting that, at least in these cohorts of IPAH patients, raised hepcidin levels were not due to inflammation. Of particular interest is BMP signaling. In vitro, *BMPR2* downregulation by a short interfering RNA increased hepcidin production. Rhodes et al. speculated that BMPR2-heritable PAH might be associated with more severe iron deficiency due to increased hepcidin levels [72].

All this evidence suggests that intravenous iron replacement could be a potential treatment in PAH patients [91,92], improving hemodynamic and clinical outcomes.

2.4. Flavonoids and Other Polyphenols

Polyphenols are a large group of plants metabolites commonly present in the human diet, specifically in vegetables, fruits, and beverages. Flavonoids comprise the major group of polyphenolic compounds. They are chemically characterized, sensu stricto, by the presence of a skeleton of 2-phenyl-4H-1-benzopyrane [93]. Isoflavonoids, neoflavonoids, chalcones, and aurones are related compounds often considered flavonoids as well. Other important polyphenols include stilbenoids.

Many studies have analyzed the influence of polyphenols in human heath [94], and more especially its positive role against cardiovascular diseases [95,96]. In addition to their antioxidant action, they also present vasodilator, antithrombotic, antiapoptotic, anti-inflammatory, hypolipidemic, and antiatherogenic effects, associated with decreased cardiovascular risk [96]. The flavonoids present in fresh fruits, vegetables, and wine are considered major contributors to the antihypertensive effects of these foodstuffs. In particular, the effects of the flavonoid quercetin, the isoflavonoid genistein, and the stilbenoid resveratrol have been studied in animal models of PAH and are reviewed herein.

Resveratrol is found in red wine, grapes, and berries. This polyphenol has been shown to attenuate right ventricular systolic pressure and pulmonary artery remodeling in monocrotaline-induced PAH in rats [97]. Moreover, this study demonstrated that resveratrol treatment (25 mg/kg per day) improved pulmonary endothelial function, assessed by increased eNOS expression, and decreased oxidative stress due to decreased of NADPH oxidase activity. Resveratrol also reduced the inflammatory cytokines IL-1β, IL-6, and TNFα, and inhibited PASMC proliferation [97]. Therefore, resveratrol exerted anti-oxidant, anti-inflammatory, and anti-proliferative effects, reducing the main hallmarks of PAH. It was speculated that ROS scavenging mediated by resveratrol may be the central process of these pleiotropic actions [98]. Several experiments have been performed to elucidate the underlying mechanisms. Chen et al. found that in vitro resveratrol treatment attenuated the hypoxia-induced proliferation in human PASMC by the inhibition of arginase II. The inhibitory effect of resveratrol on arginase II was PI3K-Akt signaling pathway-dependent [99]. Similar results were found in rat PASMC [100], in hypoxic pulmonary hypertension rats [101], and in monocrotaline-induced PAH [102].

Quercetin is probably the most widely distributed in foods and best studied flavonoid. Multiple studies have highlighted its biological activity to reduce arterial blood pressure in both human and experimental systemic hypertension [103,104]. Several animal models have also been used to examine the protective effect of quercetin in PAH. The first report analyzed the effects of quercetin as a preventive strategy for PAH (100 mg/kg from the day after monocrotaline infusion) [105]. Consecutively, our group investigated the therapeutic role of quercetin in PAH induced by monocrotaline in rats

(10 mg/kg once daily from Day 21 after PAH was established) [106]. In both studies, the authors found that quercetin administration significantly alleviated mPAP, right ventricular hypertrophy, and pulmonary artery remodeling. Furthermore, quercetin treatment significantly increased survival in monocrotaline rats. However, classic biomarkers of PAH, such as endothelial dysfunction, pulmonary artery hyperresponsiveness to 5-HT, and downregulation of BMPR2 and Kv1.5, were unaffected by quercetin [106]. These were unexpected results because quercetin has been widely reported to improve endothelial function in systemic arteries in in vivo and in vitro experiments [104,107]. Our group also demonstrated that quercetin exerted vasodilator effect in isolated pulmonary arteries, induced apoptosis and inhibited cell proliferation in PASMC [106]. The mechanism involved in the antiproliferative effects in both PASMC and endothelial cells seem to involve AKT [106,108,109], FOXO1-mTOR [110], and altered Bax/Bcl-2 ratio [108,111].

Genistein is an isoflavone abundant in soybeans. It has been widely used as a phytoestrogen substitute for hormone replacement therapy in postmenopausal women [112]. Genistein consumption is thought to reduce the incidence or severity of cardiovascular disease and of some forms of cancers [113]. It is a wide spectrum tyrosine kinase inhibitor (TKI) and it is well-known that tyrosine kinase inhibitors play an important role in the control of pulmonary vascular tone. Genistein can behave as an antioxidant and improves endothelial function in systemic and pulmonary arteries from several models of cardiovascular disease, through increasing endothelial NO synthase levels, restoring NO-mediated PA relaxation, reducing vascular superoxide production or decreasing angiotensin II receptor [114–116]. The vasodilator effect of genistein has also been studied in isolated pulmonary arteries precontracted by 5-HT [21] and ET-1 [117]. The activation of 5-HT_{2A} receptors inhibits K_V currents, and genistein treatment prevented this effect in rat PASMC [21]. In PA from chronic hypoxia rats, the contraction induced by ET-1 appeared to be mediated by the activation of tyrosine kinase, and genistein reduced the ET-1-induced response [117]. All these effects make genistein a potential therapy for PAH. In the rat model of PAH induced by monocrotaline, genistein both prevents [118] and reverses [116] the increased PAP. Moreover, genistein significantly improved pulmonary vascular remodeling, right ventricular function, and survival. It also inhibited human PASMC proliferation in vitro [116]. In addition, genistein also ameliorated pulmonary hemodynamics and vascular remodeling in a rat model of hypobaric hypoxia [119]. Some authors suggested that the mechanism underlying genistein-improved main characteristics of PAH is mediated through the improvement of PI3K/Akt/eNOS signaling pathway [119,120]. In addition, genistein also potently attenuates hypoxia-induced hypertrophy of PASMC through estrogen receptor and β-adrenoreceptor signaling [121].

2.5. Microbiota

The human gut is a bacterial ecosystem that harbors >100 trillion microbial cells and presents a symbiotic relationship with the host. Gut microbes provide help with digestion, promote gut immunity, and prevent the colonization of pathogens, while the host supplies them with a favorable environment for survival. A healthy gut microbiome is characterized in terms of diversity and richness as well as its stability and resistance to any perturbation. In contrast, gut dysbiosis is any disruption of the normal balance between the gut microbial community and the host, which can result in several diseases [122]. Gut dysbiosis is typically characterized by a lower diversity and richness of the microbial communities, an increase in Firmicutes to Bacteroidetes ratio (F/B), and altered short chain fatty acids (SCFA) producing bacteria, with an increase in lactate-producing bacteria and a decrease in acetate- and butyrate-producing bacteria [123,124]. In recent years, a growing body of evidence points to a relationship between gut dysbiosis and many diseases, including essential hypertension [124,125], obesity [126,127], inflammation [128] neurologic disorders [129], and pulmonary hypertension [130].

The diet is a critical regulator of the composition and function of the microbiota [131]. Multiple studies have focused on the effects of macronutrients (fat, carbohydrate, and protein) on the gut microbiome. Other dietary components such as soluble or insoluble fibers may be important as well [132,133]. Moreover, several food components are substrates for bacterial enzymes. These enzymatic processes lead to the production of other byproducts which can be absorbed in the gut. Importantly, SCFAs, particularly butyric and acetic acid, which derive mainly from the bacterial fermentation of fiber, are considered to promote cardiovascular health. In contrast, trimethylamine-N-oxide (TMAO), a metabolite produced by the gut microbiota from choline, betaine, and carnitine, which are abundant in meat, eggs, and fish, is associated with excess risk of heart disease [134].

In addition, it has been reported that some dietary components such as sweeteners, minerals, and vitamins can modify the microbiota. Remarkably, some of the nutrients with an impact on PAH progression, as described above, such as iron and vitamin D deficiency as well as quercetin and resveratrol significantly affect the intestinal microbiota [135–137]. Therefore, besides the aforementioned mechanisms of action of these dietary components, the changes in the gut microbiota may also be responsible of the actions of iron, vitamin D, or polyphenols. On the contrary, the composition of microbiota may affect the absorption of calcium, phosphate, iron, and zinc. Moreover, in addition to dietary sources of water-soluble vitamins, the microbiota can also synthetize some of these vitamins [132].

The role of the diet on the microbiome in the context of PAH is not known. However, it could be speculated that part of the effects of the dietary factors mentioned above in PAH might be due to changes in the microbiota. We demonstrated for the first time that there are several changes in the gut microbiota in PAH [130]. In a rat model of PAH induced by a single dose of Sugen5416 plus chronic hypoxia for two weeks, we found two main hallmarks of gut dysbiosis: a three-fold increase in F/B ratio, driven by a decrease in all Bacteroidetes families in PAH animals (2–10-fold decrease) and no changes in Firmicutes abundance. Furthermore, feces from PAH rats present a decreased in acetate-producing bacteria, accompanied by a reduced serum acetate, without changes in butyrate and lactate producing bacteria [130]. In contrast, we did not find global differences in microbial diversity and richness, as happened in other diseases [124]. Although this study is preliminary, it indicates that the abnormalities in the gut microbiota observed might play a pathophysiological role in the development and/or progression of PAH, rather than being a consequence. Likewise, Wedgwood et al. also suggested that intestinal dysbiosis may impact on distal organs including the lung, contributing to the development of PH [138]. In this study, rat pups with PH induced by postnatal growth restriction (PNGR) present gut dysbiosis and the probiotic treatment attenuates PNGR-induced PH. Considering these results, the authors suggested that PH is in part driven by the alteration of the gut microbiome [138].

It is tempting to speculate that changes in intestinal microbiota and circulating microbial products can contribute to PAH. Thenappan et al. suggested that gut dysbiosis might be involved in perivascular inflammation in the early development of PAH [139]. Gut dysbiosis can result in increased gut permeability, allowing bacteria and/or bacterial products translocation, with an increase in plasma bacterial lipopolysaccharide (LPS), the main ligand for toll-like receptor 4 (TLR4). TLR4 activation has been implicated in the pathogenesis of PAH [140]. Ranchoux et al. demonstrated that bacterial translocation occurs in PAH, suggesting a gut-lung cross-talk, in which TLR4 antagonists are plausible to be effective at disrupting this circle [141]. Gut dysbiosis also produces a pro-inflammatory environment, increasing IL-17 secretion and a downregulation of Treg cells [142]. Likewise, an increase in Th17 cells and a deficiency in normal Treg cells are observed in PAH patients, promoting vascular remodeling [26,143]. In addition to platelets, serotonin (5-HT) is also stored and produced in enterochromaffin cells. Thus, gut microbiota plays a key role in regulating 5-HT levels at colon and serum. Notably, clinical and experimental PAH showed elevated serum 5-HT levels. It is well-known that 5-HT promotes pulmonary artery remodeling, PASMC proliferation, and constriction of pulmonary arteries through the 5-HT_{1B} receptor [21,144].

3. Conclusions

Although there have been important advances in the knowledge of the pathophysiology of PAH, it remains a debilitating, limiting, and rapidly progressive disease. Targeted nutritional and lifestyle interventions could have a great clinical importance (Figure 1). Vitamin D and iron deficiency are worldwide health problems of pandemic proportions. Notably, these nutritional alterations are largely more prevalent in PAH patients than in the general population and there are several pieces of evidence suggesting that they may trigger or aggravate the disease progression. However, to date, most of this evidence is based on observational studies, animal models, and small series of uncontrolled trials. Therefore, robust randomized clinical trials are required to establish cause–effect relationships. In the meantime, it seems reasonable to study the nutritional status of all PAH patients with particular emphasis on vitamins C and D and iron. Severe nutritional deficiencies leading to scurvy, osteoporosis, or ferropenic anemia must be corrected using the appropriate supplements. Based on the above discussed evidence, the correction of these nutritional defects may be expected to have additional positive impact on the severity of the disease, the quality of life, and the prognosis of the patients.

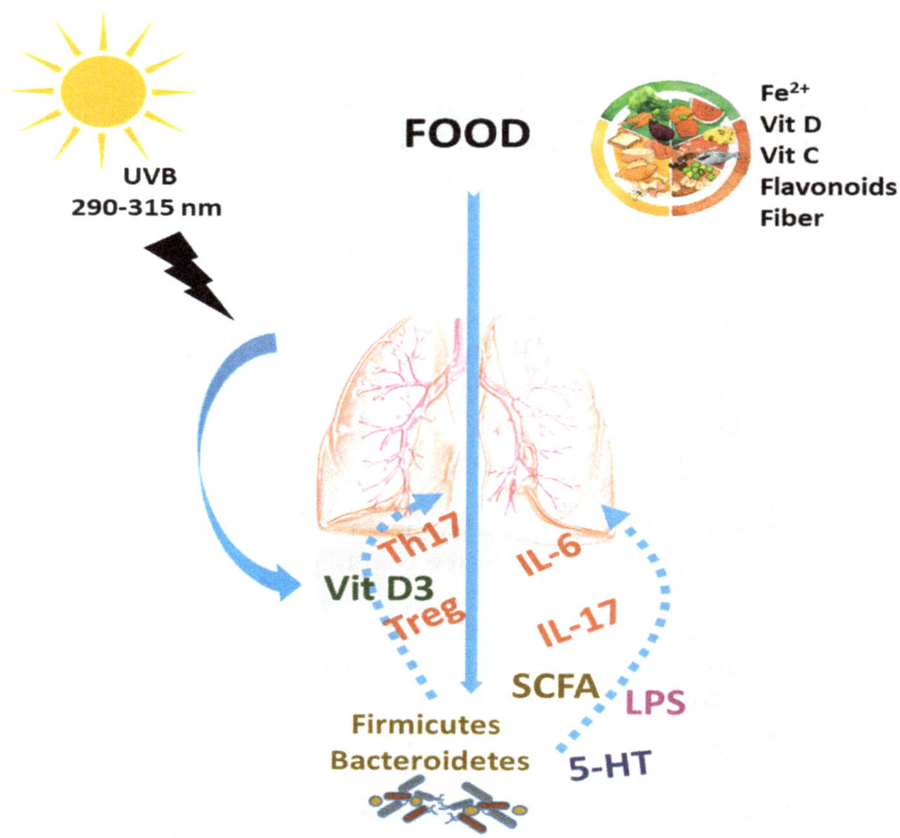

Figure 1. Impact of nutrition in PAH. Dietary components such as Fe^{2+}, vitamins C and D, flavonoids and other related polyphenols, and fiber as well as vitamin D obtained from the exposure to sunlight may have a positive impact the quality of life and prognosis of PAH patients. Each dietary factor may have its own mechanism of action. However, part of the effects of these nutrients may be related to their effect on the immune system with restoration of T cells and cytokines, changes in the microbiota and their bacterial products, and bacterial translocation.

The possible positive effects of the polyphenols quercetin, resveratrol, and genistein in PAH remain to be determined in clinical trials. The use of supplements containing these polyphenols cannot be recommended at this stage. However, given the encouraging effects of fruits and vegetables on cardiovascular health with particular impact on systemic hypertension, it seems reasonable to stimulate PAH patients to adhere to diets rich in these foods.

The role of gut dysbiosis in the pathogenesis of PAH has not been firmly established. At present, no recommendations directed to modify the gut or the lung microbiota can be established. However, if the role of dysbiosis is confirmed, several interventions may be implemented to correct or compensate the altered microbial ecosystem including the use of specific bacterial strains (probiotics), fiber and dietary polyphenols (i.e., prebiotics), fecal transplantation, antibiotics, and beta-adrenergic antagonists or replacing the deficit in specific SCFAs (e.g., acetate).

Author Contributions: F.P.-V. outlined the review, M.C. wrote a draft and J.A.B., J.D. and F.P.-V. revised and amplified the final version. All authors have read and agreed to the published version of the manuscript.

References

1. Simonneau, G.; Montani, D.; Celermajer, D.S.; Denton, C.P.; Gatzoulis, M.A.; Krowka, M.; Williams, P.G.; Souza, R. Haemodynamic definitions and updated clinical classification of pulmonary hypertension. *Eur. Respir. J.* **2019**, *53*. [CrossRef] [PubMed]
2. Humbert, M.; Guignabert, C.; Bonnet, S.; Dorfmuller, P.; Klinger, J.R.; Nicolls, M.R.; Olschewski, A.J.; Pullamsetti, S.S.; Schermuly, R.T.; Stenmark, K.R.; et al. Pathology and pathobiology of pulmonary hypertension: State of the art and research perspectives. *Eur. Respir. J.* **2019**, *53*. [CrossRef] [PubMed]
3. Galie, N.; Humbert, M.; Vachiery, J.L.; Gibbs, S.; Lang, I.; Torbicki, A.; Simonneau, G.; Peacock, A.; Vonk Noordegraaf, A.; Beghetti, M.; et al. 2015 ESC/ERS Guidelines for the diagnosis and treatment of pulmonary hypertension: The Joint Task Force for the Diagnosis and Treatment of Pulmonary Hypertension of the European Society of Cardiology (ESC) and the European Respiratory Society (ERS): Endorsed by: Association for European Paediatric and Congenital Cardiology (AEPC), International Society for Heart and Lung Transplantation (ISHLT). *Eur. Respir. J.* **2015**, *46*, 903–975. [CrossRef] [PubMed]
4. Simonneau, G.; Robbins, I.M.; Beghetti, M.; Channick, R.N.; Delcroix, M.; Denton, C.P.; Elliott, C.G.; Gaine, S.P.; Gladwin, M.T.; Jing, Z.C.; et al. Updated clinical classification of pulmonary hypertension. *J. Am. Coll. Cardiol.* **2009**, *54*, S43–S54. [CrossRef] [PubMed]
5. Lau, E.M.T.; Giannoulatou, E.; Celermajer, D.S.; Humbert, M. Epidemiology and treatment of pulmonary arterial hypertension. *Nat. Rev. Cardiol.* **2017**, *14*, 603–614. [CrossRef]
6. Badesch, D.B.; Raskob, G.E.; Elliott, C.G.; Krichman, A.M.; Farber, H.W.; Frost, A.E.; Barst, R.J.; Benza, R.L.; Liou, T.G.; Turner, M.; et al. Pulmonary arterial hypertension: Baseline characteristics from the REVEAL Registry. *Chest* **2010**, *137*, 376–387. [CrossRef]
7. Benza, R.L.; Miller, D.P.; Barst, R.J.; Badesch, D.B.; Frost, A.E.; McGoon, M.D. An evaluation of long-term survival from time of diagnosis in pulmonary arterial hypertension from the REVEAL Registry. *Chest* **2012**, *142*, 448–456. [CrossRef]
8. Humbert, M.; Sitbon, O.; Yaici, A.; Montani, D.; O'Callaghan, D.S.; Jais, X.; Parent, F.; Savale, L.; Natali, D.; Gunther, S.; et al. Survival in incident and prevalent cohorts of patients with pulmonary arterial hypertension. *Eur. Respir. J.* **2010**, *36*, 549–555. [CrossRef]
9. Morrell, N.W.; Aldred, M.A.; Chung, W.K.; Elliott, C.G.; Nichols, W.C.; Soubrier, F.; Trembath, R.C.; Loyd, J.E. Genetics and genomics of pulmonary arterial hypertension. *Eur. Respir. J.* **2019**, *53*. [CrossRef]
10. Evans, J.D.; Girerd, B.; Montani, D.; Wang, X.J.; Galie, N.; Austin, E.D.; Elliott, G.; Asano, K.; Grunig, E.; Yan, Y.; et al. BMPR2 mutations and survival in pulmonary arterial hypertension: An individual participant data meta-analysis. *Lancet Respir. Med.* **2016**, *4*, 129–137. [CrossRef]
11. Austin, E.D.; Loyd, J.E. The genetics of pulmonary arterial hypertension. *Circ. Res.* **2014**, *115*, 189–202. [CrossRef] [PubMed]

12. Ma, L.; Roman-Campos, D.; Austin, E.D.; Eyries, M.; Sampson, K.S.; Soubrier, F.; Germain, M.; Tregouet, D.A.; Borczuk, A.; Rosenzweig, E.B.; et al. A novel channelopathy in pulmonary arterial hypertension. *N. Engl. J. Med.* **2013**, *369*, 351–361. [CrossRef] [PubMed]
13. Remillard, C.V.; Tigno, D.D.; Platoshyn, O.; Burg, E.D.; Brevnova, E.E.; Conger, D.; Nicholson, A.; Rana, B.K.; Channick, R.N.; Rubin, L.J.; et al. Function of Kv1.5 channels and genetic variations of KCNA5 in patients with idiopathic pulmonary arterial hypertension. *Am. J. Physiol. Cell Physiol.* **2007**, *292*, C1837–C1853. [CrossRef] [PubMed]
14. Orcholski, M.E.; Yuan, K.; Rajasingh, C.; Tsai, H.; Shamskhou, E.A.; Dhillon, N.K.; Voelkel, N.F.; Zamanian, R.T.; de Jesus Perez, V.A. Drug-induced pulmonary arterial hypertension: A primer for clinicians and scientists. *Am. J. Physiol. Lung Cell Mol. Physiol.* **2018**, *314*, L967–L983. [CrossRef] [PubMed]
15. Southgate, L.; Machado, R.D.; Graf, S.; Morrell, N.W. Molecular genetic framework underlying pulmonary arterial hypertension. *Nat. Rev. Cardiol.* **2019**. [CrossRef] [PubMed]
16. Jaafar, S.; Visovatti, S.; Young, A.; Huang, S.; Cronin, P.; Vummidi, D.; McLaughlin, V.; Khanna, D. Impact of the revised haemodynamic definition on the diagnosis of pulmonary hypertension in patients with systemic sclerosis. *Eur. Respir. J.* **2019**, *54*. [CrossRef]
17. Jarrett, H.; Barnett, C. HIV-associated pulmonary hypertension. *Curr. Opin. HIV AIDS* **2017**, *12*, 566–571. [CrossRef]
18. Rabinovitch, M. Molecular pathogenesis of pulmonary arterial hypertension. *J. Clin. Investig.* **2012**, *122*, 4306–4313. [CrossRef]
19. Guignabert, C.; Dorfmuller, P. Pathology and pathobiology of pulmonary hypertension. *Semin. Respir. Crit. Care Med.* **2013**, *34*, 551–559. [CrossRef]
20. Mondejar-Parreno, G.; Callejo, M.; Barreira, B.; Morales-Cano, D.; Esquivel-Ruiz, S.; Moreno, L.; Cogolludo, A.; Perez-Vizcaino, F. miR-1 is increased in pulmonary hypertension and downregulates Kv1.5 channels in rat pulmonary arteries. *J. Physiol.* **2019**, *597*, 1185–1197. [CrossRef]
21. Cogolludo, A.; Moreno, L.; Lodi, F.; Frazziano, G.; Cobeno, L.; Tamargo, J.; Perez-Vizcaino, F. Serotonin inhibits voltage-gated K+ currents in pulmonary artery smooth muscle cells: Role of 5-HT2A receptors, caveolin-1, and KV1.5 channel internalization. *Circ. Res.* **2006**, *98*, 931–938. [CrossRef] [PubMed]
22. Antigny, F.; Hautefort, A.; Meloche, J.; Belacel-Ouari, M.; Manoury, B.; Rucker-Martin, C.; Pechoux, C.; Potus, F.; Nadeau, V.; Tremblay, E.; et al. Potassium Channel Subfamily K Member 3 (KCNK3) Contributes to the Development of Pulmonary Arterial Hypertension. *Circulation* **2016**, *133*, 1371–1385. [CrossRef] [PubMed]
23. Olschewski, A.; Veale, E.L.; Nagy, B.M.; Nagaraj, C.; Kwapiszewska, G.; Antigny, F.; Lambert, M.; Humbert, M.; Czirjak, G.; Enyedi, P.; et al. TASK-1 (KCNK3) channels in the lung: From cell biology to clinical implications. *Eur. Respir. J.* **2017**, *50*. [CrossRef] [PubMed]
24. Guignabert, C.; Tu, L.; Girerd, B.; Ricard, N.; Huertas, A.; Montani, D.; Humbert, M. New molecular targets of pulmonary vascular remodeling in pulmonary arterial hypertension: Importance of endothelial communication. *Chest* **2015**, *147*, 529–537. [CrossRef]
25. Budhiraja, R.; Tuder, R.M.; Hassoun, P.M. Endothelial dysfunction in pulmonary hypertension. *Circulation* **2004**, *109*, 159–165. [CrossRef]
26. Rabinovitch, M.; Guignabert, C.; Humbert, M.; Nicolls, M.R. Inflammation and immunity in the pathogenesis of pulmonary arterial hypertension. *Circ. Res.* **2014**, *115*, 165–175. [CrossRef]
27. Montani, D.; Chaumais, M.C.; Guignabert, C.; Gunther, S.; Girerd, B.; Jais, X.; Algalarrondo, V.; Price, L.C.; Savale, L.; Sitbon, O.; et al. Targeted therapies in pulmonary arterial hypertension. *Pharmacol. Ther.* **2014**, *141*, 172–191. [CrossRef]
28. O'Callaghan, D.S.; Savale, L.; Montani, D.; Jais, X.; Sitbon, O.; Simonneau, G.; Humbert, M. Treatment of pulmonary arterial hypertension with targeted therapies. *Nat. Rev. Cardiol.* **2011**, *8*, 526–538. [CrossRef]
29. Kemp, K.; Savale, L.; O'Callaghan, D.S.; Jais, X.; Montani, D.; Humbert, M.; Simonneau, G.; Sitbon, O. Usefulness of first-line combination therapy with epoprostenol and bosentan in pulmonary arterial hypertension: An observational study. *J. Heart Lung Transplant.* **2012**, *31*, 150–158. [CrossRef]
30. Richter, M.J.; Grimminger, J.; Kruger, B.; Ghofrani, H.A.; Mooren, F.C.; Gall, H.; Pilat, C.; Kruger, K. Effects of exercise training on pulmonary hemodynamics, functional capacity and inflammation in pulmonary hypertension. *Pulm. Circ.* **2017**, *7*, 20–37. [CrossRef]

31. Galie, N.; Corris, P.A.; Frost, A.; Girgis, R.E.; Granton, J.; Jing, Z.C.; Klepetko, W.; McGoon, M.D.; McLaughlin, V.V.; Preston, I.R.; et al. Updated treatment algorithm of pulmonary arterial hypertension. *J. Am. Coll. Cardiol.* **2013**, *62*, D60–D72. [CrossRef] [PubMed]
32. Cuspidi, C.; Tadic, M.; Grassi, G.; Mancia, G. Treatment of hypertension: The ESH/ESC guidelines recommendations. *Pharmacol. Res.* **2018**, *128*, 315–321. [CrossRef] [PubMed]
33. Vinke, P.; Bowen, T.S.; Boekschoten, M.V.; Witkamp, R.F.; Adams, V.; van Norren, K. Anti-inflammatory nutrition with high protein attenuates cardiac and skeletal muscle alterations in a pulmonary arterial hypertension model. *Sci. Rep.* **2019**, *9*, 10160. [CrossRef] [PubMed]
34. Carpenter, K.J. The discovery of vitamin C. *Ann. Nutr. Metab.* **2012**, *61*, 259–264. [CrossRef] [PubMed]
35. Granger, M.; Eck, P. Dietary Vitamin C in Human Health. *Adv. Food Nutr. Res.* **2018**, *83*, 281–310. [CrossRef] [PubMed]
36. Kattoor, A.J.; Pothineni, N.V.K.; Palagiri, D.; Mehta, J.L. Oxidative Stress in Atherosclerosis. *Curr. Atheroscler. Rep.* **2017**, *19*, 42. [CrossRef]
37. Incalza, M.A.; D'Oria, R.; Natalicchio, A.; Perrini, S.; Laviola, L.; Giorgino, F. Oxidative stress and reactive oxygen species in endothelial dysfunction associated with cardiovascular and metabolic diseases. *Vasc. Pharmacol.* **2018**, *100*, 1–19. [CrossRef]
38. Ye, Y.; Li, J.; Yuan, Z. Effect of antioxidant vitamin supplementation on cardiovascular outcomes: A meta-analysis of randomized controlled trials. *PLoS ONE* **2013**, *8*, e56803. [CrossRef]
39. Frank, B.S.; Runciman, M.; Manning, W.A.; Ivy, D.D.; Abman, S.H.; Howley, L. Pulmonary Hypertension Secondary to Scurvy in a Developmentally Typical Child. *J. Pediatr.* **2019**, *208*, 291. [CrossRef]
40. Dean, T.; Kaushik, N.; Williams, S.; Zinter, M.; Kim, P. Cardiac arrest and pulmonary hypertension in scurvy: A case report. *Pulm. Circ.* **2019**, *9*. [CrossRef]
41. Kupari, M.; Rapola, J. Reversible pulmonary hypertension associated with vitamin C deficiency. *Chest* **2012**, *142*, 225–227. [CrossRef] [PubMed]
42. Ghulam Ali, S.; Pepi, M. A Very Uncommon Case of Pulmonary Hypertension. *CASE* **2018**, *2*, 279–281. [CrossRef] [PubMed]
43. Taddei, S.; Virdis, A.; Ghiadoni, L.; Magagna, A.; Salvetti, A. Vitamin C improves endothelium-dependent vasodilation by restoring nitric oxide activity in essential hypertension. *Circulation* **1998**, *97*, 2222–2229. [CrossRef] [PubMed]
44. Knowles, H.J.; Raval, R.R.; Harris, A.L.; Ratcliffe, P.J. Effect of ascorbate on the activity of hypoxia-inducible factor in cancer cells. *Can. Res.* **2003**, *63*, 1764–1768.
45. Urrutia, A.A.; Aragones, J. HIF Oxygen Sensing Pathways in Lung Biology. *Biomedicines* **2018**, *6*. [CrossRef]
46. Xiang, R.P.; Sun, W.D.; Wang, J.Y.; Wang, X.L. Effect of vitamin C on pulmonary hypertension and muscularisation of pulmonary arterioles in broilers. *Br. Poult. Sci.* **2002**, *43*, 705–712. [CrossRef]
47. Jones, G. Extrarenal vitamin D activation and interactions between vitamin D(2), vitamin D(3), and vitamin D analogs. *Annu. Rev. Nutr.* **2013**, *33*, 23–44. [CrossRef]
48. Dusso, A.S.; Brown, A.J.; Slatopolsky, E. Vitamin D. *Am. J. Physiol. Ren. Physiol.* **2005**, *289*, F8–F28. [CrossRef]
49. Moore, D.D.; Kato, S.; Xie, W.; Mangelsdorf, D.J.; Schmidt, D.R.; Xiao, R.; Kliewer, S.A. International Union of Pharmacology. LXII. The NR1H and NR1I receptors: Constitutive androstane receptor, pregnene X receptor, farnesoid X receptor alpha, farnesoid X receptor beta, liver X receptor alpha, liver X receptor beta, and vitamin D receptor. *Pharmacol. Rev.* **2006**, *58*, 742–759. [CrossRef]
50. Carlberg, C.; Campbell, M.J. Vitamin D receptor signaling mechanisms: Integrated actions of a well-defined transcription factor. *Steroids* **2013**, *78*, 127–136. [CrossRef]
51. Giangreco, A.A.; Nonn, L. The sum of many small changes: microRNAs are specifically and potentially globally altered by vitamin D3 metabolites. *J. Steroid Biochem. Mol. Biol.* **2013**, *136*, 86–93. [CrossRef] [PubMed]
52. Battault, S.; Whiting, S.J.; Peltier, S.L.; Sadrin, S.; Gerber, G.; Maixent, J.M. Vitamin D metabolism, functions and needs: From science to health claims. *Eur. J. Nutr.* **2013**, *52*, 429–441. [CrossRef] [PubMed]
53. Norman, P.E.; Powell, J.T. Vitamin D and cardiovascular disease. *Circ. Res.* **2014**, *114*, 379–393. [CrossRef] [PubMed]
54. Roth, D.E.; Abrams, S.A.; Aloia, J.; Bergeron, G.; Bourassa, M.W.; Brown, K.H.; Calvo, M.S.; Cashman, K.D.; Combs, G.; De-Regil, L.M.; et al. Global prevalence and disease burden of vitamin D deficiency: A roadmap for action in low- and middle-income countries. *Ann. N. Y. Acad. Sci.* **2018**, *1430*, 44–79. [CrossRef] [PubMed]

55. Demer, L.L.; Hsu, J.J.; Tintut, Y. Steroid Hormone Vitamin D: Implications for Cardiovascular Disease. *Circ. Res.* **2018**, *122*, 1576–1585. [CrossRef]
56. Bivona, G.; Agnello, L.; Ciaccio, M. The immunological implication of the new vitamin D metabolism. *Cent. Eur. J. Immunol.* **2018**, *43*, 331–334. [CrossRef]
57. Wang, T.J.; Pencina, M.J.; Booth, S.L.; Jacques, P.F.; Ingelsson, E.; Lanier, K.; Benjamin, E.J.; D'Agostino, R.B.; Wolf, M.; Vasan, R.S. Vitamin D deficiency and risk of cardiovascular disease. *Circulation* **2008**, *117*, 503–511. [CrossRef]
58. Schottker, B.; Jorde, R.; Peasey, A.; Thorand, B.; Jansen, E.H.; Groot, L.; Streppel, M.; Gardiner, J.; Ordonez-Mena, J.M.; Perna, L.; et al. Vitamin D and mortality: Meta-analysis of individual participant data from a large consortium of cohort studies from Europe and the United States. *BMJ* **2014**, *348*, g3656. [CrossRef]
59. Tanaka, H.; Kataoka, M.; Isobe, S.; Yamamoto, T.; Shirakawa, K.; Endo, J.; Satoh, T.; Hakamata, Y.; Kobayashi, E.; Sano, M.; et al. Therapeutic impact of dietary vitamin D supplementation for preventing right ventricular remodeling and improving survival in pulmonary hypertension. *PLoS ONE* **2017**, *12*, e0180615. [CrossRef]
60. Yu, H.; Xu, M.; Dong, Y.; Liu, J.; Li, Y.; Mao, W.; Wang, J.; Wang, L. 1,25(OH)2D3 attenuates pulmonary arterial hypertension via microRNA-204 mediated Tgfbr2/Smad signaling. *Exp. Cell Res.* **2018**, *362*, 311–323. [CrossRef]
61. Ulrich, S.; Hersberger, M.; Fischler, M.; Huber, L.C.; Senn, O.; Treder, U.; Speich, R.; Schmid, C. Bone mineral density and secondary hyperparathyroidism in pulmonary hypertension. *Open Respir. Med. J.* **2009**, *3*, 53–60. [CrossRef]
62. Demir, M.; Uyan, U.; Keceoclu, S.; Demir, C. The relationship between vitamin D deficiency and pulmonary hypertension. *Prague Med. Rep.* **2013**, *114*, 154–161. [CrossRef] [PubMed]
63. Mirdamadi, A.; Moshkdar, P. Benefits from the correction of vitamin D deficiency in patients with pulmonary hypertension. *Casp. J. Intern. Med.* **2016**, *7*, 253–259.
64. Jolliffe, D.A.; Greenberg, L.; Hooper, R.L.; Griffiths, C.J.; Camargo, C.A., Jr.; Kerley, C.P.; Jensen, M.E.; Mauger, D.; Stelmach, I.; Urashima, M.; et al. Vitamin D supplementation to prevent asthma exacerbations: A systematic review and meta-analysis of individual participant data. *Lancet Respir. Med.* **2017**, *5*, 881–890. [CrossRef]
65. Jolliffe, D.A.; Greenberg, L.; Hooper, R.L.; Mathyssen, C.; Rafiq, R.; de Jongh, R.T.; Camargo, C.A.; Griffiths, C.J.; Janssens, W.; Martineau, A.R. Vitamin D to prevent exacerbations of COPD: Systematic review and meta-analysis of individual participant data from randomised controlled trials. *Thorax* **2019**, *74*, 337–345. [CrossRef]
66. Manson, J.E.; Cook, N.R.; Lee, I.M.; Christen, W.; Bassuk, S.S.; Mora, S.; Gibson, H.; Gordon, D.; Copeland, T.; D'Agostino, D.; et al. Vitamin D Supplements and Prevention of Cancer and Cardiovascular Disease. *N. Engl. J. Med.* **2019**, *380*, 33–44. [CrossRef]
67. Bolland, M.J.; Grey, A.; Gamble, G.D.; Reid, I.R. The effect of vitamin D supplementation on skeletal, vascular, or cancer outcomes: A trial sequential meta-analysis. *Lancet Diabetes Endocrinol.* **2014**, *2*, 307–320. [CrossRef]
68. Beveridge, L.A.; Khan, F.; Struthers, A.D.; Armitage, J.; Barchetta, I.; Bressendorff, I.; Cavallo, M.G.; Clarke, R.; Dalan, R.; Dreyer, G.; et al. Effect of Vitamin D Supplementation on Markers of Vascular Function: A Systematic Review and Individual Participant Meta-Analysis. *J. Am. Heart Assoc.* **2018**, *7*. [CrossRef]
69. Camaschella, C. Iron-deficiency anemia. *N. Engl. J. Med.* **2015**, *372*, 1832–1843. [CrossRef]
70. Munoz, M.; Gomez-Ramirez, S.; Besser, M.; Pavia, J.; Gomollon, F.; Liumbruno, G.M.; Bhandari, S.; Cladellas, M.; Shander, A.; Auerbach, M. Current misconceptions in diagnosis and management of iron deficiency. *Blood Transfus.* **2017**, *15*, 422–437. [CrossRef]
71. Anand, I.S.; Gupta, P. Anemia and Iron Deficiency in Heart Failure: Current Concepts and Emerging Therapies. *Circulation* **2018**, *138*, 80–98. [CrossRef] [PubMed]
72. Rhodes, C.J.; Howard, L.S.; Busbridge, M.; Ashby, D.; Kondili, E.; Gibbs, J.S.; Wharton, J.; Wilkins, M.R. Iron deficiency and raised hepcidin in idiopathic pulmonary arterial hypertension: Clinical prevalence, outcomes, and mechanistic insights. *J. Am. Coll. Cardiol.* **2011**, *58*, 300–309. [CrossRef] [PubMed]
73. Ruiter, G.; Lankhorst, S.; Boonstra, A.; Postmus, P.E.; Zweegman, S.; Westerhof, N.; van der Laarse, W.J.; Vonk-Noordegraaf, A. Iron deficiency is common in idiopathic pulmonary arterial hypertension. *Eur. Respir. J.* **2011**, *37*, 1386–1391. [CrossRef] [PubMed]

74. Ramakrishnan, L.; Pedersen, S.L.; Toe, Q.K.; Quinlan, G.J.; Wort, S.J. Pulmonary Arterial Hypertension: Iron Matters. *Front. Physiol.* **2018**, *9*, 641. [CrossRef] [PubMed]
75. Hampole, C.V.; Mehrotra, A.K.; Thenappan, T.; Gomberg-Maitland, M.; Shah, S.J. Usefulness of red cell distribution width as a prognostic marker in pulmonary hypertension. *Am. J. Cardiol.* **2009**, *104*, 868–872. [CrossRef] [PubMed]
76. Krasuski, R.A.; Hart, S.A.; Smith, B.; Wang, A.; Harrison, J.K.; Bashore, T.M. Association of anemia and long-term survival in patients with pulmonary hypertension. *Int. J. Cardiol.* **2011**, *150*, 291–295. [CrossRef]
77. Yu, X.; Zhang, Y.; Luo, Q.; Liu, Z.; Zhao, Z.; Zhao, Q.; Gao, L.; Jin, Q.; Yan, L. Iron deficiency in pulmonary arterial hypertension associated with congenital heart disease. *Scand. Cardiovasc. J.* **2018**, *52*, 378–382. [CrossRef]
78. Anker, S.D.; Comin Colet, J.; Filippatos, G.; Willenheimer, R.; Dickstein, K.; Drexler, H.; Luscher, T.F.; Bart, B.; Banasiak, W.; Niegowska, J.; et al. Ferric carboxymaltose in patients with heart failure and iron deficiency. *N. Engl. J. Med.* **2009**, *361*, 2436–2448. [CrossRef]
79. Bolger, A.P.; Bartlett, F.R.; Penston, H.S.; O'Leary, J.; Pollock, N.; Kaprielian, R.; Chapman, C.M. Intravenous iron alone for the treatment of anemia in patients with chronic heart failure. *J. Am. Coll. Cardiol.* **2006**, *48*, 1225–1227. [CrossRef]
80. Cotroneo, E.; Ashek, A.; Wang, L.; Wharton, J.; Dubois, O.; Bozorgi, S.; Busbridge, M.; Alavian, K.N.; Wilkins, M.R.; Zhao, L. Iron homeostasis and pulmonary hypertension: Iron deficiency leads to pulmonary vascular remodeling in the rat. *Circ. Res.* **2015**, *116*, 1680–1690. [CrossRef]
81. Wolin, M.S.; Patel, D.; Alhawaj, R.; Gupte, S.A.; Sun, D. Iron Metabolism and Vascular Remodeling: Novel Insights Provided by Transferrin-1 Receptor Depletion in Mice With Pulmonary Hypertension. *Am. J. Hypertens.* **2016**, *29*, 676–678. [CrossRef] [PubMed]
82. Robinson, J.C.; Graham, B.B.; Rouault, T.C.; Tuder, R.M. The crossroads of iron with hypoxia and cellular metabolism. Implications in the pathobiology of pulmonary hypertension. *Am. J. Respir. Cell Mol. Biol.* **2014**, *51*, 721–729. [CrossRef] [PubMed]
83. Smith, T.G.; Balanos, G.M.; Croft, Q.P.; Talbot, N.P.; Dorrington, K.L.; Ratcliffe, P.J.; Robbins, P.A. The increase in pulmonary arterial pressure caused by hypoxia depends on iron status. *J. Physiol.* **2008**, *586*, 5999–6005. [CrossRef] [PubMed]
84. Smith, T.G.; Talbot, N.P.; Privat, C.; Rivera-Ch, M.; Nickol, A.H.; Ratcliffe, P.J.; Dorrington, K.L.; Leon-Velarde, F.; Robbins, P.A. Effects of iron supplementation and depletion on hypoxic pulmonary hypertension: Two randomized controlled trials. *JAMA* **2009**, *302*, 1444–1450. [CrossRef]
85. Naito, Y.; Hosokawa, M.; Sawada, H.; Oboshi, M.; Iwasaku, T.; Okuhara, Y.; Eguchi, A.; Nishimura, K.; Soyama, Y.; Hirotani, S.; et al. Iron is associated with the development of hypoxia-induced pulmonary vascular remodeling in mice. *Heart Vessel.* **2016**, *31*, 2074–2079. [CrossRef]
86. Lakhal-Littleton, S.; Crosby, A.; Frise, M.C.; Mohammad, G.; Carr, C.A.; Loick, P.A.M.; Robbins, P.A. Intracellular iron deficiency in pulmonary arterial smooth muscle cells induces pulmonary arterial hypertension in mice. *Proc. Natl. Acad. Sci. USA* **2019**, *116*, 13122–13130. [CrossRef]
87. Yu, X.; Luo, Q.; Liu, Z.; Zhao, Z.; Zhao, Q.; An, C.; Huang, Z.; Jin, Q.; Gao, L.; Yan, L. Prevalence of iron deficiency in different subtypes of pulmonary hypertension. *Heart Lung* **2018**, *47*, 308–313. [CrossRef]
88. Soon, E.; Treacy, C.M.; Toshner, M.R.; MacKenzie-Ross, R.; Manglam, V.; Busbridge, M.; Sinclair-McGarvie, M.; Arnold, J.; Sheares, K.K.; Morrell, N.W.; et al. Unexplained iron deficiency in idiopathic and heritable pulmonary arterial hypertension. *Thorax* **2011**, *66*, 326–332. [CrossRef]
89. Rhodes, C.J.; Wharton, J.; Howard, L.; Gibbs, J.S.; Vonk-Noordegraaf, A.; Wilkins, M.R. Iron deficiency in pulmonary arterial hypertension: A potential therapeutic target. *Eur. Respir. J.* **2011**, *38*, 1453–1460. [CrossRef]
90. Soon, E.; Holmes, A.M.; Treacy, C.M.; Doughty, N.J.; Southgate, L.; Machado, R.D.; Trembath, R.C.; Jennings, S.; Barker, L.; Nicklin, P.; et al. Elevated levels of inflammatory cytokines predict survival in idiopathic and familial pulmonary arterial hypertension. *Circulation* **2010**, *122*, 920–927. [CrossRef]
91. Howard, L.S.; Watson, G.M.; Wharton, J.; Rhodes, C.J.; Chan, K.; Khengar, R.; Robbins, P.A.; Kiely, D.G.; Condliffe, R.; Elliott, C.A.; et al. Supplementation of iron in pulmonary hypertension: Rationale and design of a phase II clinical trial in idiopathic pulmonary arterial hypertension. *Pulm. Circ.* **2013**, *3*, 100–107. [CrossRef] [PubMed]

92. Ruiter, G.; Manders, E.; Happe, C.M.; Schalij, I.; Groepenhoff, H.; Howard, L.S.; Wilkins, M.R.; Bogaard, H.J.; Westerhof, N.; van der Laarse, W.J.; et al. Intravenous iron therapy in patients with idiopathic pulmonary arterial hypertension and iron deficiency. *Pulm. Circ.* **2015**, *5*, 466–472. [CrossRef] [PubMed]
93. Sanchez, M.; Romero, M.; Gomez-Guzman, M.; Tamargo, J.; Perez-Vizcaino, F.; Duarte, J. Cardiovascular effects of flavonoids. *Curr. Med. Chem.* **2018**. [CrossRef] [PubMed]
94. Perez-Vizcaino, F.; Fraga, C.G. Research trends in flavonoids and health. *Arch. Biochem. Biophys.* **2018**, *646*, 107–112. [CrossRef]
95. Perez-Vizcaino, F.; Duarte, J. Flavonols and cardiovascular disease. *Mol. Asp. Med.* **2010**, *31*, 478–494. [CrossRef]
96. Quinones, M.; Miguel, M.; Aleixandre, A. Beneficial effects of polyphenols on cardiovascular disease. *Pharmacol. Res.* **2013**, *68*, 125–131. [CrossRef]
97. Csiszar, A.; Labinskyy, N.; Olson, S.; Pinto, J.T.; Gupte, S.; Wu, J.M.; Hu, F.; Ballabh, P.; Podlutsky, A.; Losonczy, G.; et al. Resveratrol prevents monocrotaline-induced pulmonary hypertension in rats. *Hypertension* **2009**, *54*, 668–675. [CrossRef]
98. Chicoine, L.G.; Stewart, J.A., Jr.; Lucchesi, P.A. Is resveratrol the magic bullet for pulmonary hypertension? *Hypertension* **2009**, *54*, 473–474. [CrossRef]
99. Chen, B.; Xue, J.; Meng, X.; Slutzky, J.L.; Calvert, A.E.; Chicoine, L.G. Resveratrol prevents hypoxia-induced arginase II expression and proliferation of human pulmonary artery smooth muscle cells via Akt-dependent signaling. *Am. J. Physiol. Lung Cell Mol. Physiol.* **2014**, *307*, L317–L325. [CrossRef] [PubMed]
100. Guan, Z.; Shen, L.; Liang, H.; Yu, H.; Hei, B.; Meng, X.; Yang, L. Resveratrol inhibits hypoxia-induced proliferation and migration of pulmonary artery vascular smooth muscle cells by inhibiting the phosphoinositide 3-kinase/protein kinase B signaling pathway. *Mol. Med. Rep.* **2017**, *16*, 1653–1660. [CrossRef]
101. Xu, D.; Li, Y.; Zhang, B.; Wang, Y.; Liu, Y.; Luo, Y.; Niu, W.; Dong, M.; Liu, M.; Dong, H.; et al. Resveratrol alleviate hypoxic pulmonary hypertension via anti-inflammation and anti-oxidant pathways in rats. *Int. J. Med. Sci.* **2016**, *13*, 942–954. [CrossRef] [PubMed]
102. Shi, W.; Zhai, C.; Feng, W.; Wang, J.; Zhu, Y.; Li, S.; Wang, Q.; Zhang, Q.; Yan, X.; Chai, L.; et al. Resveratrol inhibits monocrotaline-induced pulmonary arterial remodeling by suppression of SphK1-mediated NF-kappaB activation. *Life Sci.* **2018**, *210*, 140–149. [CrossRef] [PubMed]
103. Perez-Vizcaino, F.; Duarte, J.; Jimenez, R.; Santos-Buelga, C.; Osuna, A. Antihypertensive effects of the flavonoid quercetin. *Pharmacol. Rep.* **2009**, *61*, 67–75. [CrossRef]
104. Duarte, J.; Perez-Palencia, R.; Vargas, F.; Ocete, M.A.; Perez-Vizcaino, F.; Zarzuelo, A.; Tamargo, J. Antihypertensive effects of the flavonoid quercetin in spontaneously hypertensive rats. *Br. J. Pharmacol.* **2001**, *133*, 117–124. [CrossRef]
105. Gao, H.; Chen, C.; Huang, S.; Li, B. Quercetin attenuates the progression of monocrotaline-induced pulmonary hypertension in rats. *J. Biomed. Res.* **2012**, *26*, 98–102. [CrossRef]
106. Morales-Cano, D.; Menendez, C.; Moreno, E.; Moral-Sanz, J.; Barreira, B.; Galindo, P.; Pandolfi, R.; Jimenez, R.; Moreno, L.; Cogolludo, A.; et al. The flavonoid quercetin reverses pulmonary hypertension in rats. *PLoS ONE* **2014**, *9*, e114492. [CrossRef]
107. Jimenez, R.; Lopez-Sepulveda, R.; Romero, M.; Toral, M.; Cogolludo, A.; Perez-Vizcaino, F.; Duarte, J. Quercetin and its metabolites inhibit the membrane NADPH oxidase activity in vascular smooth muscle cells from normotensive and spontaneously hypertensive rats. *Food Funct.* **2015**, *6*, 409–414. [CrossRef]
108. He, Y.; Cao, X.; Liu, X.; Li, X.; Xu, Y.; Liu, J.; Shi, J. Quercetin reverses experimental pulmonary arterial hypertension by modulating the TrkA pathway. *Exp. Cell Res.* **2015**, *339*, 122–134. [CrossRef]
109. Huang, S.; Zhu, X.; Huang, W.; He, Y.; Pang, L.; Lan, X.; Shui, X.; Chen, Y.; Chen, C.; Lei, W. Quercetin Inhibits Pulmonary Arterial Endothelial Cell Transdifferentiation Possibly by Akt and Erk1/2 Pathways. *Biomed. Res. Int.* **2017**, *2017*. [CrossRef]
110. He, Y.; Cao, X.; Guo, P.; Li, X.; Shang, H.; Liu, J.; Xie, M.; Xu, Y.; Liu, X. Quercetin induces autophagy via FOXO1-dependent pathways and autophagy suppression enhances quercetin-induced apoptosis in PASMCs in hypoxia. *Free Radic. Biol. Med.* **2017**, *103*, 165–176. [CrossRef]
111. Cao, X.; He, Y.; Li, X.; Xu, Y.; Liu, X. The IRE1alpha-XBP1 pathway function in hypoxia-induced pulmonary vascular remodeling, is upregulated by quercetin, inhibits apoptosis and partially reverses the effect of quercetin in PASMCs. *Am. J. Transl. Res.* **2019**, *11*, 641–654. [PubMed]

112. Evans, M.; Elliott, J.G.; Sharma, P.; Berman, R.; Guthrie, N. The effect of synthetic genistein on menopause symptom management in healthy postmenopausal women: A multi-center, randomized, placebo-controlled study. *Maturitas* **2011**, *68*, 189–196. [CrossRef] [PubMed]
113. Zaheer, K.; Humayoun Akhtar, M. An updated review of dietary isoflavones: Nutrition, processing, bioavailability and impacts on human health. *Crit. Rev. Food Sci. Nutr.* **2017**, *57*, 1280–1293. [CrossRef] [PubMed]
114. Vera, R.; Jimenez, R.; Lodi, F.; Sanchez, M.; Galisteo, M.; Zarzuelo, A.; Perez-Vizcaino, F.; Duarte, J. Genistein restores caveolin-1 and AT-1 receptor expression and vascular function in large vessels of ovariectomized hypertensive rats. *Menopause* **2007**, *14*, 933–940. [CrossRef]
115. Karamsetty, M.R.; Klinger, J.R.; Hill, N.S. Phytoestrogens restore nitric oxide-mediated relaxation in isolated pulmonary arteries from chronically hypoxic rats. *J. Pharmacol. Exp. Ther.* **2001**, *297*, 968–974.
116. Matori, H.; Umar, S.; Nadadur, R.D.; Sharma, S.; Partow-Navid, R.; Afkhami, M.; Amjedi, M.; Eghbali, M. Genistein, a soy phytoestrogen, reverses severe pulmonary hypertension and prevents right heart failure in rats. *Hypertension* **2012**, *60*, 425–430. [CrossRef]
117. Weigand, L.; Sylvester, J.T.; Shimoda, L.A. Mechanisms of endothelin-1-induced contraction in pulmonary arteries from chronically hypoxic rats. *Am. J. Physiol. Lung Cell. Mol. Physiol.* **2006**, *290*, L284–L290. [CrossRef]
118. Homma, N.; Morio, Y.; Takahashi, H.; Yamamoto, A.; Suzuki, T.; Sato, K.; Muramatsu, M.; Fukuchi, Y. Genistein, a phytoestrogen, attenuates monocrotaline-induced pulmonary hypertension. *Respir. Int. Rev. Thorac. Dis.* **2006**, *73*, 105–112. [CrossRef]
119. Kuriyama, S.; Morio, Y.; Toba, M.; Nagaoka, T.; Takahashi, F.; Iwakami, S.; Seyama, K.; Takahashi, K. Genistein attenuates hypoxic pulmonary hypertension via enhanced nitric oxide signaling and the erythropoietin system. *Am. J. Physiol. Lung Cell. Mol. Physiol.* **2014**, *306*, L996–L1005. [CrossRef]
120. Zheng, Z.; Yu, S.; Zhang, W.; Peng, Y.; Pu, M.; Kang, T.; Zeng, J.; Yu, Y.; Li, G. Genistein attenuates monocrotaline-induced pulmonary arterial hypertension in rats by activating PI3K/Akt/eNOS signaling. *Histol. Histopathol.* **2017**, *32*, 35–41. [CrossRef]
121. Zhang, M.; Wu, Y.; Wang, M.; Wang, Y.; Tausif, R.; Yang, Y. Genistein rescues hypoxia-induced pulmonary arterial hypertension through estrogen receptor and beta-adrenoceptor signaling. *J. Nutr. Biochem.* **2018**, *58*, 110–118. [CrossRef] [PubMed]
122. Levy, M.; Kolodziejczyk, A.A.; Thaiss, C.A.; Elinav, E. Dysbiosis and the immune system. *Nat. Rev. Immunol.* **2017**, *17*, 219–232. [CrossRef] [PubMed]
123. Yang, T.; Santisteban, M.M.; Rodriguez, V.; Li, E.; Ahmari, N.; Carvajal, J.M.; Zadeh, M.; Gong, M.; Qi, Y.; Zubcevic, J.; et al. Gut dysbiosis is linked to hypertension. *Hypertension* **2015**, *65*, 1331–1340. [CrossRef] [PubMed]
124. Marques, F.Z.; Mackay, C.R.; Kaye, D.M. Beyond gut feelings: How the gut microbiota regulates blood pressure. *Nat. Rev. Cardiol.* **2018**, *15*, 20–32. [CrossRef] [PubMed]
125. Robles-Vera, I.; Toral, M.; Romero, M.; Jimenez, R.; Sanchez, M.; Perez-Vizcaino, F.; Duarte, J. Antihypertensive Effects of Probiotics. *Curr. Hypertens. Rep.* **2017**, *19*, 26. [CrossRef] [PubMed]
126. Ley, R.E.; Turnbaugh, P.J.; Klein, S.; Gordon, J.I. Microbial ecology: Human gut microbes associated with obesity. *Nature* **2006**, *444*, 1022–1023. [CrossRef]
127. Mariat, D.; Firmesse, O.; Levenez, F.; Guimaraes, V.; Sokol, H.; Dore, J.; Corthier, G.; Furet, J.P. The Firmicutes/Bacteroidetes ratio of the human microbiota changes with age. *BMC Microbiol.* **2009**, *9*, 123. [CrossRef]
128. Pascale, A.; Marchesi, N.; Govoni, S.; Coppola, A.; Gazzaruso, C. The role of gut microbiota in obesity, diabetes mellitus, and effect of metformin: New insights into old diseases. *Curr. Opin. Pharmacol.* **2019**, *49*, 1–5. [CrossRef]
129. Strati, F.; Cavalieri, D.; Albanese, D.; De Felice, C.; Donati, C.; Hayek, J.; Jousson, O.; Leoncini, S.; Renzi, D.; Calabro, A.; et al. New evidences on the altered gut microbiota in autism spectrum disorders. *Microbiome* **2017**, *5*, 24. [CrossRef]
130. Callejo, M.; Mondejar-Parreno, G.; Barreira, B.; Izquierdo-Garcia, J.L.; Morales-Cano, D.; Esquivel-Ruiz, S.; Moreno, L.; Cogolludo, A.; Duarte, J.; Perez-Vizcaino, F. Pulmonary Arterial Hypertension Affects the Rat Gut Microbiome. *Sci. Rep.* **2018**, *8*, 9681. [CrossRef]
131. Quigley, E.M.M. Nutraceuticals as Modulators of Gut Microbiota: Role in Therapy. *Br. J. Pharmacol.* **2019**. [CrossRef] [PubMed]

132. Biesalski, H.K. Nutrition meets the microbiome: Micronutrients and the microbiota. *Ann. N. Y. Acad. Sci.* **2016**, *1372*, 53–64. [CrossRef] [PubMed]
133. Skrypnik, K.; Suliburska, J. Association between the gut microbiota and mineral metabolism. *J. Sci. Food Agric.* **2018**, *98*, 2449–2460. [CrossRef] [PubMed]
134. Janeiro, M.H.; Ramirez, M.J.; Milagro, F.I.; Martinez, J.A.; Solas, M. Implication of Trimethylamine N-Oxide (TMAO) in Disease: Potential Biomarker or New Therapeutic Target. *Nutrients* **2018**, *10*. [CrossRef]
135. Robles-Vera, I.; Callejo, M.; Ramos, R.; Duarte, J.; Perez-Vizcaino, F. Impact of Vitamin D Deficit on the Rat Gut Microbiome. *Nutrients* **2019**, *11*. [CrossRef]
136. Yilmaz, B.; Li, H. Gut Microbiota and Iron: The Crucial Actors in Health and Disease. *Pharmaceuticals* **2018**, *11*. [CrossRef]
137. Zhao, L.; Zhang, Q.; Ma, W.; Tian, F.; Shen, H.; Zhou, M. A combination of quercetin and resveratrol reduces obesity in high-fat diet-fed rats by modulation of gut microbiota. *Food Funct.* **2017**, *8*, 4644–4656. [CrossRef]
138. Wedgwood, S.; Warford, C.; Agvatisiri, S.R.; Thai, P.N.; Chiamvimonvat, N.; Kalanetra, K.M.; Lakshminrusimha, S.; Steinhorn, R.H.; Mills, D.A.; Underwood, M.A. The developing gut-lung axis: Postnatal growth restriction, intestinal dysbiosis, and pulmonary hypertension in a rodent model. *Pediatr. Res.* **2019**. [CrossRef]
139. Thenappan, T.; Khoruts, A.; Chen, Y.; Weir, E.K. Can Intestinal Microbiota and Circulating Microbial Products Contribute to Pulmonary Arterial Hypertension? *Am. J. Physiol. Heart Circ. Physiol.* **2019**. [CrossRef]
140. Bauer, E.M.; Chanthaphavong, R.S.; Sodhi, C.P.; Hackam, D.J.; Billiar, T.R.; Bauer, P.M. Genetic deletion of toll-like receptor 4 on platelets attenuates experimental pulmonary hypertension. *Circ. Res.* **2014**, *114*, 1596–1600. [CrossRef]
141. Ranchoux, B.; Bigorgne, A.; Hautefort, A.; Girerd, B.; Sitbon, O.; Montani, D.; Humbert, M.; Tcherakian, C.; Perros, F. Gut-Lung Connection in Pulmonary Arterial Hypertension. *Am. J. Respir. Cell Mol. Biol.* **2017**, *56*, 402–405. [CrossRef] [PubMed]
142. Lee, Y.K.; Mazmanian, S.K. Has the microbiota played a critical role in the evolution of the adaptive immune system? *Science* **2010**, *330*, 1768–1773. [CrossRef] [PubMed]
143. Huertas, A.; Phan, C.; Bordenave, J.; Tu, L.; Thuillet, R.; Le Hiress, M.; Avouac, J.; Tamura, Y.; Allanore, Y.; Jovan, R.; et al. Regulatory T Cell Dysfunction in Idiopathic, Heritable and Connective Tissue-Associated Pulmonary Arterial Hypertension. *Chest* **2016**, *149*, 1482–1493. [CrossRef] [PubMed]
144. Hood, K.Y.; Mair, K.M.; Harvey, A.P.; Montezano, A.C.; Touyz, R.M.; MacLean, M.R. Serotonin Signaling Through the 5-HT1B Receptor and NADPH Oxidase 1 in Pulmonary Arterial Hypertension. *Arterioscler. Thromb. Vasc. Biol.* **2017**, *37*, 1361–1370. [CrossRef]

6

Maternal Obesity in Mice Exacerbates the Allergic Inflammatory Response in the Airways of Male Offspring

Rodrigo Rodrigues e-Lacerda [1], Caio Jordão Teixeira [1], Silvana Bordin [2], Edson Antunes [1] and Gabriel Forato Anhê [1,*]

[1] Department of Pharmacology, Faculty of Medical Sciences, State University of Campinas, 13083-881 Campinas, SP, Brazil; rodrigofarmapb@gmail.com (R.R e.-L.); caiojteixeira@gmail.com (C.J.T.); edson.antunes@uol.com.br (E.A.)

[2] Department of Physiology and Biophysics, Institute of Biomedical Sciences, University of Sao Paulo, 05508-900 Sao Paulo, SP, Brazil; sbordin@icb.usp.br

* Correspondence: anhegf@fcm.unicamp.br

Abstract: It was previously demonstrated that non-allergen-sensitized rodents born to mothers exposed to a high-fat diet (HFD) spontaneously develop lower respiratory compliance and higher respiratory resistance. In the present study, we sought to determine if mice born to mothers consuming HFD would exhibit changes in inflammatory response and lung remodeling when subjected to ovalbumin (OVA) sensitization/challenge in adult life. Mice born to dams consuming either HFD or standard chow had increased bronchoalveolar lavage (BAL) levels of IL-1β, IL-4, IL-5, IL-10, IL-13, TNF-α and TGF-β1 after challenge with OVA. IL-4, IL-13, TNF-α and TGF-β1 levels were further increased in the offspring of HFD-fed mothers. Mice born to obese dams also had exacerbated values of leukocyte infiltration in lung parenchyma, eosinophil and neutrophil counts in BAL, mucus overproduction and collagen deposition. The programming induced by maternal obesity was accompanied by increased expression of miR-155 in peripheral-blood mononuclear cells and reduced miR-133b in trachea and lung tissue in adult life. Altogether, the present data support the unprecedented notion that the progeny of obese mice display exacerbated responses to sensitization/challenge with OVA, leading to the intensification of the morphological changes of lung remodeling. Such changes are likely to result from long-lasting changes in miR-155 and miR-133b expression.

Keywords: obesity; pregnancy; allergic airway disease; offspring; high fat diet

---

1. Introduction

The global prevalence of allergic asthma has continuously increased since the last decade of the 20th century [1]. From a clinical perspective, distinct types of asthma are commonly hallmarked by chronic airway inflammation, remodeling of the airway wall and airway hyperresponsiveness. The inflammatory response of allergic asthma is classically recognized as a predominantly T_H2 activation that leads to IgE production and eosinophil development and infiltration in the lung parenchyma. Such features are granted by T_H2 cytokines such as interleukin (IL)-4 and IL-5 [2]. IL-13 has also been shown to play a role in airways hyperresponsiveness, mucous secretion and eosinophil recruitment [3–5]. More recent is the notion that exacerbation of allergic asthma is also supported by lung neutrophil accumulation, increased production of acute phase proteins, such as the proinflammatory cytokines tumor necrosis factor-α (TNF-α) and IL-1β, and activation of nuclear factor-κB (NF-κB) [6,7].

Along with the history of exposure to the allergen, the incidence of asthma has other determinants. Prospective cohort studies have revealed that increased body mass index (BMI) is significantly related to the risk of asthma in adults [8,9]. A causal relationship between asthma and obesity has been further demonstrated by the improvement of pulmonary function in asthmatic obese patients subjected to weight loss [10]. Obese asthmatic patients have also been described to display exacerbated eosinophilic activation compared to their non-obese counterparts [11]. Accordingly, mice rendered obese by the consumption of a high-fat diet (HFD) and subjected to the model of sensitization and challenge with ovalbumin (OVA) display increased lung eosinophil infiltration and elevated production of both T_H2 cytokines and acute phase proteins such as IL-6, TNF-α and IL-1β [12–15].

The impacts of obesity on the intensity and frequency of asthma also have a transgenerational aspect. Human studies have shown that maternal obesity during pregnancy and increased gestational weight gain were positively associated with the risk of childhood asthma [16,17]. In accordance with those findings, it was also described that non-allergen-sensitized mice and rats born to mothers exposed to HFD during pregnancy and lactation spontaneously develop lower respiratory system compliance and higher respiratory system resistance [18,19]. Similar data were found in adult non-allergen-sensitized offspring of mice breastfed by dams consuming HFD [20].

The current study was conducted to evaluate if maternal obesity also affects the inflammatory response in offspring subjected to a model of allergic airway disease. We investigated multiple aspects of eosinophilic inflammation and lung remodeling after sensitization and challenge with OVA in the offspring of mice born to mothers fed HFD. The expression of intracellular signaling proteins and miRNAs associated with the inflammatory response were also evaluated as candidate mechanisms for immune programming.

2. Materials and Methods

2.1. Animals and Experimental Design

Four-week-old female C57BL/6J mice were obtained from the Animal Breeding Center at the University of Campinas (CEMIB, Campinas, Sao Paulo, Brazil) and were housed at 22 ± 2 °C under a 12:12 hours light:dark cycle (lights on at 7:00 a.m.) with free access to standard chow (SC) and water for 2 weeks. Two weeks later, female mice were either kept on SC or offered a HFD ad libitum with 22.36 kJ·g^{-1} (60% fat, 15% protein, 25% carbohydrates). Six weeks later, both SC- and HFD-fed mice were mated (housing one male with two females for 3 days). The same diet offered before mating was kept for both groups throughout pregnancy and lactation. The number of pups was adjusted to 5–6 per litter no later than 24 h after delivery. Twenty-one days after delivery, the male offspring of SC- and HFD-fed dams were weaned to the SC diet (originating SC offspring and HFD offspring, respectively).

We used two independent cohorts of pregnant mice in this study. In the first cohort, we generated six litters from HFD-fed mice and six litters of SC-fed mice. Two male littermates per litter belonging to the progenies of both SC- and HFD-fed mothers were sensitized with OVA (cat. no. A5503; Sigma-Aldrich Co; St Louis, MO, USA) by reaching 6 weeks of age. Sensitization consisted of one (i.p.) injection with OVA (30 µg of OVA plus 0.9 mg $Al(OH)_3$ diluted in 400 µL of 0.9% NaCl) followed by two additional injections performed 7 and 11 days after the first injection. Three days after the last i.p. injection, one sensitized mouse from each litter was challenged with intranasal installations containing OVA (10 µg/40 µL) (two instillations per day for two consecutive days). Sensitized/challenged mice were thereafter identified as SC/OVA or HFD/OVA. The remaining sensitized littermates were kept unchallenged and received intranasal installations containing vehicle only. These mice were thereafter identified as SC/SHAM or HFD/SHAM. The results showing four different groups were therefore obtained with the mice of the first cohort.

The second cohort was consisted with 12 pregnant HFD-fed mice and 12 pregnant SC-fed mice. One mouse of each litter was allocated in the SC/OVA or in the HFD/OVA subgroup. The remaining littermates were discarded. Therefore, the results showing two different groups were obtained with the mice of the second cohort.

The same weight balance was used throughout the experiments to assess body mass of the dams and of the offspring.

All the experiments were performed 48 h after the beginning of the intranasal challenge, and the procedures were approved by the State University of Campinas Committee for Ethics in Animal Experimentation (protocol no. 3875-1) and were conducted in accordance with the guidelines of the Brazilian College for Animal Experimentation.

2.2. Bronchoalveolar Lavage (BAL) Sampling

The mice were euthanized with sodium thiopental (80 mg/kg), and the trachea was exposed and subsequently cannulated with a polyethylene catheter. The lungs were washed with three flushes containing 500 µL of 0.9% NaCl solution. The volumes were recovered together to produce one BAL sample of approximately 1.5 mL. BAL samples were centrifuged for 10 min at 4 °C (500× *g*) and the supernatants were collected and stored at −80 °C for cytokine determination. The pellets were resuspended in 1.5 mL of 0.9% NaCl solution and used either for flow cytometry or for staining and differential counting of leukocytes as previously described [12].

2.3. Flow Cytometry

Aliquots containing 200 µL of BAL samples were centrifuged, and the pellets were suspended in staining buffer (SB) (cat. #554656; BD Biosciences, San Jose, CA, USA) and incubated with Alexa Fluor 647-conjugated anti-mouse CCR3 (cat. #557974; BD Biosciences, San Jose, CA, USA) (0.4 µg per 200 µL) and PE-conjugated anti-mouse VLA4 (cat. #557420; BD Biosciences, San Jose, CA, USA) (0.36 µg per 200 µL) for 20 min at 4 °C. After incubation, the samples were washed three times with SB and fixed (cat. #554655; BD Biosciences, San Jose, CA, USA) for 20 min at RT. After fixation, cells were subjected to an additional washing and reconstituted in SB to a final volume of 300 µL. Samples were added with 50 µL of CountBright beads (54,000 beads/µL) (cat. #C36950; Life Technologies, Carlsbad, CA, USA) for absolute cell counting and then analyzed in a BD FACSCalibur Cytometer (San Jose, CA, USA). Final volume of every sample was 350 µL.

FSC and SSC parameters were acquired in linear scale, while fluorescent signals were acquired in logarithmic scales. Two gates were placed in the FSC versus SSC dot plot. A gate excluding the beads and encompassing the leukocytes was used to evaluate fluorescence (R1). A total of 10,000 events were acquired in R1. The second gate placed in the FSC versus SSC dot plot encompassed the beads population (R2). The absolute number of beads in R2 was used to calculate the volume of each sample that was consumed by the cytometer (consumed volume).

In parallel, we assessed the fluorescent signal of the events acquired in R1 gate. Fluorescent signals were placed in the dot plot of FL2-H (VLA4-positive cells) against FL4-H (CCR3-positive cells). The fluorescence dot plots were divided into four quadrants and the events appearing in the upper right quadrant were considered $CCR3^+/VLA4^+$ events. The absolute number of $CCR3^+/VLA4^+$ events acquired in the consumed volume, the consumed volume and the final volume were used to estimate the whole number $CCR3^+/VLA4^+$ events in each sample. The fluorescent signal obtained from samples stained with Alexa Fluor 647-conjugated (cat. #557690; BD Biosciences, San Jose, CA, USA) and PE-conjugated (cat. #552784; BD Biosciences, San Jose, CA, USA) negative isotypes were previously used to set unspecific fluorescence, and therefore, the dimensions of the lower left quadrant in the fluorescence dot plots. All acquisitions, plots and analyses were obtained using the BD CellQuest Pro software (San Jose, CA, USA).

2.4. Cytokine and IgE Determinations

Cytokines were measured in the supernatants of BAL samples using commercially available Enzyme-Linked Immunosorbent Assay (ELISA) kits. The kits for IL-4 (cat. #555232), IL-5 (cat. #555236) and IL-10 (cat. #555252) were from BD Biosciences (San Jose, CA, USA), and the kits for IL-13 (cat. #M1300CB), IL-1β (cat. #DY401), TNF-α (cat. #DY410) and transforming growth factor-β1 (TGF-β1) (cat. #DY1679-05) were from R&D Systems (Minneapolis, MN, USA). IgE levels were determined in plasma samples using ELISA kits (cat. 555248; BD Biosciences, San Jose, CA, USA). Leptin levels were determined in plasma samples using EIA kit (EZML-82K; Merck Millipore, Billerica, MA, USA). Triglycerides, glucose and cholesterol concentrations were determined in plasma samples using colorimetric enzymatic assays (respectively, Cat. No. 1770290, 1770130 and 1770080; LaborLab, Sao Paulo, Brazil).

2.5. Lung Histology and Immunohistochemistry

The inferior lobes of the right lungs were excised, immersed in 10% (wt/vol) formalin fixative solution for 72 h and embedded in paraffin. Serial sections (5 μm thick) were mounted onto aminopropyltriethoxysilane-coated glass slides and sequentially processed for paraffin removal with xylol followed by rehydration. Sections were subjected either to different staining protocols or to immunohistochemical detection of phosphorylated NF-κB and tumor necrosis factor alpha-induced protein 3 (TNFAPI3).

Staining with hematoxylin and eosin (H&E) was performed to assess leukocyte infiltrated area. Two random pictures (20× magnification) from each section were analyzed (one random section per animal). The fields were chosen to contain one or two bronchioles. The peribronchiolar leukocyte infiltrated area was manually outlined and its value (excluding the bronchiolar lumen) in μm^2 was automatically determined with the ImageJ software (http://imagej.nih.gov/ij). To estimate the area of neutrophils and eosinophils within the leukocyte infiltrated area, we used the following approach. The perimeters of the bronchioles were carefully examined using a light microscope equipped with 100× objective lens for use with immersion oil (Nikon Eclipse E200; Nikon, Tokyo, Japan). The percentage of eosinophil and neutrophils in the first layer of leukocytes adjacent to the bronchiolar epithelial cells was estimated. Next, it was assumed that the eosinophil and neutrophil infiltrated areas were a fraction of the leukocyte infiltrated area that were directly proportional to the percentage of eosinophil and neutrophils found in the first layer of leukocytes adjacent to the bronchiolar epithelial cells.

The Masson's trichrome protocol was performed to determine collagen accumulation. The presence of blue-stained collagen fibers was visualized by optical microscopy under 20× magnification. Images were acquired under 20× magnification using a Leica DM4500 B optical microscope coupled to a digital camera (Leica Microsystems; Wetzlar, Germany) and analyzed with Image-Pro Plus software (version 2.0, Media Cybernetics; Rockville, MD, USA). The blue-stained area with collagen fibers was automatically detected by the software and expressed as the percentage of the tissue section area. The tissue section area was calculated by the software and was defined as the picture area subtracted of the bronchioles and vessels lumen area (empty bronchioles and vessels lumen area was automatically outlined by the software).

The periodic acid-Schiff (PAS) method was performed to determine the mucus content in the epithelial layer. The presence of purple-magenta stained mucus was visualized by optical microscopy under 20× magnification. Images were acquired under 20× magnification using a Leica DM4500 B optical microscope coupled to a digital camera and analyzed with Image-Pro Plus software. The purple-magenta stained area containing mucus was automatically detected by the software and expressed as the percentage of the tissue section area. Calculations were performed as for collagen stained area. Pictures of sections subjected to the PAS method were also used to determine the number of globet cells around the bronchiole perimeter. To this end, the perimeters of the bronchioles were carefully by applying a 2× digital zoom to the images. The number of globet cells (defined as cells containing unstained vacuoles) were manually counted around the bronchiole perimeter and expressed as number of cells per 100 μm.

Sections used for immunohistochemistry were washed with 0.05 M Tris buffered saline (TBS) (pH 7.4) and then incubated with 0.1 M sodium citrate buffer containing 0.05% Tween-20 (pH 6.0) for 24 min at 98 °C for antigen retrieval. Endogenous peroxidase activity was blocked with 0.3% hydrogen peroxide followed by permeabilization with TBS containing 0.1% Tween-20 and 0.5% bovine serum albumin (BSA) at room temperature. Primary antibodies against TNFAIP3 (cat. no. bs-2803R-B; InsightTech; Woburn, MS, USA) or against phospho-NF-κB p65 (S536) (cat. no. ab86299; Abcam; Cambridge, UK) were used at a final dilution of 1:200. Incubations were performed in TBS containing 0.5% BSA overnight at 4 °C. Subsequently, sections were washed with TBS and incubated with biotinylated mouse anti-rabbit IgG, avidin and biotinylated HRP (cat. no. SC-2018; St. Cruz Biotechnology; St. Cruz, CA, USA) following the manufacturer's instructions. These antibodies have been previously tested in lung sections in parallel to primary omission controls. The area stained for A20 or NF-κB was detected with 3,3′-diaminobenzidine (Sigma Chemical, St Louis, MO, USA) solution. All slides were counterstained with hematoxylin and mounted for observation by microscopy. Images were acquired under a final magnification of 20× using a Leica DM4500 B optical microscope coupled to a digital camera and analyzed with Image-Pro Plus software. The brown-stained areas present both in the sections stained with phospho-NF-κB p65 or in the sections stained with TNFAIP3 were automatically detected by the software and expressed as the percentage of the tissue section area. The tissue section area was calculated by the software and was defined as the picture area subtracted of the bronchioles and vessels lumen area (empty bronchioles and vessels lumen area was automatically outlined by the software).

Two random pictures for each section (one random section per animal) were analyzed in order to originate the data for collagen, mucus, TNFAIP3 and phospho-NF-κB p65 stained area. One bronchiole per picture (two pictures per section, one section per animal) were analyzed to originate the data on globet cell numbers.

2.6. *RNA Extraction and mRNA and miRNA Detections*

A fragment of lung weighing approximately 100 mg, a segment of the trachea and mononuclear cells from whole blood and from spleen were immediately processed for total RNA extraction with Qiazol following the manufacturer's instructions. PBMCs were obtained from 1 mL of whole blood using Ficoll-Paque PLUS (cat no. 17-1440-02; GE Life Sciences; Uppsala, Sweden) manufacturer's instructions. For SMCs, whole spleen cells were subjected to hemolysis followed by washing in Dulbecco's Minimum Essential Medium (DMEM). After washing, the remaining cells were subjected to the Ficoll-Paque method for mononuclear separation exactly as for whole-blood samples.

RNA purity (260/280 and 260/230 ratios) and concentration were calculated using a NanoDrop 2000 spectrophotometer (Thermo Scientific, Waltham, MA, USA) and subjected to poly(A) tailing and reverse transcription with an annealed adaptor (5′-GGCCACGCGTCGACTAGTAC(T)12-3′) as previously described [21]. PCRs were conducted using KAPA SYBR® FAST qPCR Master Mix (Kapa Biosystems, Inc., Boston, MA, USA) in a StepOnePlus Real-Time PCR System (Applied Biosystems, Foster City, CA, USA), using adhesive-sealed plates. The primer sequences were as follows: miRNA antisense (universal): 5′-GGCCACGCGTCGACTAGTAC-3′; miR-133b (miR-133-3p) sense: 5′-TTTGGTCCCCTTCAACCAGCTA-3′; miR-155 (miR-155-5p) sense: 5′-TTAATGCTAATTGTGATAGGGGT-3′; *Rpl37a* (NM_009084) sense: 5′-GTACACTT GCTCCTTCTGTGGC-3′ and antisense: 5′-AGGTGGTGTTGTAGGTCCAGG-3′; *Il4* (NM_021283) sense: 5′-AGCAACGAAGAACACCACAGA-3′ and antisense: 5′-AAGCACCTTGGAAGCCC.

TAC-3′; *Il5* (NM_010558) sense: 5′-TCAAACTGTCCGTGGGGGTA-3′ and antisense: 5′-CTCG CCACACTTCTCTTTTTGG-3′; *Il10* (NM_010548) sense: 5′-AGGCGCTGTCATCGATTTCTC-3′ and antisense: 5′-CTCTTCACCTGCTCCACTGC-3′; *Il13* (NM_008355) sense: 5′-GGCCCCCA CTACGGTCT-3′ and antisense: 5′-TCCTCATTAGAAGGGGCCGT-3′. miRNA primer sequences were based on their respective seed sequences; mRNA primers were designed with GeneRunner software. Specificity of the primers were checked by melting profiles and agarose gel electrophoresis of the amplicons. The miRNA and mRNA expression values were normalized using the geometric mean calculated from the reference gene *Rpl37a*. The fold changes were calculated via the $2^{-\Delta\Delta CT}$ method. Ct values of targets and reference genes were <35, and of the negative control (non-template reactions) were ≥40.

2.7. Statistical Analysis

The results are presented as the mean ± standard error of the mean (SEM). D'Agostino and Pearson normality test was used to check for parametric distribution. Comparisons of data from different offspring were made with two-way ANOVA considering (i) type of maternal diet (SC or HFD) and (ii) exposure to challenge with OVA (challenged or unchallenged). Tukey's multiple comparison test was used as a post-test. Data from SC- and HFD-fed mothers or from parameters assessed exclusively in challenged offspring were compared with Student's *t*-test (for parametric distribution) or Mann Whitney test (for non-parametric distribution). Pearson or Spearman correlations were used for parametric or non-parametric data, respectively (GraphPad Prism, Version 8.0, San Diego, CA, USA). Results with p values that were less than 0.05 were considered significant. The number of independent measures (n) indicated throughout the text refers to animals from different progenies.

3. Results

3.1. Weight and Biochemical Characteristics of Mice Before Mating and Pregnancy Outcomes

We initially assessed biochemical and body weight parameters to demonstrate that our experimental approach was efficient in inducing obesity and its metabolic consequences just before the beginning of pregnancy. Mice fed either SC or HFD were evaluated one day before mating (except for leptin level, which was assessed 21 days after delivery). Our data revealed that body weight, blood glucose and serum triglycerides, cholesterol and leptin were increased in pregnant mice fed a HFD (respectively, 24%, 33%, 38%, 49% and 611% higher than in SC-fed mice; $p < 0.05$) (Table 1).

Table 1. Body weight and biochemical characteristics of Standard chow (SC) and High Fat Diet (HFD) fed dams.

	SC Dams	HFD Dams	P
N	12	12	-
Body mass (g)	21.68 ± 1.24	27.03 ± 3.89	***
Triglycerides (mg/dL)	114.3 ± 27.4	158.1 ± 36.6	**
Glucose (mg/dL)	128.8 ± 14.9	170.5 ± 15.54	****
Cholesterol (mg/dL)	94.15 ± 7.9	141.2 ± 32.9	***
Leptin (ng/mL)	1.555 ± 0.297	11.070 ± 2.130	***
Number of pups per litter	6.1 ± 1.6	5 ± 1.9	nd

Body mass, blood glucose and serum triglycerides and cholesterol were assessed 1 day before mating. Serum leptin was evaluated 21 days after delivery. The number of pups per litter was evaluated during the first 24 h after delivery. Data are shown as mean ± SEM. ** $p < 0.01$ versus SC dams; *** $p < 0.001$ versus SC dams; **** $p < 0.0001$ versus SC dams. nd: Not detected.

We found no differences between the numbers of siblings within the progenies born to SC- and HFD-fed dams. The body weight of the offspring born to HFD-fed mice was reduced on the 3rd day and at the end of the 3rd week of life (21% and 17%, respectively, lower than that of the offspring born to SC-fed mice; $p < 0.05$). This difference in body weight was no longer detected at the end of the 8th week of life. Serum triglyceride, cholesterol, leptin and blood glucose levels were also similar between 8-week-old offspring born to HFD- and SC-fed mice (Table 2).

Table 2. Body weight and biochemical characteristics of the offspring born to SC- and HFD-fed dams.

	SC Offspring	HFD Offspring	*P*
N	8	8	-
Triglycerides (mg/dL)	82.02 ± 29.5	67.16 ± 24.87	nd
Glucose (mg/dL)	150.4 ± 24.29	142.4 ± 18.28	nd
Cholesterol (mg/dL)	78.36 ± 12.24	67.07 ± 12.08	nd
Leptin (ng/mL)	0.588 ± 0.162	0.587 ± 0.064	nd
Body mass at the 3rd day of life (g)	3.17 ± 0.14	2.52 ± 0.14	**
Body mass at the 21st day of life (g)	9.36 ± 0.61	7.56 ± 0.19	*
Body mass at the 8th week of life (g)	26.13 ± 2.34	24.38 ± 0.73	nd

Blood glucose and serum triglycerides, cholesterol and leptin were assessed at the 8th week of life. Data are shown as mean ± SEM. * $p < 0.05$ versus SC offspring; ** $p < 0.01$ versus SC offspring. nd: Not detected.

3.2. Increased Eosinophil Accumulation in BAL of OVA-Challenged Mice born to HFD-Fed Mice

We conducted multiple measurements to assess if mice born to obese mothers would display an exacerbation of eosinophilic infiltration in BAL and lung parenchyma. A scheme illustrating the protocol for sensitization and challenge with OVA is shown in Figure 1a. Both SC/OVA and HFD/OVA mice had more leukocytes in BAL compared to their unchallenged counterparts (respectively, 20- and 41-fold higher; $p < 0.0001$). However, the number of leukocytes in BAL of HFD/OVA was higher than in that of SC/OVA (2.0-fold; $p < 0.0001$) ($p < 0.0001$ for interaction) (Figure 1b).

Differential counting revealed that eosinophils were only present in the BAL of SC/OVA and HFD/OVA. As observed for total leukocytes, the number of eosinophils in the BAL of HFD/OVA was higher than in that of SC/OVA (1.9-fold; $p < 0.0001$) ($p < 0.0001$ for interaction). Although a prevalence of eosinophils was noted in both challenged groups, challenge with OVA also resulted in an increased number of neutrophils exclusively in BAL of HFD/OVA (6.0-fold higher than in HFD/SHAM and 3.0-fold higher than in SC/OVA; $p < 0.0001$) ($p = 0.0006$ for interaction) (Figure 1c).

Changes in the number of eosinophils in BAL samples were also evaluated by flow cytometry quantification of $CCR3^+/VLA4^+$ cells. In agreement with the results of the differential counting, the flow cytometry experiments revealed that the number of $CCR3^+/VLA4^+$ cells was increased in BAL of HFD/OVA (28% higher than in SC/OVA; $p = 0.0048$) (Figure 1d,e).

The exacerbation of leukocyte migration to BAL seen in HFD/OVA was paralleled by a more pronounced accumulation of leukocytes in the lung parenchyma, as evidenced by H&E-stained lung sections. H&E staining also revealed that leukocytosis in the peri-bronchoalveolar and peri-vascular spaces, partial destruction of the epithelial layer, smooth muscle hypertrophy and hyperplasia and the development of a subepithelial layer were more pronounced in the HFD/OVA than in the SC/OVA (Figure 2a). The leukocyte infiltrated area in lung parenchyma was increased in HFD/OVA (4.0-fold higher than in SC/OVA; $p < 0.0001$) (Figure 2b). Both the area infiltrated with neutrophils and eosinophils were increased in HFD/OVA (respectively, 3.3- and 4.3-fold higher than SC/OVA; $p < 0.0001$) (Figure 2c).

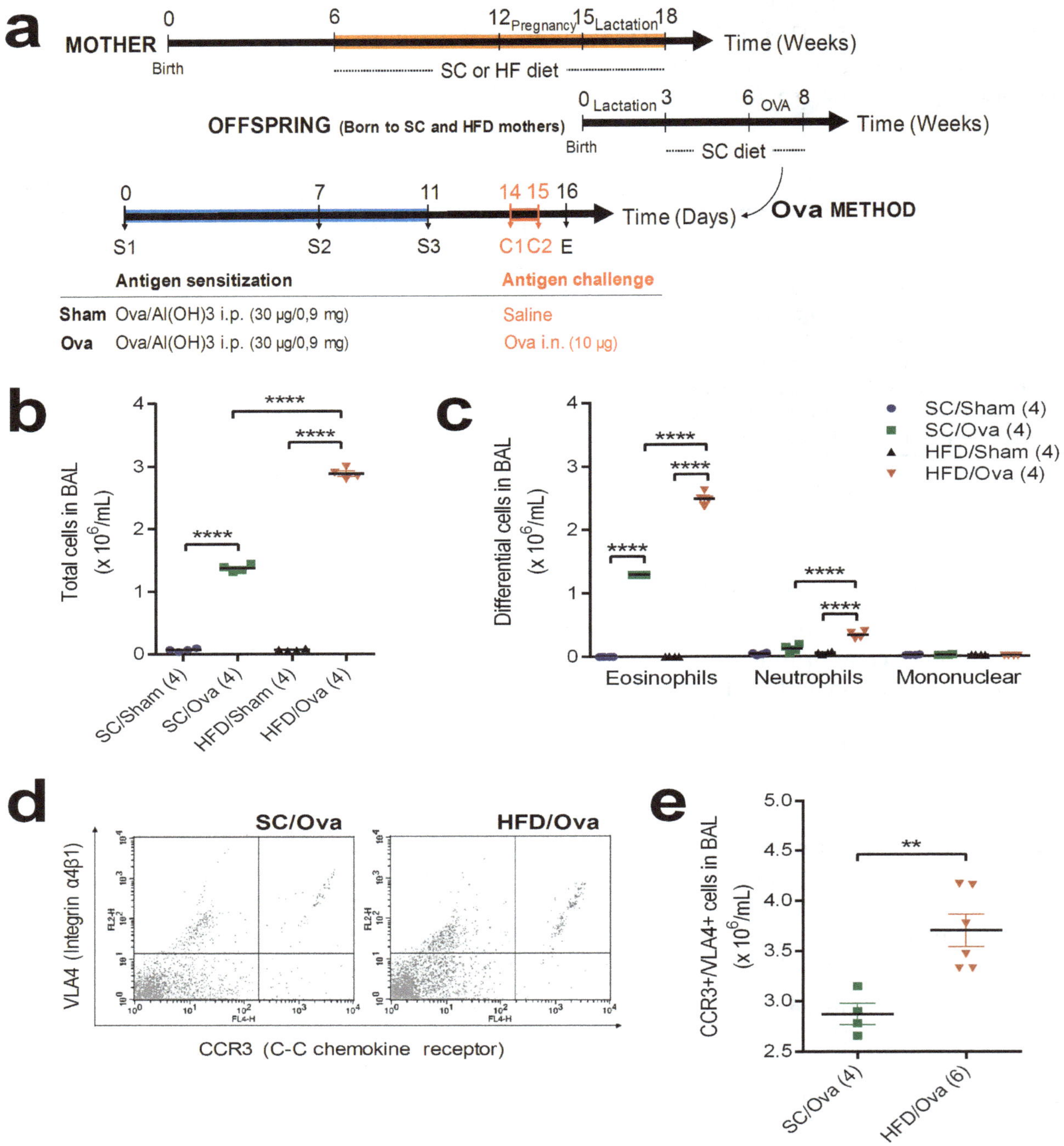

Figure 1. Leukocyte infiltration in the bronchoalveolar lavage (BAL) of mice born to HFD-fed mothers. The offspring born to SC- and HFD-fed mothers were subjected to sensitization only (SHAM) or sensitization and challenge with ovalbumin (OVA) (**a**). BAL samples were obtained from SC/SHAM, SC/OVA, HFD/SHAM and HFD/OVA and processed for total (**b**) and differential leukocyte counting (**c**). BAL samples from SC/OVA and HFD/OVA were also processed for flow cytometry quantification of $CCR3^+/VLA4^+$ cells (**d**,**e**). Data are shown as mean ± SEM. ** $p < 0.01$ and **** $p < 0.0001$.

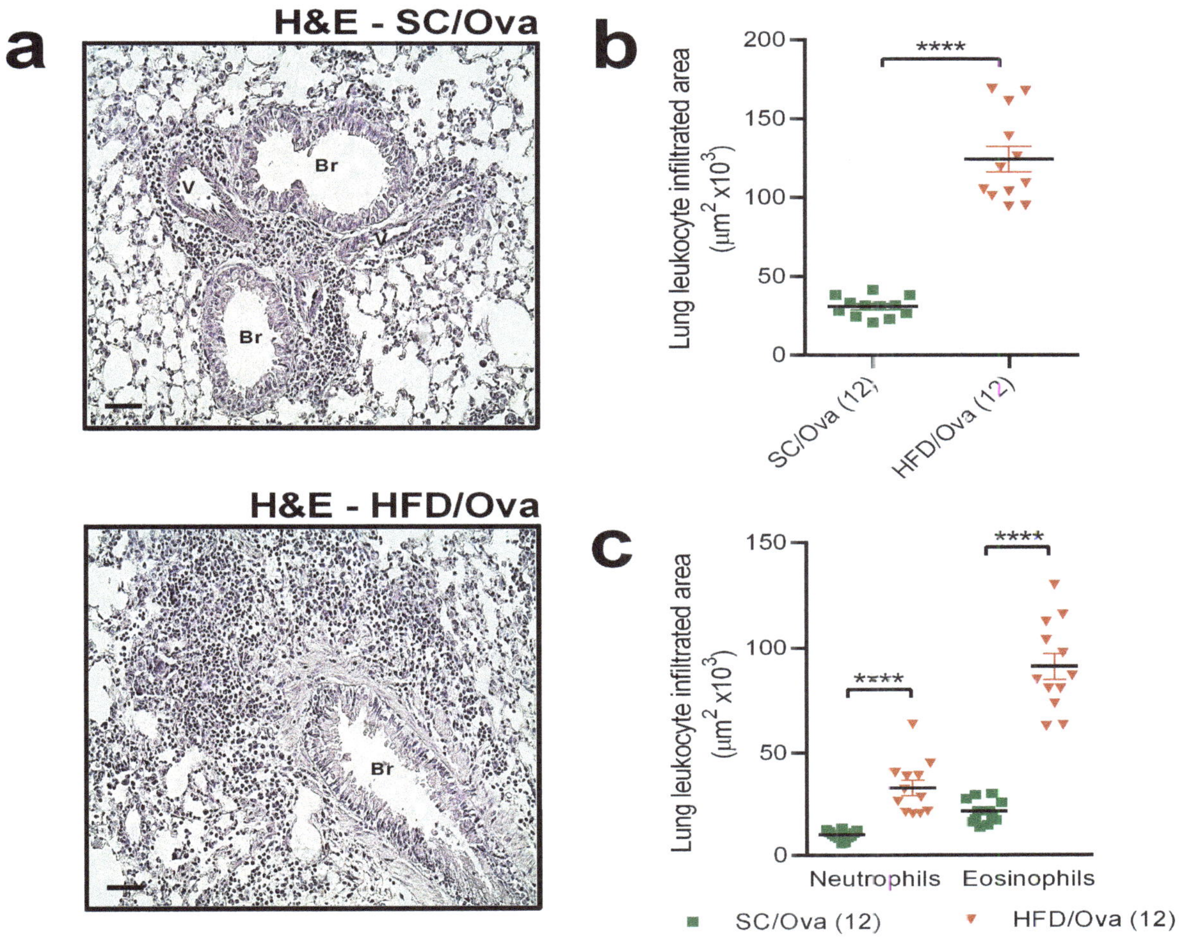

Figure 2. Leukocyte infiltration in the lung parenchyma of mice born to HFD-fed mothers. Lung tissue samples from SC/OVA and HFD/OVA were processed for hematoxylin and eosin (H&E) staining to visualize morphological aspects (**a**). The total leukocyte infiltrated area (**b**) and the neutrophil and eosinophil infiltrated area around the bronchial alveolar space (**c**) were determined using ImageJ software. Horizontal bars represent 50 μm. Data are shown as mean ± SEM. **** $p < 0.0001$. Br: Bronchiole; V: Vessel.

3.3. Increased BAL Levels of Interleukins of the T_H2 *Response and Serum Level of IgE in OVA-Challenged Mice Born to HFD-Fed Mice*

We next evaluated IL-4, IL-5, IL-10 and IL-13 BAL levels to elucidate if increased accumulation of eosinophils in BAL and lung of mice born to HFD-fed mice challenged with OVA was associated with a widespread exacerbation of the T_H2 response. IL-4 level in BAL samples was elevated by challenge with OVA in the SC/OVA and in the HFD/OVA (respectively, 272% and 369% higher than in SC/SHAM and HFD/SHAM; $p = 0.03$ and $p < 0.0001$). IL-4 level in BAL samples of HFD/OVA, however, was higher than in those of SC/OVA (125% higher; $p = 0.0007$) ($p = 0.0067$ for interaction) (Figure 3a).

Although a trend towards an increase in IL-5 in BAL samples was noted in OVA-challenged mice ($p = 0.06$), no specific change was seen when the comparison was made between SC/OVA and HFD/OVA ($p = 0.43$ for interaction) (Figure 3b). Similarly, challenge with OVA equally increased IL-10 in BAL samples from SC/OVA and HFD/OVA (36% higher than in unchallenged mice; $p = 0.01$). However, no specific changes were found when comparing the IL-10 levels of SC/OVA and HFD/OVA ($p = 0.72$ for interaction) (Figure 3c). IL-13 was only detected in BAL samples of challenged mice, but its level in HFD/OVA was higher than in SC/OVA (214% higher; $p = 0.0005$) ($p = 0.0032$ for interaction) (Figure 3d).

As with the BAL level of IL-4, the serum level of IgE was elevated by challenge with OVA in the SC/OVA and in the HFD/OVA (respectively, 575% and 981% higher than in SC/SHAM and HFD/SHAM; $p = 0.03$ and $p < 0.0001$). However, the IgE level of HFD/OVA was higher than in SC/OVA (119% higher; $p = 0.004$) ($p = 0.012$ for interaction) (Figure 3e).

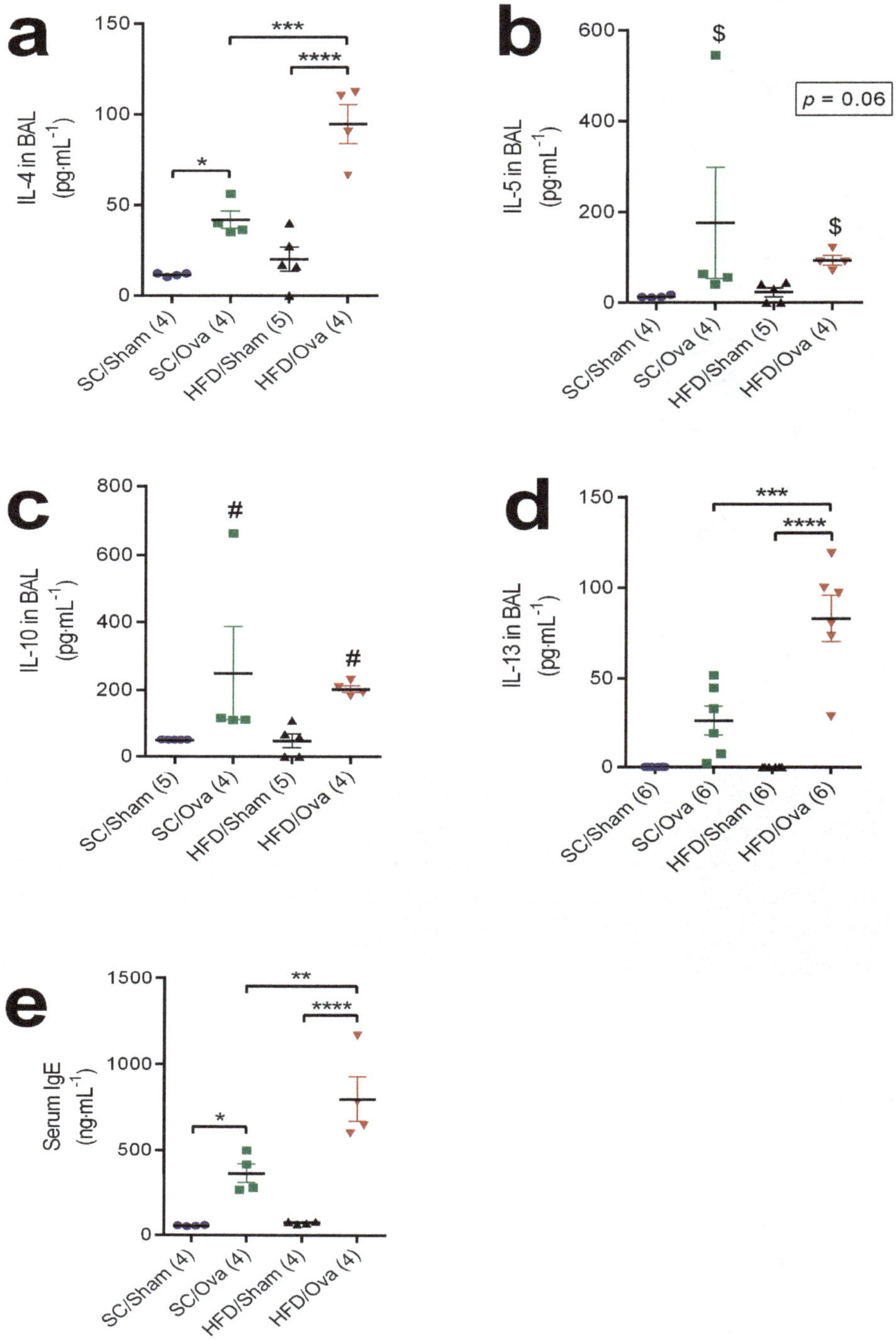

Figure 3. T_H2 cytokine and IgE levels in mice born to HFD-fed mothers. BAL and serum samples were obtained from SC/SHAM, SC/OVA, HFD/SHAM and HFD/OVA. BAL samples were processed for IL-4 (**a**), IL-5 (**b**), IL-10 (**c**) and IL-13 quantification (**d**). Serum samples were used for IgE determination (**e**). Data are shown as mean ± SEM. * $p < 0.05$; ** $p < 0.01$; *** $p < 0.001$; **** $p < 0.0001$; \$ $p = 0.06$ indicating the effect of challenge with OVA and # $p < 0.05$ indicating the effect of challenge with OVA.

3.4. Intensification of Lung Remodeling in OVA-Challenged Mice Born to HFD-Fed Mice

We next evaluated if the overproduction of some T_H2 interleukins induced by challenge with OVA in mice born to HFD-fed mice could impact the changes associated with lung remodeling in the allergic asthma. Masson's trichrome staining revealed that both SC/OVA and HFD/OVA had evident collagen deposition in the peri-bronchoalveolar space that was partially located over the subendothelial smooth muscle layer. The percentage of the area stained for collagen was, however, 60% higher in HFD/OVA than in SC/OVA ($p < 0.0001$) (Figure 4a,b). TGF-β1 was not detected in BAL samples of unchallenged mice. On the other hand, TGF-β1 level in BAL samples of HFD/OVA was 255% higher than in those of SC/OVA ($p < 0.001$) ($p = 0.004$ for interaction) (Figure 4c).

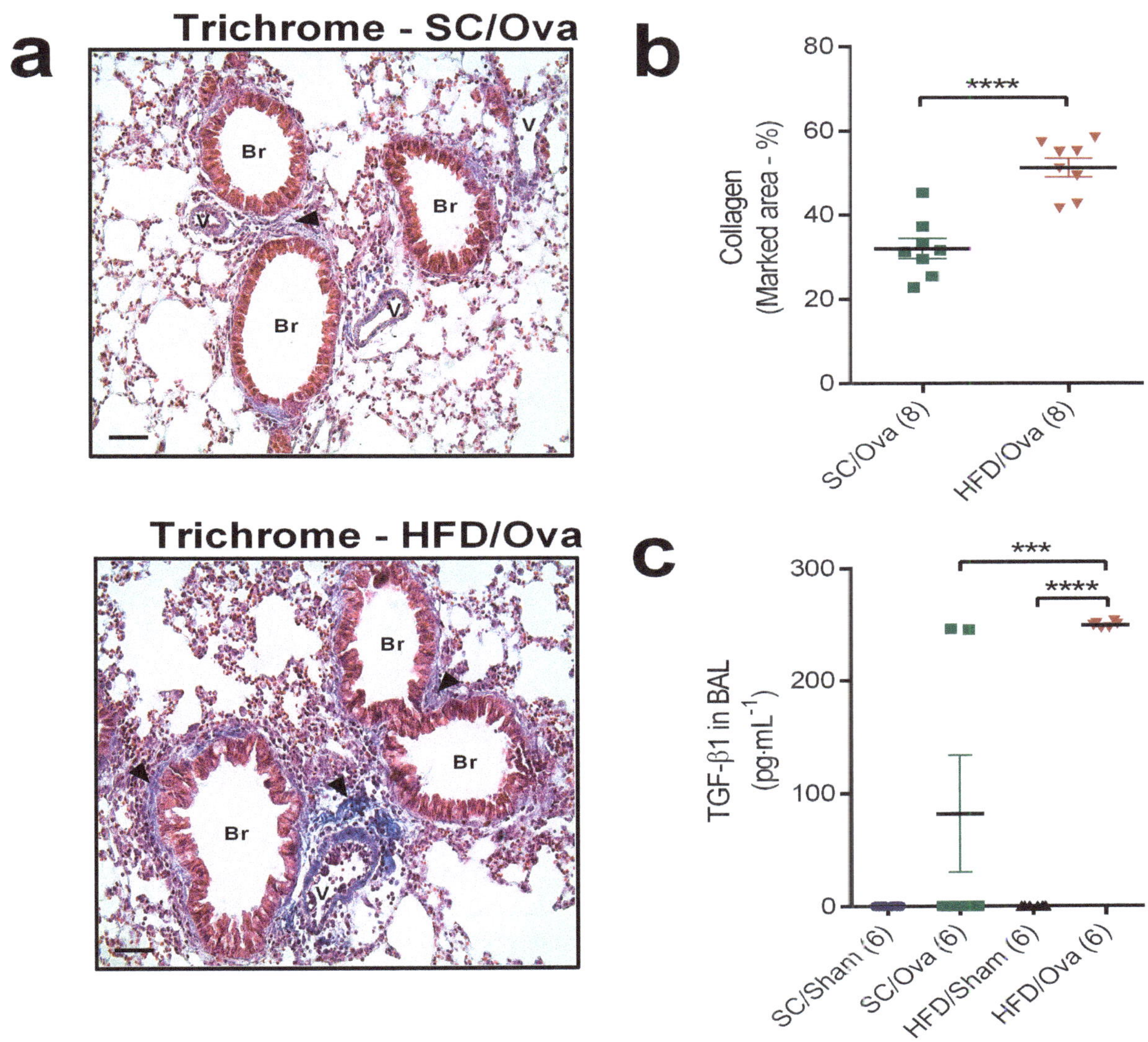

Figure 4. Lung collagen deposition and TGF-β1 level in mice born to HFD-fed mothers. Lung tissue samples from SC/OVA and HFD/OVA were subjected to the Masson's trichrome staining protocol to assess collagen deposition. Representative images show peri-bronchoalveolar blue-stained collagen fibers (black arrows) (**a**). The percentage of stained area was assessed with Image-Pro Plus software (**b**). BAL samples were obtained from SC/SHAM, SC/OVA, HFD/SHAM and HFD/OVA mice and processed for TGF-β1 quantification (**c**). Horizontal bars represent 50 μm. Data are shown as mean ± SEM. *** $p < 0.001$ and **** $p < 0.0001$. Br: Bronchiole; V: Vessel.

The PAS method also revealed that both groups of mice challenged with OVA presented purple-magenta staining for mucus over the epithelial layer. This indication of mucus production was exacerbated in HFD/OVA, as evidenced by the quantification of the percentage of purple-magenta-stained area (214% higher than in SC/OVA; $p < 0.0001$) (Figure 5a,b). The number of globet cells in the bronchioles was also increased in HFD/OVA mice (150% higher than in those of SC/OVA; $p < 0.0001$) (Figure 5c).

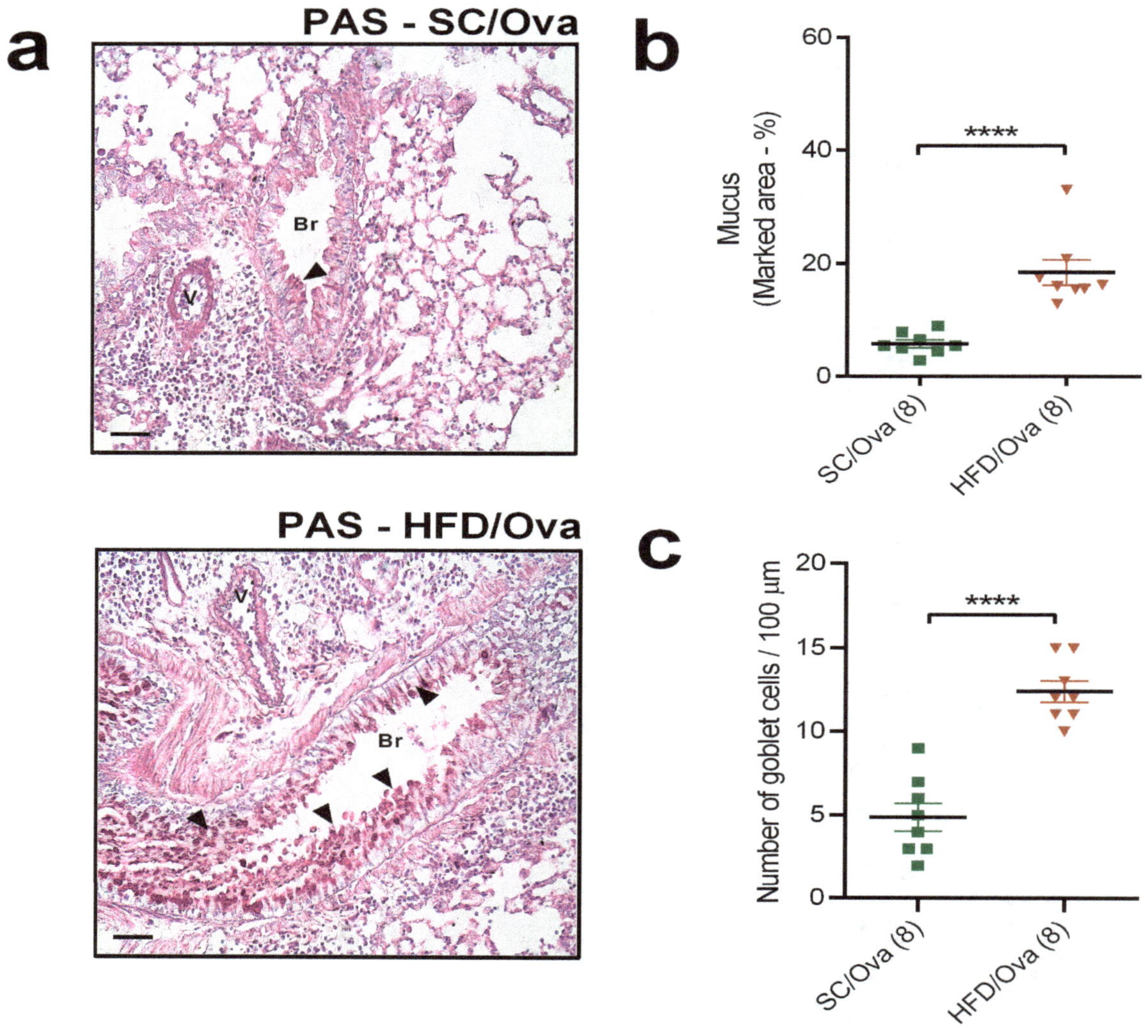

Figure 5. Mucus production in mice born to HFD-fed mothers. Lung tissue samples from SC/OVA and HFD/OVA were subjected to the PAS staining method to assess mucus production. Representative images show purple-magenta-stained mucus over the epithelial layer (black arrows) (**a**). The percentage of stained area was assessed with Image-Pro Plus software (**b**). The number of goblet cells in the broncho epithelial layer was determined by morphological criteria (**c**). Horizontal bars represent 50 µm. Data are shown as mean ± SEM. **** $p < 0.0001$. Br: Bronchiole; V: Vessel.

3.5. Mice Born to HFD-Fed Mothers Have Exacerbated TNF-α level and Increased TNF-α Signaling after Being Challenged with OVA

To evaluate if the exacerbation of the inflammatory response to allergic asthma in mice born to HFD-fed mothers was not restricted to the T_H2/eosinophil axis, we also assessed the production of proinflammatory cytokines that act as acute phase proteins. BAL IL-1β was only detected in samples of OVA-challenged mice, but no difference was noted between HFD/OVA and SC/OVA ($p = 0.72$ for interaction) (Figure 6a). TNF-α concentration was also elevated in BAL samples of SC/OVA and

HFD/OVA mice (respectively, 172% and 177% higher than in SC/SHAM and HFD/SHAM; $p = 0.006$ and $p < 0.0001$). In contrast to IL-1β, the level of TNF-α in BAL of HFD/OVA was higher than in those of SC/OVA (86% higher; $p = 0.0008$) ($p = 0.01$ for interaction) (Figure 6b).

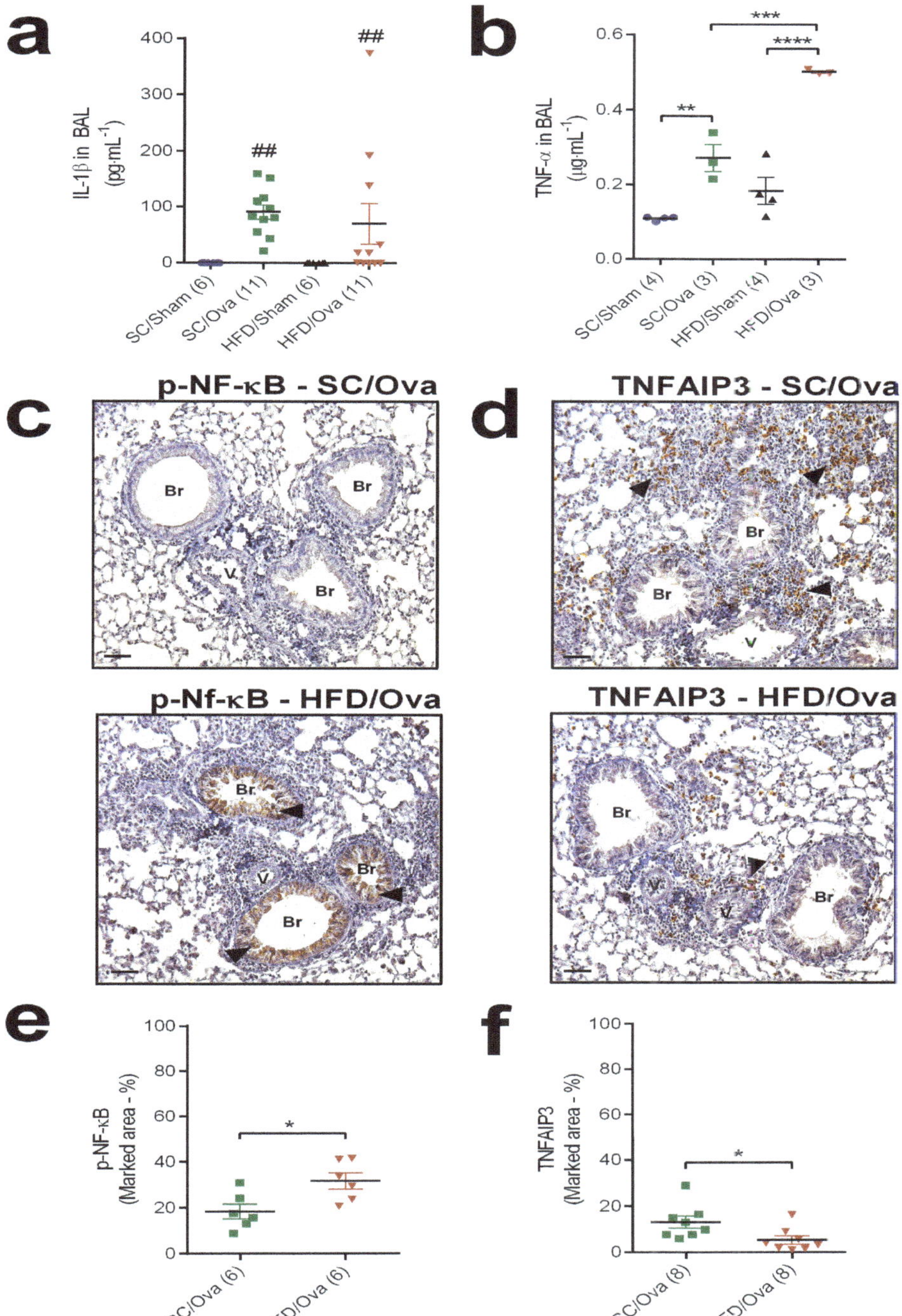

Figure 6. Acute phase protein levels and TNF-α signaling in mice born to HFD-fed mothers. BAL samples were obtained from SC/SHAM, SC/OVA, HFD/SHAM and HFD/OVA mice and processed for IL-1β (**a**) and TNF-α quantification (**b**). Lung tissue samples from SC/OVA and HFD/OVA were subjected to immunohistochemistry detection of phospho-NF-κB (**c**) and TNFAIP3 (**d**) (black arrows). The percentages of phospho-NF-κB- (**e**) and TNFAIP3-stained areas (**f**) were assessed with Image-Pro Plus software. Horizontal bars represent 50 μm. Data are shown as mean ± SEM. * $p < 0.05$; ** $p < 0.01$; *** $p < 0.001$; **** $p < 0.0001$ and ## $p < 0.01$ indicating the effect of challenge with OVA. Br: Bronchiole; V: Vessel.

We also evaluated two intracellular proteins that take part in the cellular signaling evoked by TNF-α. The area stained for phosphorylated NF-κB was higher in lung sections of HFD/OVA than in SC/OVA (71% higher; $p = 0.02$) (Figure 6c,e). On the other hand, the area stained for TNFAIP3, a repressor of TNF-α signaling, was reduced in lung sections of HFD/OVA (60% lower than in SC/OVA; $p = 0.03$) (Figure 6d,f).

3.6. Mice Born to HFD-Fed Mice Have Increased miRNAs That Are Associated with the Exacerbation of the T_H2 Response and IL-13 Signaling

The present investigation also sought to clarify the mechanisms underlying the exacerbated allergic airway inflammation detected later in the life of the progeny born to obese mothers. We chose to study miR-133b based on the following reasons. A study profiling several circulating miRNAs in serum samples has shown that miR-133b was one miRNA that was downregulated in asthmatic patients [22]. Evidence showing that miR-133b is more than only a biomarker for allergic asthma came from studies with mice demonstrating that the model of sensitization and challenge with OVA leads to a reduction in miR-133b expression in nasal mucosa. It was further demonstrated that upregulation of miR-133b with an specific agomir was able to abrogate OVA-induced increased in IgE, IL-4, IL-5 and TNF-α levels and lung eosinophil infiltration [23].

Investigating the expression of miR-133b in our model was also of particular interest because this microRNA was described to modulate the proliferation of smooth muscle cells in different territories. Increased expression of miR-133b was associated to reduced proliferation and calcium levels in vascular smooth muscle cells [24,25]. Additionally, it was also shown that TGF-β1-induced reduction of miR-133b expression in bladder smooth muscle cells was pivotal for collagen accumulation in these cells [26].

Due to the reasons stated above, and based on our data on collagen deposition and TGF-β1 levels in BAL, we decided to evaluate miR-133b expression in the lung and in the trachea of HFD/OVA and SC/OVA mice.

The choice for the study of miR-155 was based on consistent literature showing its participation in the T_H2 response of allergic airway disease. Mice knockout for miR-155 exhibited attenuated eosinophil infiltration in the lung parenchyma, reduced mucus production and lower IL-4, IL-5 and IL-13 levels when subjected to OVA sensitization and challenge [27]. Concordant data using mice knockout for miR-155 were found by other groups [28,29]. Accordingly, miR-155 overexpression resulted in increased mucus production, lung eosinophil infiltration and IL-4, IL-5 and IL-13 levels [30]. Directly inhibiting miR-155 expression in T_H2 cells prevents T_H2-mediated airway allergy (airway eosinophilia, IL-13 production and airway mucus production [31]). miR-155 expression was also described to be positively associated in IL-4, IL-5 and IL-13 production by $CD4^+$ cells isolated from allergic patients [32]. On the other hand, miR-155 was reported to reduce IL-13-induced bronchial smooth muscle cells proliferation and migration [33]. Therefore, we decided to evaluate miR-155 expression not only in peripheral-blood mononuclear cells (PBMCs) and in splenic mononuclear cells (SMC), but also in lung and trachea of HFD/OVA and SC/OVA mice.

The expression of miR-155 was upregulated in PBMCs of HFD/OVA mice (483% higher than in SC/OVA; $p = 0.003$). No significant changes were found in SMC or trachea or lung samples (Figure 7a). The expression of miR-133b was not detected in PBMCs or in SMCs, but its level was reduced in the trachea and in the lung samples of the HFD/OVA (respectively, 87% and 58% lower than in SC/OVA; $p = 0.03$) (Figure 7b).

In order to explore the relevance for the increased miR-155 in PBMC of HFD/OVA mice, we evaluated the mRNA expression of *Il4*, *Il5*, *Il10* and *Il13*. In agreement with our data on interleukin concentration in BAL, we found that HFD/OVA mice had increased *Il4* and *Il13* expressions in PBMC (respectively, 175% and 212% higher than in SC/OVA; $p = 0.027$ and $p = 0.007$). No changes were found in *Il5* and *Il10* expression when comparing PBMC samples of HFD/OVA and SC/OVA (Figure 7c).

The relevance for the reduced miR-133b in trachea and lung samples of HFD/OVA mice was explored by measuring the *Il13* mRNA expression in these samples. The expression of *Il13* was increased both in trachea and lung samples of HFD/OVA (respectively, 67% and 190% higher than in SC/OVA; $p = 0.019$ and $p = 0.003$) (Figure 7c).

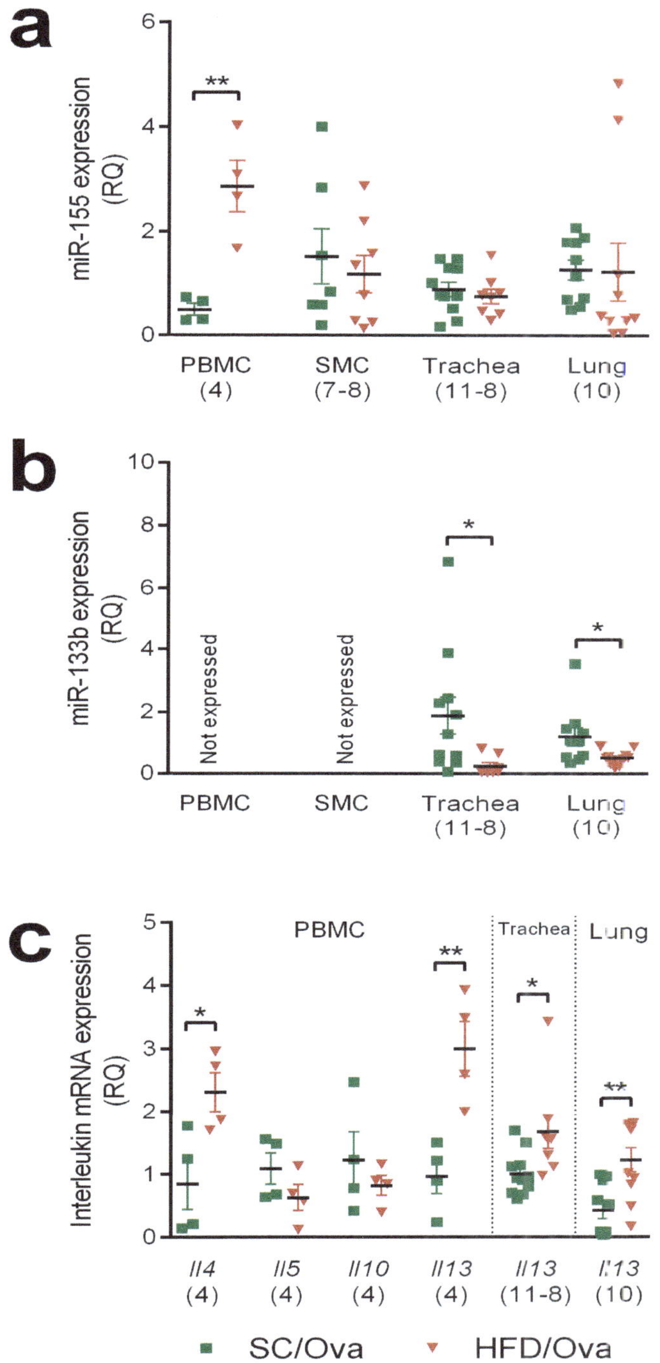

Figure 7. miR-155, miR-133b and interleukins expression in mice born to HFD-fed mothers. PBMC, SMC, trachea and lung tissue samples were obtained from SC/OVA and HFD/OVA and processed for RNA extraction and miR-155 (**a**) and miR-133b detection (**b**) by Quantitative polymerase chain reaction (qPCR). Expression of interleukins *Il4*, *Il5*, *Il10* and *Il13* mRNA in PBMC, and *Il13* mRNA in trachea and lung were also determined. (**c**) *Rpl37a* was used as an internal control. Data are shown as mean ± SEM. * $p < 0.05$ and ** $p < 0.01$.

We also tested whether the levels of miR-155 and miR-133b would correlate with the levels *Il4* and *Il13* expressions. We detected a trend towards a positive correlation between miR-155 and *Il4* expressions in PBMC ($r = 0.6721$; $p = 0.0679$) and a positive correlation between miR-155 and *Il13* expressions in PBMC ($r = 0.9272$; $p = 0.0009$) (Figure 8a,b). On the other hand, a negative correlation between miR-133b and *Il13* expressions were found in trachea ($r = -0.5789$; $p = 0.0094$) and lung samples ($r = -0.4648$; $p = 0.039$) (Figure 8c,d).

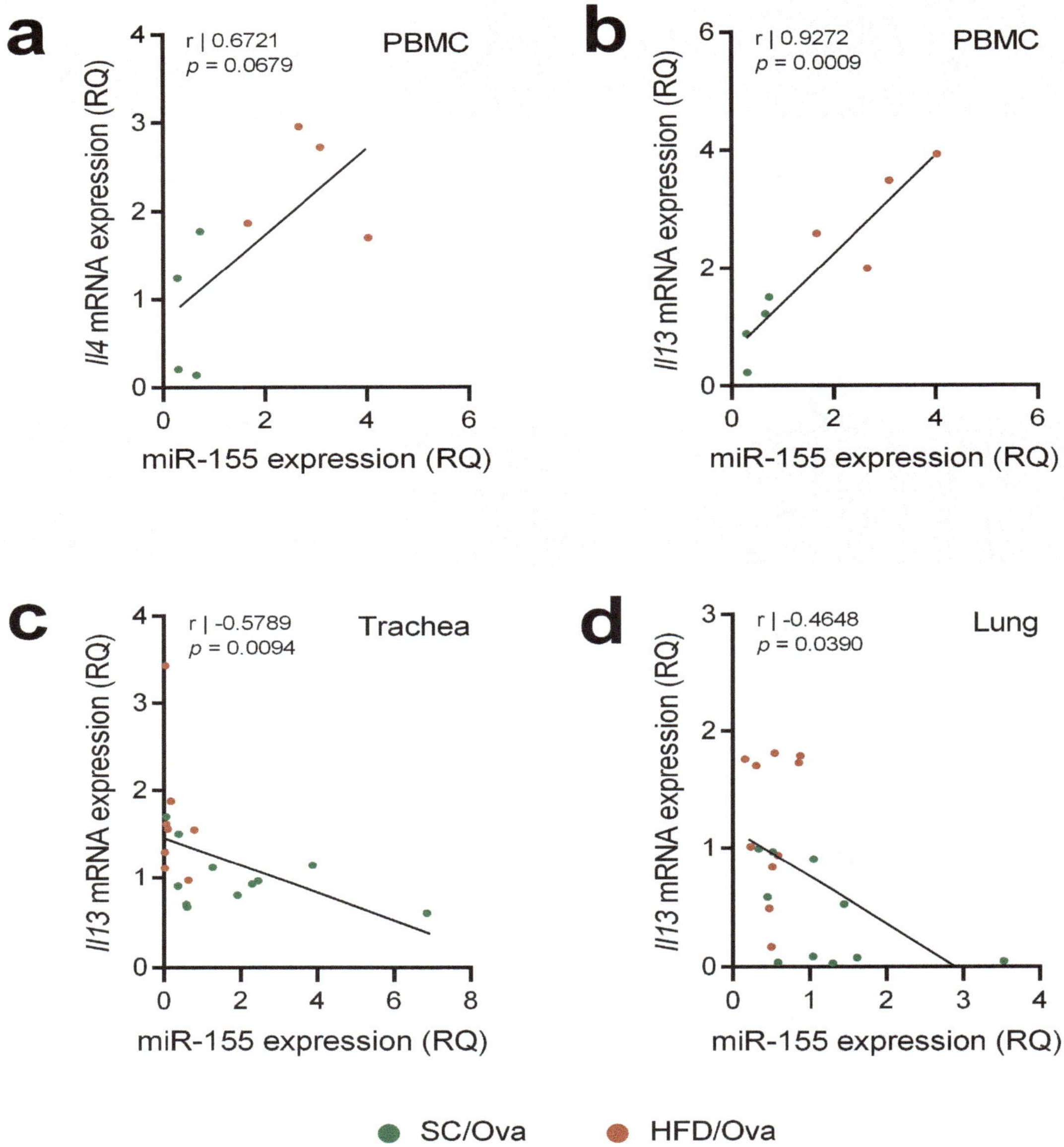

Figure 8. Correlation of interleukin expression with miRNAs in mice subjected to sensitization and challenge with OVA. The expression miR-155 in PBMC of SC/OVA and HFD/OVA was correlated with *Il4* (**a**) and *Il13* (**b**) expressions. The expression miR-133b in trachea (**c**) and in lung (**d**) of SC/OVA and HFD/OVA was correlated with *Il13* expression.

4. Discussion

Recent observational studies have shown that children born to obese women are more prone to develop asthma [16,17]. The increased risk for asthma in children born to obese mothers was observed using models that were adjusted for several co-varieties including mother's race, maternal age and child's sex [34]. Apart from these studies, no clear mechanism for this relationship has been suggested thus far. To the best of our knowledge, this is the first study to demonstrate that mice born to and breastfed by obese mothers exhibit exacerbated activation of inflammatory parameters when subjected to the model of allergic airway inflammation characterized by sensitization followed by challenge with OVA.

The present data are in accordance with previously published papers showing persistent respiratory abnormalities in offspring born to HFD-fed dams. Using OVA-naive offspring, a previous report by Griffiths et al. demonstrated that rats born to mothers fed a HFD during pregnancy and lactation display increased levels of acute phase proteins, such as IL-1α, IL-1β and TNF-α, along with an increase in the T_H2 cytokine IL-5, during the first days of life. Some changes were persistently observed at the moment of weaning and in the adult offspring. Those authors have also demonstrated that weanling rats born to and breastfed by HFD-fed dams had higher basal respiratory resistance and lower respiratory compliance, although some of these changes disappeared when the progeny reached adult life [19].

MacDonald et al. have demonstrated that the male and female offspring of BALB/cByJ mice born to and breastfed by mothers receiving HFD manifest increased methacholine-induced respiratory resistance and increased neutrophil count and IL-6 level in BAL samples [18]. Dinger et al., instead, used C57B6 mice to show that feeding dams with HFD during lactation caused greater airway resistance in the male offspring not exposed to OVA [20]. Given the data published by Dinger et al. [20], we decided to carry our experiments in the male offspring of C57BL/6J mice.

The present study further contributes to this field of investigation by demonstrating that sensitization followed by challenge with OVA leads to an exacerbated increase in IL-4, IL-13 and TNF-α in BAL of male C57BL/6J mice born to and breastfed by HFD-fed dams. Such findings support the notion that changes imprinted on the immune system may play an important role in the respiratory programming induced by maternal obesity.

We have found no differences in leukocytes in BAL when comparing SC/SHAM to HFD/SHAM mice. This is in apparent contrast to the study published by MacDonald et al. [18]. Those researchers found increased leukocytes in BAL of mice born to HFD-fed mice. However, there are two important differences between the study by MacDonald et al. and the present experiments that may contribute such different results. The offspring in the study by MacDonald et al. were naive to OVA while our SHAM animals were sensitized with the allergen. The study by MacDonald et al. used a strain of BALB/c mice, while we used C57Bl/6J mice.

Interestingly, our data show that, in contrast to IL-4 and IL-13, challenge with OVA did not promote a further increase in IL-10 and IL-5 levels in BAL of mice born to HFD-fed dams. Such selective modulation demonstrates that the programming induced by maternal obesity is not characterized by a widespread activation of the T_H2 response in the offspring. On the other hand, it is noteworthy that published evidence clearly supports the proposition that overproduction of IL-4 and IL-13 may be responsible for the features of allergic asthma that are exacerbated in the offspring born to HFD-fed mice after challenge with OVA.

IL-4 is known to act in uncommitted B cells, promoting their switch to an IgG1- and IgE-secreting phenotype [35]. Therefore, an exacerbated IL-4 level in BAL samples explains the increased serum IgE found in HFD/OVA mice. Moreover, IL-4 has been shown to boost the airway eosinophilia induced by IL-5 in mice sensitized/challenged with OVA [36]. Accordingly, we found increased eosinophils in the lung parenchyma and in the BAL of HFD/OVA mice. Evidence also exists supporting the proposition that exacerbated IL-13 level in BAL of OVA-challenged mice born to HFD-fed dams may contribute to their increased lung eosinophilia [3].

IL-10, instead, is produced by Treg cells and exerts regulatory function of T_H1 and T_H2 cells [37]. It was already described that IL-10 production by thymic Foxp3-negative Treg cells alleviates the lung eosinophil infiltration, globet cell hyperplasia and IgE and production in mice subjected to the OVA model of allergic asthma [38]. Our data revealed that the male offspring born to either HFD-fed or SC-fed mothers exhibit a similar increase in BAL IL-10 levels when challenged with OVA. Thus, we can conclude that the exacerbated features of allergic airway inflammation seen in the offspring born to HFD-fed mothers are probably not due to an impaired IL-10 production by Treg cells.

The exacerbated presence of eosinophils in BAL of OVA-challenged mice born to HFD-fed dams was also evidenced by the increased concentration of CCR3^{+}/VLA4^{+} cells. CCR3, also known as CD193, was described to play a pivotal role in the transendothelial migration of activated eosinophils [39]. VLA4, also known as $\alpha 4\beta 1$ integrin, is highly expressed in eosinophils of asthmatic individuals and contributes to their increased adhesion to airway smooth muscle [40].

Another features induced by challenge with OVA that were intensified in mice born to obese mothers were mucus hypersecretion and globet cells hyperplasia. As we understand, it is reasonable to assume that excessive IL-4 and IL-13 may account for mucus hypersecretion in mice born to HFD-fed mice. Accordingly, previous studies have demonstrated that IL-13 and IL-4 can stimulate mucus production in vivo and in vitro by acting directly in goblet cells [5,41–43] stimulating the expression of different mucins such as Muc2 and Muc5-ac [44,45]. IL-4, in turn, was also described to induce structural changes, such as epithelial hypertrophy of the airways, a feature also noted in the offspring born to obese dams [46].

The present study also reveals that exacerbation of the inflammatory response induced by OVA in the offspring born to obese dams has consequences for lung remodeling, as evidenced by increased collagen deposition and BAL TGF-β1 level. Interestingly, TGF-β1 produced by airway smooth muscle cells was described to act in an autocrine fashion to stimulate collagen expression [47,48].

Another aspect revealed by the present study is that OVA-challenged mice born to obese mothers manifested exacerbated TNF-α level along with neutrophils in BAL and increased NF-κB phosphorylation in lung. We also found reduced TNFAIP3 level in the lung of HFD/OVA mice. TNFAIP3 is an inhibitor of NF-κB that was reported to reduce airway leukocyte recruitment, peribronchoalveolar inflammation and mucus production and airway hyperresponsiveness (AHR) in mice subjected to OVA sensitization/challenge [49,50]. Interestingly, TNF-α, by activating NF-κB, was described to play a role in the steroid-resistant neutrophilic inflammation and AHR that occur in chronically sensitized (four weeks) mice subjected to a single moderate OVA challenge [6]. Furthermore, neutrophils and TNF-α levels in the lung were implicated in NF-κB activation in distinct models of lung injury [51,52]. Accordingly, as our data with BAL samples were obtained by washing the entire lungs, it is plausible to assume that, even assessing one random section per animal, our immunohistochemistry data represent phenomena that are taking place in the whole lung.

Our data showing reduced miR-133b in the trachea and in the lung and increased miR-155 in the PBMC indicates a putative mechanism by which the exacerbated response to OVA develops in the adult progeny. Several lines of evidence indicate that miR-133b is relevant to the inflammatory response and lung remodeling in allergic asthma. Lower levels of circulating miR-133b have been detected in asthmatic patients [22], and its overexpression in nasal mucosa was shown to target the Nlrp3 inflammasome and reduce eosinophil infiltration and IgE, TNF-α, IL-4, IL-5 and IFN-γ levels in mice sensitized/challenged with OVA [23].

The reduction in miR-133b was also shown to mediate TGF-β1-induced collagen accumulation in bladder smooth muscle cells [26]. Notably, IL-13-induced collagen synthesis was reported to be dependent on TGF-β1 production [53]. In vivo IL-13 neutralization also resulted in lower collagen deposition in lung of mice subjected to experimental asthma [54]. Our data showing a negative correlation of IL-13 with miR-133b in trachea and lung of the mice belonging to the OVA subgroups further suggest that the downregulation of miR-133b may play a role in the increased collagen deposition seen in the HFD/OVA group.

As we understand, the increased expression of miR-155 in PBMCs found in the offspring born to obese mothers also helps to explain their increased IL-4 and IL-13 levels. It has been demonstrated that allergen stimulation of CD4^{+} cells in vitro increases miR-155 expression and IL-13 production [32]. miR-155-knockout mice subjected to OVA sensitization/challenge showed reduced levels of IL-4, IL-5 and IL-13 as well as lower lung eosinophil/neutrophil infiltration compared to wild-type [27].

Accordingly, miR-155 was described to stimulate the T_H2 response and mucus hypersecretion by directly targeting sphingosine-1-phosphate receptor 1 and cytotoxic T lymphocyte–associated antigen 4 in $CD4^+$ cells in experimental models of asthma [30,31]. The positive correlation between miR-155 with IL-13 and a trend towards a significant correlation with IL-4 in PBMCs of the mice belonging to the OVA subgroups favors the interpretation that elevated miR-155 may be relevant for the increased levels of IL-4 and IL-13 in HFD/OVA.

It is still challenging to determine the mechanism by which maternal obesity increases the intensity allergic outcomes in the offspring. It is now clear that changes in gut microbiota play a crucial role in metabolic adaptations to obesity [55]. Feeding mice with a HFD has been show to induce changes in gut microbiota in parallel to a reduction in fecal content of short chain fatty acids (SCFAs) [56]. SCFAs are produced by the intestinal microbiota fermentation of indigestible dietary carbohydrates such dietary fiber. It has been shown that treatment with several SCFAs including acetate is capable of preventing HFD-induced metabolic outcomes [57]. In this context, a recent study in mice has suggested that diet-induced changes gut microbial diversity in the mother may play a crucial role in the programming of allergic asthma in the offspring. Exposure of pregnant mice to a high fiber diet or to the SCFA acetate in the drinking water resulted in an attenuation of allergic airway disease in the offspring subjected to sensitization/challenge with house dust mite challenge [58].

In summary, our study reveals unprecedented data showing that progeny born to obese mice display exacerbated responses to sensitization/challenge with OVA. This exacerbation is hallmarked by overproduction of IL-4, IL-13, TNF-α and TGF-β1, which is paralleled by increased circulating IgE. Mice born to obese mothers also display accentuated eosinophil/neutrophil infiltration in the lung parenchyma, increased collagen deposition and increased mucus hypersecretion. From the mechanistic point of view, our data suggest that increased miR-155 in PBMCs and reduced miR-133b in lung tissue and trachea are likely to mediate the programming events described herein.

Author Contributions: G.F.A. and R.R.e.-L. designed the research. R.R.e.-L. and C.J.T. performed the experiments and analyzed the data. G.F.A, R.R.e.-L., E.A. and S.B. wrote the paper.

Acknowledgments: The authors are grateful for the technical assistance of Miguel Borges da Silva, Agnaldo Fernando de Azevedo and Ivani Franco Correia dos Santos. The authors also thank Clive P. Page and Yanira Riffo-Vasquez from the Sackler Institute of Pulmonary Pharmacology, Institute of Pharmaceutical Science (King's College, London, UK) for kindly providing the antibodies and Caroline M. Ferreira (Federal University of Sao Paulo) for providing part of the primers used in the present experiments.

References

1. Backman, H.; Räisänen, P.; Hedman, L.; Stridsman, C.; Andersson, M.; Lindberg, A.; Lundbäck, B.; Rönmark, E. Increased prevalence of allergic asthma from 1996 to 2006 and further to 2016—results from three population surveys. *Clin. Exp. Allergy* **2017**, *47*, 1426–1435. [CrossRef] [PubMed]
2. Foster, P.S.; Maltby, S.; Rosenberg, H.F.; Tay, H.L.; Hogan, S.P.; Collison, A.M.; Yang, M.; Kaiko, G.E.; Hansbro, P.M.; Kumar, R.K.; et al. Modeling T H 2 responses and airway inflammation to understand fundamental mechanisms regulating the pathogenesis of asthma. *Immunol. Rev.* **2017**, *278*, 20–40. [CrossRef] [PubMed]
3. Grünig, G.; Warnock, M.; Wakil, A.E.; Venkayya, R.; Brombacher, F.; Rennick, D.M.; Sheppard, D.; Mohrs, M.; Donaldson, D.D.; Locksley, R.M.; et al. Requirement for IL-13 independently of IL-4 in experimental asthma. *Science* **1998**, *282*, 2261–2263. [CrossRef] [PubMed]

4. Wills-Karp, M.; Luyimbazi, J.; Xu, X.; Schofield, B.; Neben, T.Y.; Karp, C.L.; Donaldson, D.D. Interleukin-13: Central mediator of allergic asthma. *Science* **1998**, *282*, 2258–2261. [CrossRef] [PubMed]
5. Zhu, Z.; Homer, R.J.; Wang, Z.; Chen, Q.; Geba, G.P.; Wang, J.; Zhang, Y.; Elias, J.A. Pulmonary expression of interleukin-13 causes inflammation, mucus hypersecretion, subepithelial fibrosis, physiologic abnormalities, and eotaxin production. *J. Clin. Investig.* **1999**, *103*, 779–788. [CrossRef] [PubMed]
6. Ito, K.; Herbert, C.; Siegle, J.S.; Vuppusetty, C.; Hansbro, N.; Thomas, P.S.; Foster, P.S.; Barnes, P.J.; Kumar, R.K. Steroid-resistant neutrophilic inflammation in a mouse model of an acute exacerbation of asthma. *Am. J. Respir. Cell Mol. Biol.* **2008**, *39*, 543–550. [CrossRef]
7. Herbert, C.; Scott, M.M.; Scruton, K.H.; Keogh, R.P.; Yuan, K.C.; Hsu, K.; Siegle, J.S.; Tedla, N.; Foster, P.S.; Kumar, R.K. Alveolar macrophages stimulate enhanced cytokine production by pulmonary CD4+ T-lymphocytes in an exacerbation of murine chronic asthma. *Am. J. Pathol.* **2010**, *177*, 1657–1664. [CrossRef]
8. Romieu, I.; Avenel, V.; Leynaert, B.; Kauffmann, F.; Clavel-Chapelon, F. Body mass index, change in body silhouette, and risk of asthma in the E3N cohort study. *Am. J. Epidemiol.* **2003**, *158*, 165–174. [CrossRef]
9. Camargo, C.A.; Weiss, S.T.; Zhang, S.; Willett, W.C.; Speizer, F.E. Prospective study of body mass index, weight change, and risk of adult-onset asthma in women. *Arch. Intern. Med.* **1999**, *159*, 2582–2588. [CrossRef]
10. Baltieri, L.; Cazzo, E.; de Souza, A.L.; Alegre, S.M.; de Paula Vieira, R.; Antunes, E.; de Mello, G.C.; Claudio Martins, L.; Chaim, E.A. Influence of weight loss on pulmonary function and levels of adipokines among asthmatic individuals with obesity: One-year follow-up. *Respir. Med.* **2018**, *145*, 48–56. [CrossRef]
11. Grotta, M.B.; Squebola-Cola, D.M.; Toro, A.A.D.C.; Ribeiro, M.A.G.O.; Mazon, S.B.; Ribeiro, J.D.; Antunes, E. Obesity increases eosinophil activity in asthmatic children and adolescents. *BMC Pulm. Med.* **2013**, *13*. [CrossRef] [PubMed]
12. Calixto, M.C.; Lintomen, L.; Schenka, A.; Saad, M.J.; Zanesco, A.; Antunes, E. Obesity enhances eosinophilic inflammation in a murine model of allergic asthma. *Br. J. Pharmacol.* **2010**, *159*, 617–625. [CrossRef] [PubMed]
13. Dietze, J.; Böcking, C.; Heverhagen, J.T.; Voelker, M.N.; Renz, H. Obesity lowers the threshold of allergic sensitization and augments airway eosinophilia in a mouse model of asthma. *Allergy Eur. J. Allergy Clin. Immunol.* **2012**, *67*, 1519–1529. [CrossRef] [PubMed]
14. Everaere, L.; Ait-Yahia, S.; Molendi-Coste, O.; Vorng, H.; Quemener, S.; LeVu, P.; Fleury, S.; Bouchaert, E.; Fan, Y.; Duez, C.; et al. Innate lymphoid cells contribute to allergic airway disease exacerbation by obesity. *J. Allergy Clin. Immunol.* **2016**, *138*, 1309–1318.e11. [CrossRef] [PubMed]
15. Zheng, H.; Wu, D.; Wu, X.; Zhang, X.; Zhou, Q.; Luo, Y.; Yang, X.; Chock, C.J.; Liu, M.; Yang, X.O. Leptin Promotes Allergic Airway Inflammation through Targeting the Unfolded Protein Response Pathway. *Sci. Rep.* **2018**, *8*, 8905. [CrossRef]
16. Forno, E.; Young, O.M.; Kumar, R.; Simhan, H.; Celedón, J.C. Maternal Obesity in Pregnancy, Gestational Weight Gain, and Risk of Childhood Asthma. *Pediatrics* **2014**, *134*, e535–e546. [CrossRef]
17. Godfrey, K.M.; Reynolds, R.M.; Prescott, S.L.; Nyirenda, M.; Jaddoe, V.W.V.; Eriksson, J.G.; Broekman, B.F.P. Influence of maternal obesity on the long-term health of offspring. *Lancet Diabetes Endocrinol.* **2017**, *5*, 53–64. [CrossRef]
18. MacDonald, K.D.; Moran, A.R.; Scherman, A.J.; McEvoy, C.T.; Platteau, A.S. Maternal high-fat diet in mice leads to innate airway hyperresponsiveness in the adult offspring. *Physiol. Rep.* **2017**, *5*, e13082. [CrossRef]
19. Griffiths, P.S.; Walton, C.; Samsell, L.; Perez, M.K.; Piedimonte, G. Maternal high-fat hypercaloric diet during pregnancy results in persistent metabolic and respiratory abnormalities in offspring. *Pediatr. Res.* **2016**, *79*, 278–286. [CrossRef]
20. Dinger, K.; Kasper, P.; Hucklenbruch-Rother, E.; Vohlen, C.; Jobst, E.; Janoschek, R.; Bae-Gartz, I.; Van Koningsbruggen-Rietschel, S.; Plank, C.; Dötsch, J.; et al. Early-onset obesity dysregulates pulmonary adipocytokine/insulin signaling and induces asthma-like disease in mice. *Sci. Rep.* **2016**, *6*, 24168. [CrossRef]
21. Pantaleão, L.C.; Murata, G.; Teixeira, C.J.; Payolla, T.B.; Santos-Silva, J.C.; Duque-Guimaraes, D.E.; Sodré, F.S.; Lellis-Santos, C.; Vieira, J.C.; De Souza, D.N.; et al. Prolonged fasting elicits increased hepatic triglyceride accumulation in rats born to dexamethasone-Treated mothers. *Sci. Rep.* **2017**, *7*, 10367. [CrossRef] [PubMed]
22. Panganiban, R.P.; Wang, Y.; Howrylak, J.; Chinchilli, V.M.; Craig, T.J.; August, A.; Ishmael, F.T. Circulating microRNAs as biomarkers in patients with allergic rhinitis and asthma. *J. Allergy Clin. Immunol.* **2016**, *137*, 1423–1432. [CrossRef] [PubMed]

23. Xiao, L.; Jiang, L.; Hu, Q.; Li, Y. MicroRNA-133b Ameliorates Allergic Inflammation and Symptom in Murine Model of Allergic Rhinitis by Targeting Nlrp3. *Cell. Physiol. Biochem.* **2017**, *42*, 901–912. [CrossRef] [PubMed]
24. Liu, H.; Xiong, W.; Liu, F.; Lin, F.; He, J.; Liu, C.; Lin, Y.; Dong, S. MicroRNA-133b regulates the growth and migration of vascular smooth muscle cells by targeting matrix metallopeptidase 9. *Pathol. Res. Pract.* **2019**, *215*, 1083–1088. [CrossRef] [PubMed]
25. Panizo, S.; Naves-Díaz, M.; Carrillo-López, N.; Martínez-Arias, L.; Fernández-Martín, J.L.; Ruiz-Torres, M.P.; Cannata-Andía, J.B.; Rodríguez, I. MicroRNAs 29b, 133b, and 211 regulate vascular smooth muscle calcification mediated by high phosphorus. *J. Am. Soc. Nephrol.* **2016**, *27*, 824–834. [CrossRef] [PubMed]
26. Duan, L.J.; Qi, J.; Kong, X.J.; Huang, T.; Qian, X.Q.; Xu, D.; Liang, J.H.; Kang, J. MiR-133 modulates TGF-β1-induced bladder smooth muscle cell hypertrophic and fibrotic response: Implication for a role of microRNA in bladder wall remodeling caused by bladder outlet obstruction. *Cell. Signal.* **2015**, *27*, 215–227. [CrossRef] [PubMed]
27. Malmhäll, C.; Alawieh, S.; Lu, Y.; Sjöstrand, M.; Bossios, A.; Eldh, M.; Rådinger, M. MicroRNA-155 is essential for TH2-mediated allergen-induced eosinophilic inflammation in the lung. *J. Allergy Clin. Immunol.* **2014**, *133*. [CrossRef]
28. Zech, A.; Ayata, C.K.; Pankratz, F.; Meyer, A.; Baudiß, K.; Cicko, S.; Yegutkin, G.G.; Grundmann, S.; Idzko, M. MicroRNA-155 modulates P2R signaling and Th2 priming of dendritic cells during allergic airway inflammation in mice. *Allergy Eur. J. Allergy Clin. Immunol.* **2015**, *70*, 1121–1129. [CrossRef]
29. Johansson, K.; Malmhäll, C.; Ramos-Ramírez, P.; Rådinger, M. MicroRNA-155 is a critical regulator of type 2 innate lymphoid cells and IL-33 signaling in experimental models of allergic airway inflammation. *J. Allergy Clin. Immunol.* **2017**, *139*, 1007–1016.e9. [CrossRef]
30. Zhang, Y.; Sun, E.; Li, X.; Zhang, M.; Tang, Z.; He, L.; Lv, K. miR-155 contributes to Df1-induced asthma by increasing the proliferative response of Th cells via CTLA-4 downregulation. *Cell. Immunol.* **2017**, *314*, 1–9. [CrossRef]
31. Okoye, I.S.; Czieso, S.; Ktistaki, E.; Roderick, K.; Coomes, S.M.; Pelly, V.S.; Kannan, Y.; Perez-Lloret, J.; Zhao, J.L.; Baltimore, D.; et al. Transcriptomics identified a critical role for Th2 cell-intrinsic miR-155 in mediating allergy and antihelminth immunity. *Proc. Natl. Acad. Sci. USA* **2014**, *111*, E3081–E3090. [CrossRef] [PubMed]
32. Daniel, E.; Roff, A.; Hsu, M.-H.; Panganiban, R.; Lambert, K.; Ishmael, F. Effects of allergic stimulation and glucocorticoids on miR-155 in CD4+ T-cells. *Am. J. Clin. Exp. Immunol.* **2018**, *7*, 57–66. [PubMed]
33. Shi, Y.; Fu, X.; Cao, Q.; Mao, Z.; Chen, Y.; Sun, Y.; Liu, Z.; Zhang, Q. Overexpression of miR-155-5p inhibits the proliferation and migration of IL-13-induced human bronchial smooth muscle cells by suppressing TGF-ß-activated kinase 1/MAP3K7-binding protein 2. *Allergy Asthma Immunol. Res.* **2018**, *10*, 260–267. [CrossRef] [PubMed]
34. Polinski, K.J.; Liu, J.; Boghossian, N.S.; McLain, A.C. Maternal Obesity, Gestational Weight Gain, and Asthma in Offspring. *Prev. Chronic Dis.* **2017**, *14*, 170196. [CrossRef]
35. Bergstedt-Lindqvist, S.; Moon, H.-B.; Persson, U.; Möller, G.; Heusser, C.; Severinson, E. Interleukin 4 instructs uncommitted B lymphocytes to switch to IgGl and IgE. *Eur. J. Immunol.* **1988**, *18*, 1073–1077. [CrossRef]
36. Hogan, S.P.; Mould, A.; Kikutani, H.; Ramsay, A.J.; Foster, P.S. Aeroallergen-induced eosinophilic inflammation, lung damage, and airways hyperreactivity in mice can occur independently of IL-4 and allergen-specific immunoglobulins. *J. Clin. Investig.* **1997**, *99*, 1329–1339. [CrossRef]
37. Jutel, M.; Akdis, M.; Budak, F.; Aebischer-Casaulta, C.; Wrzyszcz, M.; Blaser, K.; Akdis, C.A. IL-10 and TGF-β cooperate in the regulatory T cell response to mucosal allergens in normal immunity and specific immunotherapy. *Eur. J. Immunol.* **2003**, *33*, 1205–1214. [CrossRef]
38. Böhm, L.; Maxeiner, J.; Meyer-Martin, H.; Reuter, S.; Finotto, S.; Klein, M.; Schild, H.; Schmitt, E.; Bopp, T.; Taube, C. IL-10 and Regulatory T Cells Cooperate in Allergen-Specific Immunotherapy To Ameliorate Allergic Asthma. *J. Immunol.* **2015**, *194*, 887–897. [CrossRef]
39. Shahabuddin, S.; Ponath, P.; Schleimer, R.P. Migration of Eosinophils Across Endothelial Cell Monolayers: Interactions Among IL-5, Endothelial-Activating Cytokines, and C-C Chemokines. *J. Immunol.* **2014**, *164*, 3847–3854. [CrossRef]

40. Januskevicius, A.; Gosens, R.; Sakalauskas, R.; Vaitkiene, S.; Janulaityte, I.; Halayko, A.J.; Hoppenot, D.; Malakauskas, K. Suppression of eosinophil integrins prevents remodeling of airway smooth muscle in asthma. *Front. Physiol.* **2017**, *7*, 680. [CrossRef]

41. Yang, M.; Hogan, S.P.; Henry, P.J.; Matthaei, K.I.; McKenzie, A.N.J.; Young, I.G.; Rothenberg, M.E.; Foster, P.S. Interleukin-13 mediates airways hyperreactivity through the IL-4 receptor-alpha chain and STAT-6 independently of IL-5 and eotaxin. *Am. J. Respir. Cell Mol. Biol.* **2001**, *25*, 522–530. [CrossRef]

42. Alimam, M.Z.; Piazza, F.M.; Selby, D.M.; Letwin, N.; Huang, L.; Rose, M.C. Muc-5/5ac mucin messenger RNA and protein expression is a marker of goblet cell metaplasia in murine airways. *Am. J. Respir. Cell Mol. Biol.* **2000**, *22*, 253–260. [CrossRef]

43. Shim, J.J.; Dabbagh, K.; Takeyama, K.; Burgel, P.R.; Dao-Pick, T.P.; Ueki, I.F.; Nadel, J.A. Suplatast tosilate inhibits goblet-cell metaplasia of airway epithelium in sensitized mice. *J. Allergy Clin. Immunol.* **2000**, *105*, 739–745. [CrossRef]

44. Dabbagh, K.; Takeyama, K.; Lee, H.M.; Ueki, I.F.; Lausier, J.A.; Nadel, J.A. IL-4 induces mucin gene expression and goblet cell metaplasia in vitro and in vivo. *J. Immunol.* **1999**, *162*, 6233–6237.

45. Narala, V.R.; Ranga, R.; Smith, M.R.; Berlin, A.A.; Standiford, T.J.; Lukacs, N.W.; Reddy, R.C. Pioglitazone is as effective as dexamethasone in a cockroach allergen-induced murine model of asthma. *Respir. Res.* **2007**, *8*, 90. [CrossRef]

46. Rankin, J.A.; Picarella, D.E.; Geba, G.P.; Temann, U.A.; Prasad, B.; DiCosmo, B.; Tarallo, A.; Stripp, B.; Whitsett, J.; Flavell, R.A. Phenotypic and physiologic characterization of transgenic mice expressing interleukin 4 in the lung: Lymphocytic and eosinophilic inflammation without airway hyperreactivity. *Proc. Natl. Acad. Sci. USA* **2002**, *93*, 7821–7825. [CrossRef]

47. Coutts, A.; Chen, G.; Stephens, N.; Hirst, S.; Douglas, D.; Eichholtz, T.; Khalil, N. Release of biologically active TGF-β from airway smooth muscle cells induces autocrine synthesis of collagen. *Am. J. Physiol. Cell. Mol. Physiol.* **2017**, *280*, L999–L1008. [CrossRef]

48. Ma, Y.; Huang, W.; Liu, C.; Li, Y.; Xia, Y.; Yang, X.; Sun, W.; Bai, H.; Li, Q.; Peng, Z. Immunization against TGF-β1 reduces collagen deposition but increases sustained inflammation in a murine asthma model. *Hum. Vaccines Immunother.* **2016**, *12*, 1876–1885. [CrossRef]

49. Kang, N.-I.; Yoon, H.-Y.; Lee, Y.-R.; Won, M.; Chung, M.J.; Park, J.-W.; Hur, G.M.; Lee, H.-K.; Park, B.-H. A20 Attenuates Allergic Airway Inflammation in Mice. *J. Immunol.* **2009**, *183*, 1488–1495. [CrossRef]

50. Sasse, S.K.; Altonsy, M.O.; Kadiyala, V.; Cao, G.; Panettieri, R.A.; Gerber, A.N. Glucocorticoid and TNF signaling converge at A20 (TNFAIP3) to repress airway smooth muscle cytokine expression. *Am. J. Physiol. Lung Cell. Mol. Physiol.* **2016**, *311*, L421–L432. [CrossRef]

51. Lentsch, A.B.; Czermak, B.J.; Bless, N.M.; Ward, P.A. NF-κB activation during IgG immune complex-induced lung injury: Requirements for TNF-α and IL-1β but not complement. *Am. J. Pathol.* **1998**, *152*, 1327. [PubMed]

52. Fei, M.; Bhatia, S.; Oriss, T.B.; Yarlagadda, M.; Khare, A.; Akira, S.; Saijod, S.; Iwakura, Y.; Fallert Junecko, B.A.; Reinhart, T.A.; et al. TNF-α from inflammatory dendritic cells (DCs) regulates lung IL-17A/IL-5 levels and neutrophilia versus eosinophilia during persistent fungal infection. *Proc. Natl. Acad. Sci. USA* **2011**, *108*, 5360–5365. [CrossRef] [PubMed]

53. Firszt, R.; Francisco, D.; Church, T.D.; Thomas, J.M.; Ingram, J.L.; Kraft, M. Interleukin-13 induces collagen type-1 expression through matrix metalloproteinase- 2 and transforming growth factor-β1 in airway fibroblasts in asthma. *Eur. Respir. J.* **2014**, *43*, 464–473. [CrossRef] [PubMed]

54. Blease, K.; Jakubzick, C.; Westwick, J.; Lukacs, N.; Kunkel, S.L.; Hogaboam, C.M. Therapeutic Effect of IL-13 Immunoneutralization During Chronic Experimental Fungal Asthma. *J. Immunol.* **2001**, *166*, 5219–5224. [CrossRef] [PubMed]

55. Gohir, W.; Ratcliffe, E.M.; Sloboda, D.M. Of the bugs that shape us: Maternal obesity, the gut microbiome, and long-term disease risk. *Pediatr. Res.* **2015**, *77*, 196–204. [CrossRef] [PubMed]

56. Kimura, I.; Ozawa, K.; Inoue, D.; Imamura, T.; Kimura, K.; Maeda, T.; Terasawa, K.; Kashihara, D.; Hirano, K.; Tani, T.; et al. The gut microbiota suppresses insulin-mediated fat accumulation via the short-chain fatty acid receptor GPR43. *Nat. Commun.* **2013**, *4*, 1829. [CrossRef]

57. Lu, Y.; Fan, C.; Li, P.; Lu, Y.; Chang, X.; Qi, K. Short chain fatty acids prevent high-fat-diet-induced obesity in mice by regulating g protein-coupled receptors and gut Microbiota. *Sci. Rep.* **2016**, *6*, 37589. [CrossRef]
58. Thorburn, A.N.; McKenzie, C.I.; Shen, S.; Stanley, D.; MacIa, L.; Mason, L.J.; Roberts, L.K.; Wong, C.H.Y.; Shim, R.; Robert, R.; et al. Evidence that asthma is a developmental origin disease influenced by maternal diet and bacterial metabolites. *Nat. Commun.* **2015**, *6*, 7320. [CrossRef]

7

Nutrients and Microbiota in Lung Diseases of Prematurity: The Placenta-Gut-Lung Triangle

Fiammetta Piersigilli [1], Bénédicte Van Grambezen [1], Catheline Hocq [1] and Olivier Danhaive [1,2,*]

[1] Division of Neonatology, St-Luc University Hospital, Catholic University of Louvain, Brussels 1200, Belgium; fiammetta.piersigilli@uclouvain.be (F.P.); Benedicte.vangrambezen@uclouvain.be (B.V.G.); Catheline.hocq@uclouvain.be (C.H.)

[2] Department of Pediatrics, Benioff Children's Hospital, University of California San Francisco, San Francisco, CA 94158, USA

* Correspondence: olivier.danhaive@uclouvain.be

Abstract: Cardiorespiratory function is not only the foremost determinant of life after premature birth, but also a major factor of long-term outcomes. However, the path from placental disconnection to nutritional autonomy is enduring and challenging for the preterm infant and, at each step, will have profound influences on respiratory physiology and disease. Fluid and energy intake, specific nutrients such as amino-acids, lipids and vitamins, and their ways of administration —parenteral or enteral—have direct implications on lung tissue composition and cellular functions, thus affect lung development and homeostasis and contributing to acute and chronic respiratory disorders. In addition, metabolomic signatures have recently emerged as biomarkers of bronchopulmonary dysplasia and other neonatal diseases, suggesting a profound implication of specific metabolites such as amino-acids, acylcarnitine and fatty acids in lung injury and repair, inflammation and immune modulation. Recent advances have highlighted the profound influence of the microbiome on many short- and long-term outcomes in the preterm infant. Lung and intestinal microbiomes are deeply intricated, and nutrition plays a prominent role in their establishment and regulation. There is an emerging evidence that human milk prevents bronchopulmonary dysplasia in premature infants, potentially through microbiome composition and/or inflammation modulation. Restoring antibiotic therapy-mediated microbiome disruption is another potentially beneficial action of human milk, which can be in part emulated by pre- and probiotics and supplements. This review will explore the many facets of the gut-lung axis and its pathophysiology in acute and chronic respiratory disorders of the prematurely born infant, and explore established and innovative nutritional approaches for prevention and treatment.

Keywords: microbiome; nutrients; prematurity; lung development; respiratory distress syndrome; bronchopulmonary dysplasia

1. Introduction

Acute and chronic lung disease of the premature infant have multiple origins spanning from fetal life to perinatal and postnatal exposures. Genomic variations have a profound influence on critical pathways involved in lung development, maturation and adaptation to various environmental challenges [1]. On the other hand, nutrients supply both the fuel and building blocks for these essential processes, and they have a profound influence on the homeostasis and responses of the developing lung. Deficiencies, excesses or imbalances of nutrients lead to developmental, functional and inflammatory lung disorders (Table 1).

Table 1. Evidence-based recommendations on selected nutrients for premature lung disease prevention.

	Nutrient	Mechanisms of Action	Effect on Lung Disease	RCT/Meta-Analyses	Recommendations
Vitamins	Vitamin A	Organogenesis, differentiation, lung development and growth, alveolar maturation	Low levels associated with decreased alveolarization and susceptibility to injury [2]	Antenatal supplementation in VitA deficit 7000 UI PO (RCT, [3])	Improved lung function—decreased morbidity **R (high)**
				Postnatal supplementation 5-10,000 UI IM (META–4 studies) [4]	Decreased BPD at 36 weeks **R (moderate)**
	Vitamin D	Pre/postnatal type II cell maturation, surfactant, immune system	Low levels associated with BPD, asthma, RTI	Postnatal supplementation 400–800 UI PO (2 RCT, [5,6])	No change in RDS and BPD NR (low) Decreased wheezing **R (moderate)**
	Vitamin E	Early lung development, antioxidant	Low levels associated with BPD	Postnatal supplementation 20–150 mg/kg IM/TV/PO (Cochrane [7]–25 studies)	No effect on BPD **NR (low)**
Lipids	LCPUFA	Organogenesis Modulation of inflammation	DHA/AA deficit increases BPD [8]	Postnatal ω-3 LCPUFA supplementation (META 26 14 RCT [9])	No effect on BPD **NR (high)**
			LCPUFA-rich emulsions increase DHA and EPA but decrease AA levels [10]	SMOF vs. Clinoleic-RCT-2 studies	Equivocal: BPD prevention [11] vs. no effect [12] **Unknown (low)**
				SMOF vs. Intralipid (Cochrane–15 studies [13])	Trend to BPD prevention **R (low)**
Glucides	Inositol	Surfactant synthesis	Improves early mortality and death/BPD [14]	Supplementation (80 mg/kg/day) (Cochrane–6 studies [15])	No effect on BPD **NR (high)**
Peptides	Lactoferrin	Bactericidal, innate immunity	Prevents NEC and LOS; unclear on BPD [16]	Supplementation 150 mg/kg 24–33 weeks (RCT [17]	No effect on BPD **NR (high)**
Human milk	Various	Various	MBM vs. formula decreased BPD; DBM vs. formula: trend to decreased BPD [18]	Combined exclusive vs. partial; MBM vs. DBM META 22 studies including 5 RCT [19]	Trend to BPD prevention (OR 0.73–1.03) **R (moderate)**
Microbiome	HMO (prebiotics)	Beneficial microbiota, gut maturation, immune system	HMO formula supplementation decreases bronchiolitis in term [20]; limited effects on immature organs [21]	No data on premature lung diseases	n/a
	Probiotics	Immune system, gut permeability, bacterial metabolites	Probiotics decrease NEC [22]	Supplementation for NEC as primary outcome META 15 studies [23]	No effect on BPD **NR (moderate)**

Abbreviations: LCPUFA: long chain polyinsaturatyed fatty acid; HMO: human milk oligosaccharide; BPD: bronchopulmonary dysplasia; RTI: respiratory tract infection; DHA: docosahexenoic acid; AA: arachidonic acid; NEC: necrotizing enterocolitis; LOS: late-onset sepsis; META: meta-analysis; MBM: maternal breast milk; DBM: donor breast milk; RCT: randomized controlled trial; RDS: respiratory distress syndrome; R: recommended; NR not recommended; high, moderate, low: level of recommendation.

The concept of the gut-lung axis has emerged as a cross talk between the two systems, mediated by the microbiome, with bilateral influences on health and disease. Initial studies have highlighted the role of the intestinal microbiome on the metabolic functions of various organs as well as immune responses. Only recently, the development of genomics and metagenomic approaches (including 16S ribosomal RNA profiling and shotgun-sequencing technology) has allowed a more detailed and extensive definition of organ-specific microbiomes. These technologies have permitted the discovery and exploration of a distinct microbiome of the airway and the lung, but its origin and timeframe around birth are still incompletely understood. The paradigm of a sterile fetal environment preserved by the amnion is now challenged by the emergence of intrauterine microbiota influencing fetal programming and development [24] and its relation to premature birth and neonatal respiratory diseases [25,26].

Premature birth causes an interruption of lung development and maturation, and at the same time exposes the neonate to profound alterations of these systems. Abrupt interruption of placental nutrition, lung exposure to a highly oxidant environment, disruption of the nascent microbiome by invasive procedures, hospital microbiota, broad-spectrum antibiotics and many other factors lead to acute and chronic lung disease. Bronchopulmonary dysplasia (BPD), a major cause of chronic lung disease and mortality in preterm infants, is characterized by impaired alveolar and vascular development determined by a combination of genetic factors [1], antenatal exposures and postnatal insults, with a central role played by inflammation. The goal of this review is to summarize the current concepts on nutrition, microbiomes and lung disease in the premature infant, and to delineate strategies and potential opportunities for prevention and treatment by acting on the nutritional and microbiotic balance.

2. Role of Antenatal and Postnatal Nutrition

2.1. Global Substrate Deficiency and Growth Failure

Global nutritional intake, both antenatal and postnatal, has a critical importance on lung development and the pathogenesis of respiratory disorders in the preterm infant. Intrauterine growth restriction (IUGR), a consequence of placental insufficiency and suboptimal transfer of oxygen and nutrients to the fetus, is associated with chronic lung disease of prematurity and altered lung function during infancy, which may last throughout adulthood [27]. In the infant born prematurely with an immature lung at risk of developmental disruption and highly vulnerable to exposures, IUGR is an additional contributor to acute/chronic lung disease. In a prospective cohort of preterm infants <30 weeks monitored during pregnancy, those with abnormal fetal doppler velocimetry and fetal growth failure had a 33% incidence of BPD compared to 7% in controls [28]. Postnatal growth failure is also a critical factor that contributes to chronic lung disease. Early alteration of body composition can be found starting in the first weeks of life for infants who will develop BPD compared to matched controls [29], which suggests ante- or perinatal metabolic reprogramming. In a large cohort study of 600 preterm infants 500–1000 g, a twofold higher incidence of BPD was observed between the first and fourth postnatal weight gain quartile, among other adverse outcomes [30]. Recommendations regarding global energy supply and amounts of specific macro- and micronutrients in healthy and sick preterm infants are multiple, sometimes controversial or contradictory, and abundantly discussed in the literature (e.g., [31,32]).

2.2. Carbohydrates

Glucose supply through the placenta directly influences lung maturation processes. High fetal glucose exposure due to maternal insulin-dependent diabetes mellitus (DM) increases the risk for respiratory distress syndrome (RDS) in late preterm and term infants [33]. This may be explained by altered glucocorticoid-mediated fetal lung development and delayed surfactant maturation due to insulin resistance in late gestation [34]. Conversely, suboptimal postnatal carbohydrate intake and delayed enteral nutrition predisposes to BPD in preterm infants [35].

2.3. Lipids

The effect of undernutrition on respiratory outcome is well established. In animals, 72 h fasting results in RDS, and induces a decrease of dipalmitoylsulfatidylcholine (DPPC) content in lung lavage fluid and an increase in minimal surface tension, indicating surfactant dysfunction [36]. Using the elegant methodology of simultaneous stable isotope tracers using plasma glucose, free palmitate and body water to quantify surfactant disaturated-phosphatidylcholine (DSPC) kinetics in-vivo,

P. Cogo et al. showed the importance of dietary and endogenous fatty acids (FA) in surfactant homeostasis, and the role of kinetics alteration in the pathogenesis of BPD [37].

Whether excess FA intake in a high-fat diet and obesity in pregnancy (a condition increasingly prevalent in developed and developing countries) has any effect on neonatal respiratory function is still poorly established. In a large study on women with preterm premature rupture of membranes, maternal obesity was not associated with adverse neonatal outcome after adjustment for gestational age at birth [38]. Some animal data suggest that a maternal high-fat diet affects fetal lung development through an inflammation-induced placental insufficiency mechanism [39].

Specific fatty acid deficiencies, both antenatal and postnatal, may lead to respiratory disorders. Long-chain polyunsaturated fatty acids (LCPUFAs), in particular docosahexaenoic acid (DHA) and arachidonic acid (AA), are critical for organogenesis during fetal life and for retina and brain development, and are major regulators of inflammation prior to and following birth [10]. In an endotoxin animal model of acute respiratory distress syndrome (ARDS), a high-LCPUFA diet had detrimental effect on lung function, potentially by disrupting surfactant homeostasis [40]. In an animal hyperoxia-induced BPD model, both ante- and postnatal DHA supplementation decreased inflammation and improved alveolarization [41].

LCPUFAs are acquired during fetal life mostly through passive and carrier-mediated placental transfer, a process peaking during the third trimester of pregnancy. Premature birth disrupts this process and results in lower DHA and AA systemic levels and adipose tissue storage, rendering the preterm infant even more dependent on postnatal nutritional strategies. This congenital deficit can further deepen after birth in parenterally and enterally fed preterm infants. Parenteral lipid solutions are not tailored for the preterm infant's needs and, since human milk LCPUFAs are highly variable, enteral feedings rarely reach full volume prior to the second or third weeks after delivery, with limited bioavailability due to impaired intestinal absorption and lipolysis [42]. In a retrospective human cohort study of <30 weeks premature infants, every 1% decline in DHA was associated with a 2.5-fold increased risk of BPD [8]. However, in the largest randomized controlled trial (RCT) to date including 1237 infants <29 weeks, postnatal DHA supplementation failed to prevent BPD, illustrating the complexity of the mechanisms involved [43]. A recent meta-analysis of 15 RCTs involving various LCPUFAs and mixtures lead to the same conclusion [9].

Intravenous lipid emulsions are composed of three elements: triglycerides, glycerol and phospholipids. Both saturated and monounsaturated fatty acids are synthesized from acetyl CoA derived from the metabolism of fat, carbohydrate or protein. Linoleic acid (C 18:2ω-6) and α-linolenic acid (C 18:3ω-3) are considered essential fatty acids from which most other LCPUFAs are metabolized. Total parenteral nutrition based on soybean lipid emulsion, which provides essential linoleic acid (LA) and gamma-linolenic acid, may not be adequate for preterm infants due to deficient downstream metabolic enzymes, and does not allow levels comparable to third trimester fetuses and term-born infants to be sustained [10]. However, 100% fish oil-based emulsions (Omegaven, Fresenius-Kabi, Bad Homburg, Germany) result in elevated DHA and EPA plasma levels, but negatively affect the level of AA, which is essential for brain and retina development as well as growth [13,44]. Newer-generation fish oil-based compound (SMOFLipid, Fresenius-Kabi) showed a benefit in decreasing BPD severity compared to an olive oil-based compound (ClinOleic, Baxter Healthcare SA, Wallisellen, Switzerland) in one small RCT [11], although another RCT failed to show any difference in BPD incidence [12]. A retrospective cohort study comparing SMOFLipid with an older, soybean oil-based product (Intralipid, Baxter Healthcare SA) showed no difference in BPD prevalence [44]. LCPUFAs also influence lung pathology through their effects on surfactant and inflammation (see the "inflammation and BPD" section). In conclusion, human data are too scarce to provide conclusive evidence favoring one specific intravenous lipid compound versus another one in regards to preterm lung disease at this stage.

2.4. Micronutrients

Vitamin A. Vitamin A (VitA) and, more specifically, its principal bioactive metabolite retinoic acid, is important in regulating early lung development and alveolar formation, contributing to branching morphogenesis, adequate formation and maintenance of the alveoli type II pneumocyte proliferation and synthesis of surfactant-associated proteins B and C through complex pathways modulating extracellular matrix proteins, most importantly elastin [27]. Recent animal data suggest that IUGR exerts its deleterious effects on lung development and alveolarization in part through disruption of the retinol pathway [45]. In extremely low-birth-weight humans (ELBW), postnatal intramuscular VitA supplementation reduces the incidence of BPD or death significantly, albeit slightly [2,46]. In a recent meta-analysis of four trials, VitA supplementation for ELBW showed significant benefits in oxygen dependency at the postmenstrual age of 36 weeks in survivors (841 infants, pooled risk ratio, 0.88) and length of hospital stay [4]. In a large RCT, antenatal oral VitA supplementation in vitamin-deficient mothers resulted in improved lung functional tests in offspring with 9–13 years follow-up compared to controls, indicating the longstanding beneficial potential of VitA for the fetus and newborn [3]. High pharmacy costs of intramuscular VitA preparations and the high number needed to treat have led certain neonatal intensive care units not to adopt this regimen; however, VitA prophylaxis may prevent BPD-related morbidity throughout infancy and childhood, and thus lead to numerous other long-term potential health benefits [47]. Disruption of the retinol pathway by genetic variants is a major contributor of congenital diaphragmatic hernia (CDH) [48]. Single-gene mutations or large genomic alterations may be involved in the non-isolated forms or subtle primary or secondary gene alterations in the isolated forms [49]. In a Japanese observational cohort, maternal dietary intake of VitA during pregnancy was inversely associated with congenital diaphragmatic hernia [50], suggesting that prenatal VitA supplementation may contribute to preventing this severe pulmonary disease.

Vitamin D. The role of vitamin D (VitD) in non-skeletal health is increasingly recognized. Vitamin D plays relevant roles in placental development, in lung maturation processes and in the development of the innate and adaptive immune systems, and thus has the potential to influence neonatal lung pathophysiology through these various fundamental mechanisms. VitD receptor expression in the lung peaks in late gestation in animals, highlighting the role of vitamin D in alveolar maturation. VitD promotes AECII differentiation, enhances surfactant phospholipid and SP-B biosynthesis and stimulates surfactant release; in addition, VitD may be involved in postnatal lung growth and alveolarization, but evidence is limited (for review, see [51]). Preterm babies have lower levels of 25-OH-vitD at birth and are at a higher risk than term infants for postnatal deficiency due to intestinal immaturity and co-morbidities, which theoretically puts them at risk of acute and ch ronic lung disease [52]. However, the clinical impact of VitD on prematurity-related lung disease is not clear so far, with only a few studies linking RDS with VitD insufficiency (125-OH VitD 2–20 ng/mL) or deficiency (<12 ng/mL) [53,54]. Some epidemiological studies have associated neonatal hypovitaminosis D with risk of wheezing, asthma and respiratory tract infections later in infancy [55]. A prospective observational study correlating cord blood and 36-weeks corrected age 25OH-vitD levels in extremely preterm infants with odds of BPD failed to show any association, although most enrolled subjects did not reach vitamin D insufficiency levels (30/33 ng/mL at birth in the BPD and no-BPD groups, respectively) [56]. Interestingly, a similar study conducted in another environment with low/insufficient maternal and neonatal levels yielded opposite results (i.e., a significant correlation between maternal and neonatal levels between BPD/noBPD groups (19/28 and 15/7 ng/mL, respectively) [57]). One small RCT showed no difference in RDS or BPD in extremely preterm infants receiving low- or high-dose VitD supplementation [5]. Regarding the role of VitD on immunity, in one large RCT, 28–36 week preterm infants receiving high-dose VitD for six months had less wheezing than low-dose controls (OR 0.66) [6]. Altogether, these studies suggest that vitamin D insufficiency plays a role in BPD, but no clear evidence has emerged so far regarding the benefits and modalities of VitD supplementation for the purpose of neonatal lung disease prevention.

Vitamin E. Vitamin E (VitE) influences fetal growth and early lung development [58] and is a potent antioxidant, but its relevance in preterm lung disease and the effects of supplementation are unclear to date. In a murine model of CDH and lung hypoplasia, maternal supplementation of α- and γ-tocopherol have led to increased lung complexity, accelerated alveolar growth and increased air surface [59]. In premature infants with respiratory distress syndrome, lower levels of VitE were associated with increased risk of developing BPD [60]. Unfortunately, trials of regular- and high-dose VitE supplementation in very low birth-weight infants showed variable results for BPD prevention and, potentially, an increased risk of sepsis and necrotizing enterocolitis. A Cochrane meta-analysis of these same studies reported no association between VitE and BPD, although wide confidence intervals suggest that these studies, even combined, are underpowered for drawing definitive conclusions [7]. However, none of these trials were conducted after 1991, and the nature and epidemiology of BPD has since profoundly evolved. No human trial has investigated antenatal supplementation and neonatal outcomes so far (for review, see [61]).

3. Lung Disease Mechanisms and Nutrients

3.1. Fetal Growth and Lung Development

In a large prospective cohort of very premature, very low-birth-weight neonates, intrauterine growth restriction increased the risk of death and BPD up to fourfold [62] through various mechanisms including impaired vascular and alveolar development [63] independently from RDS and acute lung disease severity [62]. These findings were confirmed, among others, in another large epidemiological study on extremely low gestational age neonates (the Extremely Low Gestational Age Newborn ELGAN study) in which the incidence of BPD was 74% vs. 49% in infants with z scores < -1 and ≥ -1 respectively, with an odd ratio of 3.2, showing the primordial importance of IUGR on BPD pathogenesis [64]. The relative contribution of impaired substrate and oxygen delivery in IUGR is unclear, as well as their specific contribution in BPD pathogenesis. IUGR-related placental dysfunction translates into significantly decreased expression and activity of the amino-acid system A and system L transporters, of lipoprotein lipase and of lipoprotein receptors, but not of the glucose transporters GLUT1-4, which is either unaltered or increased [65]. In a mouse IUGR model combining altered diet and stress, alveolar simplification similar to BPD and decreased expression of the vascular endothelial growth factor (VEGF) pathway were observed, reflecting disrupted airway and vascular development [66].

3.2. Respiratory Distress Syndrome (RDS) and Surfactant Dysfunction

Surfactant is a complex mixture of lipids (90%) and four specific proteins (10%), surfactant proteins-A (SP-A), -B, -C and -D (10%). Of the surfactant lipids, 80–90% are phospholipids, the most abundant of which is the phosphatidylcholine (PC) class, the di-saturated dipalmitoylhosphatidylcholine (DPPC) and other phospholipids with saturated fatty acids in the one and two position of the glycerol moiety being the most critical for surfactant tension-active properties [67]. Glycerol is the main substrate for PC synthesis in the early neonatal period, when its concentration in circulation increases markedly, whereas later in life, glucose is the major source [68]. The fatty acids of surfactant phospholipids are synthesized in type II cells, taken up from the blood or derived from recycling.

Primary surfactant deficiency due to alveolar epithelium immaturity is the cause of respiratory distress syndrome of prematurity (RDS). In adults and children, qualitative or quantitative surfactant dysfunction plays a major role in acute respiratory distress syndrome (ARDS), affecting phospholipids and surfactant-specific proteins associated with extensive lung tissue inflammation. The same secondary surfactant inactivation also exists in several post-natal conditions both in term and preterm infants, such as meconium aspiration syndrome, sepsis, pulmonary hemorrhage and others [69]. A delayed-onset surfactant dysfunction associated with transient SP-B deficiency has been observed in preterm infants with severe RDS protracted beyond the first week of life [70], highlighting the importance of postnatal surfactant disruption in the pathogenesis of BPD.

IUGR also leads to surfactant dysfunction at birth. In an experimental placental reduction model (global oxygen/substrate depletion), the expression of SP-A, -B, and -C protein and mRNA was reduced in growth-restricted fetal animals compared to controls at ages corresponding to severe and late prematurity in humans [71]. Interestingly, IUGR induction by maternal hypoxia yielded divergent effects, increasing the levels of many hypoxia-inducible genes in the fetus including SP-B and -D as well as ABCA3, a lamellar body phospholipid carrier, and aquaporin-4, which is in part responsible for the airway absorption of fetal lung fluid at birth [34]. Maternal undernutrition during late gestation directly affects surfactant lipid levels in the immediate postnatal period and alters lung structural development [72] as well as decreasing the surfactant pool size [73]. Together, these results illustrate a specific role of fetal nutritional deficiency in IUGR-related respiratory complications in humans.

Maternal diabetes mellitus and excessive fetal carbohydrate exposure alters surfactant synthesis in term and near-term infants. Animals born from induced-DM mothers show impaired lung development and maturation, with decreased expression of surfactant proteins B and C and their regulatory factor FOXA2 associated with inducible nitric oxide synthase induction and generation of reactive oxygen species [74], a possible mechanism explaining respiratory failure in infants of diabetic mothers.

The composition of dietary fats plays a role in RDS and ARDS. In a model of endotoxin-triggered ARDS, adult animals fed with an unsaturated fatty acid diet (either LA or fish-oil) showed more severe vascular congestion, intra-alveolar edema and alveolar septa thickening than those fed with a saturated fatty acid diet (palmitate), suggesting that different substrates may influence lung pathophysiology through different mechanisms [40]. In animal models of premature lung disease, maternal DHA supplementation improved lung growth and enhanced fetal surfactant composition and synthesis [75].

The specific protein fraction of surfactant is also dependent on dietary substrates. Maternal protein intake may directly affect surfactant protein synthesis. Surfactant protein-A (SP-A) levels in the fetal lungs and amniotic fluid from protein-malnourished pregnant rats are lower than in those with normal protein intake [76]. Prenatal and postnatal serum SP-D concentrations are higher in IUGR newborns than in controls, inversely correlating with birthweight percentiles [77] and potentially reflecting the well-established intrauterine hypercortisolemia characterizing the IUGR state rather than specific protein intake deficiency.

Inositol, a key component of membrane phospholipids originating from diet or endogenous synthesis, is contained in high concentration in colostrum and breast milk. In a 1992 RCT, parenteral administration of inositol to premature infants 26–32 weeks with RDS significantly increased the odds of survival without BPD (71% vs. 55%) [14]. However, these results were not confirmed in subsequent studies, and a recent Cochrane meta-analysis encompassing 1177 infants concluded in not recommending its use [15].

3.3. Pulmonary Vascular Disease

Pulmonary arterial hypertension is a major factor contributing to morbidity and mortality in BPD [78] and other forms of neonatal chronic lung disease such as CDH [79]. Recent animal studies show that postnatal malnutrition associated with hyperoxia induces right ventricle and pulmonary arterial remodeling in growth-restricted pups [80]. Interestingly, the same authors showed that intestinal dysbiosis is associated with postnatal malnutrition in this model, and that probiotic supplementation prevents the onset of pulmonary hypertension in the growth-restricted group [81]. In a mouse model of hyperoxia-induced BPD, maternal DHA supplementation resulted in reduced inflammation and decreased pulmonary vascular disease [82] in the offspring. In a retrospective cohort of 138 infants born <28 weeks, the birth-weight-for-gestational age ration was a strong independent predictor of pulmonary hypertension in those with moderate-to-severe BPD, with an odd ratio of 4.2 in the <25th percentile group [83], highlighting the importance of antenatal substrate supply in the fetal onset of pulmonary vascular disease.

3.4. *Inflammation and BPD*

Bronchopulmonary dysplasia (BPD), the main cause of chronic lung disease and respiratory morbidity and morbidity in preterm infants, is characterized by impaired alveolar and vascular development determined by a combination of genetic factors [1], antenatal exposures and postnatal insults to the developing lung, with a central role played by inflammation (Figure 1). BPD most strongly correlates with lower gestational age [84], and low maternal DHA levels are associated with premature birth [85]. In a simplified view, ω-6 FA are pro-inflammatory whereas ω-3 FA are anti-inflammatory. ω-3 FA, found in fish oil, in particular DHA, are capable of partly inhibiting many aspects of inflammation including leucocyte chemotaxis, adhesion molecule expression and leucocyte–endothelial adhesive interactions, production of eicosanoids like prostaglandins and leukotrienes from the ω-6 FA arachidonic acid and production of pro-inflammatory cytokines. Enriching diets with DHA can change the inflammatory balance, modulating cell function and suppressing inflammatory responses [86]. In a retrospective observational study in preterm infants <30 weeks of gestation, decreased DHA levels in the first weeks of life were associated with an increased risk of BPD [8]. In a multicenter prospective randomized control trial (RCT) aimed at comparing neurological outcomes in maternal breast milk-fed preterm infants <33 weeks of gestation whose mothers had received either a high- or standard-DHA diet (the DHA for the Improvement of Neurodevelopmental Outcome in preterm infants DINO trial [87]), a lower incidence of BPD was observed in the high-DHA diet group for some subsets of cases (males and for <1250 g infants) [88]. These preliminary human data led to an adequately targeted and powered RCT involving over 1200 infants <29 weeks (the N3RO trial), which, surprisingly, showed no benefit of postnatal DHA supplementation for BPD prevention [43]. These contrasting data illustrate the complexity of the interactions between lipid nutrients and the developing lung, supporting the need for further translational research and clinical trials.

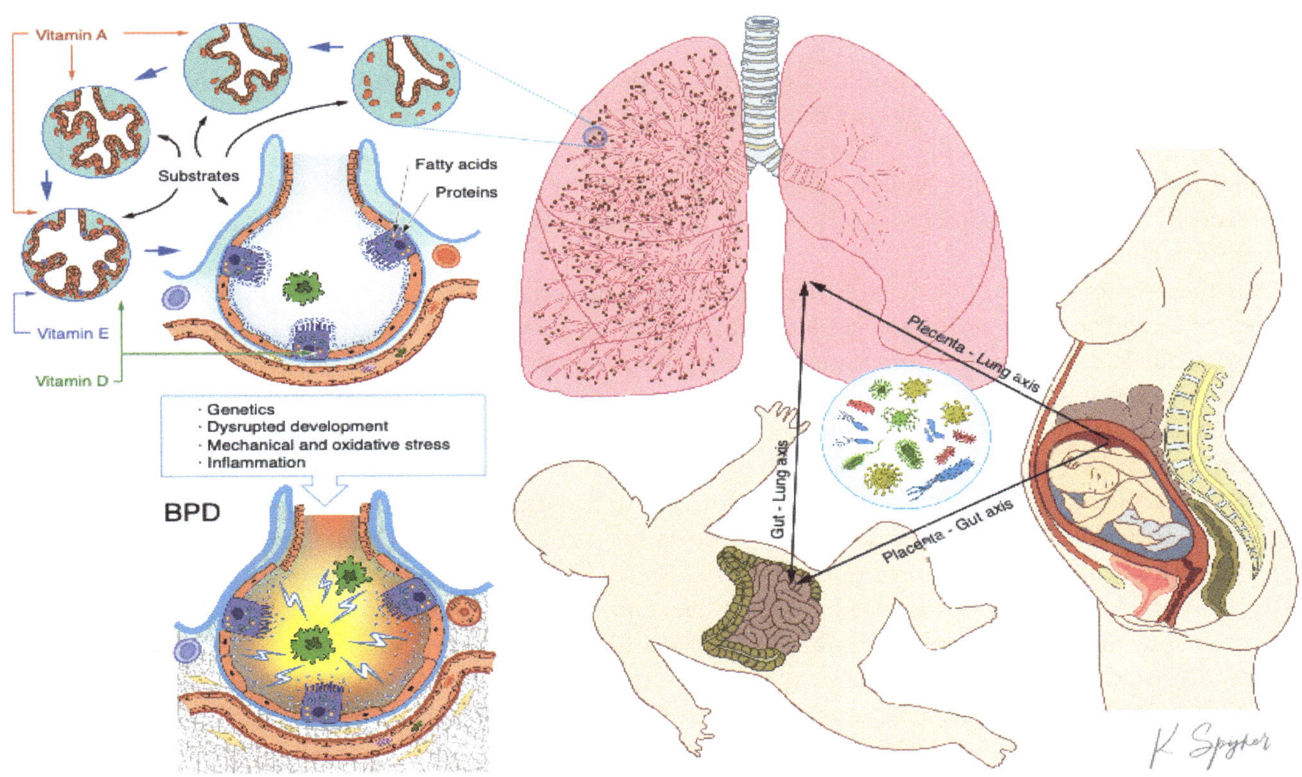

Figure 1. The placenta-gut-lung triangle. The figure illustrates the potential sources of the lung microbiome and the role of substrate supplies and specific nutrients in alveolar homeostasis, and their role in the pathway towards chronic lung disease.

Lactoferrin, an iron-binding glycoprotein secreted by many epithelial cells and contained at high concentration in breastmilk (~1 mg/mL) with various antimicrobial properties, is a key component of innate immunity together with defensins, IgA and other peptides [89]. Supplementation with bovine lactoferrin, which is 70% analogue to human, significantly decreased late-onset sepsis and necrotizing enterocolitis but not BPD in preterm infants [90]. Six subsequent trials, meta-analyzed in a 2017 Cochrane review, confirmed these findings acknowledging low-quality results and the need for better data [16]. Subsequently, a recent multicenter, adequately powered RCT including 2203 infants <34 weeks (the Enteral Lactoferrin supplementation For very preterm INfants ELFIN trial) showed no difference in any of the measured morbidities, including necrotizing enterocolitis (NEC), late onset sepsis and BPD [17], dismissing lactoferrin for BPD prevention.

4. Microbiomics of the Lungs—The Gut-Lung Axis in BPD

All the microorganisms inhabiting the body (both symbiotic and pathogenic) are defined as microbiota, whereas the whole genome of all the microbial communities that colonize the body are referred to as the microbiome. The number of microbial cells is 10 times more the number of human cells. Furthermore, the number of bacterial genes is more than 100 times that of human genes. Microbiota have a pivotal role in the development of the immune system and the metabolic homeostasis of their host.

Most of the microorganisms that inhabit the human body do not grow in vitro, and therefore the whole microbiome could be thoroughly explored only when high-throughput genomic sequencing technologies became available. The Human Microbiome Project [91] was launched in 2008 by the National Institute of Health with the goal of characterizing the entire bacterial community colonizing the human body. This would allow the determination of whether there was an association between microbiome alterations and the onset of specific diseases.

In neonatology, most microbiome studies have focused on the relation of necrotizing enterocolitis with a particular microbiome [92,93]. It is now clear that there is a strict association between the type of microbial community of the gut and the risk of developing NEC. Indeed, in order to prevent the development of NEC it is now recommended to provide probiotics as soon as possible, so to restore a beneficial commensal flora [22]. Contrarily, the lower respiratory tract of healthy individuals was considered sterile in the past. Nevertheless, the presence of a resident microbial community in healthy lungs recently emerged, and research currently focuses on correlating particular lung microbiome profiles with disease.

Studies exploring the neonatal lung microbiome have mostly used bronchoalveolar lavage fluid samples or lung biopsies acquired via surgical sterile explants. In older children and adults, the lung microbiota has been defined in various pulmonary diseases, such as cystic fibrosis, asthma or chronic obstructive pulmonary disease [94]. In the preterm infant, a specific lung microbiome is present from the first days of life, and is dominated by *staphylococcus* and *ureaplasma* species [26]. At first clinicians considered fetal lungs to be sterile, and the acquisition of a microbial community in the lungs was attributed to a colonization occurring in the immediate post-delivery period, depending on the mode of delivery. Intuitively, vaginally delivered infants would acquire bacterial communities resembling the microbial vaginal environment (*Lactobacillus, Prevotella*), whereas C-section infants would acquire mostly skin microbiota (*Staphylococcus, Corynebacterium, Propionibacterium*) [95]. Actually, the immature lung's microbiome origin is controversial. Several studies have shown that airway bacterial colonization is already detectable at birth, suggesting an antenatal origin [25]. When bacterial DNA sequencing techniques became widely available, the detection of microbiota in the placenta, amniotic fluid and fetus became possible both in mice and human [96–98], challenging the concept of the sterile womb. One human study reported the presence of DNA from the common intestinal bacteria *Lactobacillus* and *Bifidobacterium* in placental biopsies collected at term after an elective C-section without rupture of membranes or chorioamnionitis [99]. Very recently, combining metagenomic shotgun sequencing and targeted 16S techniques, Al Alam et al. demonstrated the presence of diverse and overlapping taxa in placenta, lung and intestine from 31 human fetuses harvested from 10 to 18 weeks of gestation [100]. However, a recent study based on placenta samples from two large cohorts of complicated and uncomplicated pregnancies showed that most bacterial signatures were acquired during labor and delivery or resulted from technical contamination, with the exception of the pathogen *Streptococcus agalactiae*, which was observed in 5% of pre-labor placentas [101,102], as echoed by others [103].

After birth, maternal breastfeeding influences the colonization and maturation of an infant's intestinal microbiome, depending on early or late lactation stage, gestational age, maternal health and mode of delivery (Figure 1). The same *Bifidobacterium* and *Lactobacillus* strains identified in an infant's gut microbiome are also found in mother's milk, indicating that breastfeeding is a postnatal route of mother–child microbial exchange. However, the origin of these microbes, the complex dynamics of their transmission and their site specificities remain to be determined [104].

Can lung microbiota influence lung diseases? Inflammation can predispose to BPD, and lower respiratory tract infections are a recognized inflammatory trigger [105]. Thus, it is foreseeable that certain bacterial infections can predispose to BPD. For example, *Ureaplasma urealyticum* infections have been associated with the development of BPD [26,106]. Indeed, several small RCTs of postnatal prophylactic macrolide therapy in preterm infants for BPD prevention have been conducted, showing some efficacy in a meta-analysis [107].

Is the susceptibility to developing BPD only associated with pathogenic bacteria, or also with dysbiosis? In fact, it is been demonstrated that neonates with a reduced diversity of the lung microbiome have an increased risk of developing BPD [108]. In their systematic review, Pammi et al. evaluated six studies relating the lung microbiome with BPD development [26]. Infants who would later develop BPD had a different concentration of *Proteobacteria* and *Firmicutes*, a reduced number of *Lactobacilli* and an increased microbial turnover in the first weeks of life compared to those with no BPD. Since lactobacilli have established anti-inflammatory properties [109], such BPD predisposition could result in part from a shift to predominantly pro-inflammatory taxa. Lal et al. studied the airway microbiome at birth in 23 preterm infants (10 evolving to BPD and 13 not) and found that *Lactobacilli* were less abundant at birth in preterm neonates predisposed to BPD [110]. They then compared the microbiome examined at birth with the microbiome examined after diagnosis of BPD and found a subsequent increase in *Proteobacteria* phylum (with a predominance of *enterobacteriaceae*) and a decrease in the *Firmicutes* and *Fusobacteria* phyla. Lactobacilli were also less abundant in neonates born from mothers with chorioamnionitis. The composition of the fecal microbiota in a recent cohort of infants born at <29 weeks and diagnosed with BPD had significant differences in the relative abundance of *Klebsiella*, *Salmonella*, *Escherichia/Shigella* and *Bifidobacterium* species associated with down-regulation of immune-related genes by transcriptome sequencing analysis [111]. Lal et al. described an alternative mechanism by investigating pulmonary metabolome and correlating it with the microbiome [112]. The authors compared bronchoalveolar fluid samples of 30 preterm neonates at birth with and without BPD, showing an increase in *Proteobacteria* and a reduction in *Lactobacilli* associated with a decrease in the ratio acetyl-CoA/propionyl-CoA carboxylase, indicating a reduced fatty acid β-oxidation pathway and an increase in airway inflammation in the BPD group. Targeting specific microbiomes that lead to the metabolomic changes contributing to BPD with specific antimicrobial therapies could represent a novel preventive or therapeutic approach. Nevertheless, attempts made to decrease *Ureaplasma urealyticum* colonization by antibiotic prophylaxis did not result in the reduction of BPD rates [113].

5. Host and Microbiome Genetic Factors

Early small fingerprinting-based twin studies showed a greater similarity of microbiota in monozygotic vs heterozygotic twins [114], suggesting an influence of the host's genetic background, but these results were not confirmed in 16S rRNA sequencing studies. Animal studies comparing microbiome diversity in different mouse strains showed that environmental factors were stronger determinants than the genetic background. Quantitative trait locus (QTL) analysis identified immunity-related genes influencing relative abundance of certain microbiota species, such as IRAK3 (regulating the toll-like receptor pathway), LYZ1/2, IFNγ and IL22. Single-gene approaches have identified the role of immune genes (MEFV, MYD88, NOD2, defensin-encoding genes, RELMB, HLA genes, the IgA locus), and metabolic genes (APOA1-encoding apolipoprotein, LEP and LEPR-encoding leptin and its receptor) (for review, see [115]). Subsequent host and microbiota genome-wide association studies (GWAS) confirmed the importance of immune gene variants (HLA-DRA, TLR1) but yielded divergent results, supporting the need for more omics research in this field [116].

6. Mechanisms Involved in the Placenta-Gut-Lung Cross-Talk

6.1. Antenatal Reciprocal Lung-Placenta Signaling

There is a subtle balance between maternal tolerance of the fetal immune system and resistance towards pathogens susceptible to infect the amnion and lead to premature labor and various neonatal morbidities, in which the genital tract microbiome plays a key role [117]. The transplacental mechanisms through which maternal taxonomy translates into the offspring is still poorly understood. Microbial metabolites may play a role in this exchange (see below).

Exosomes have emerged as mediators of cell-to-cell, organ-to-organ and system-to-system cross talk. Arterial cord blood obtained from neonates born at term after spontaneous labor compared to term and preterm cesarean-section-born infants, was shown to contain high levels of exosome-embedded complement component 4B-binding protein alpha chain (C4BPA). C'BPA originating from the fetal lung turns on several pro-labor placental genes such as corticotropin-releasing hormone (CRH), cyclo-oxygenase 2 (COX-2) and pro-inflammatory cytokines (TNFα, IL1, IL6, IL8) through CD40 interaction and NFκB activation [118]. A similar fetal–maternal interaction was demonstrated in mice by the induction of parturition through lung-derived steroid receptor coactivators 1 and 2 (SRC-1, -2) endogenous steroid pathway activation [119]. Preterm infant's early dysbiosis, characterized by the predominance of gram-negative, potentially pathogenic *gammaproteobacteria,* is strongly associated with antenatal exogenous steroids exposure as well as inflammation [120]. Taken together, these studies suggest that the fetal/neonatal lung has the capacity of influencing the establishment and development of local and remote microbiomes, a process in which exosomes may play a key role.

6.2. Postnatal Immunity and Microbiomes

Respiratory and digestive mucosal surfaces are part of an integrated network of tissues, cells and effectors that constitute a global immunological organ in which stimulation of one compartment can lead to changes in distal areas. Oral, intestinal, airway and genital mucosae are interconnected through circulating lymphocytes [121]. The exposure to specific antigens, sensed by local dendritic cells, shape future immune response such as Th1 vs. Th2, with a longstanding impact on the health and diseases of the subject [122], a process in which the nature and composition of local microbiomes play a central role. As microbiota in each compartment have an influence on immune system development, the immune system plays a role in shaping and maintaining microbial communities, as demonstrated in germ-free zebrafish and mice [123]. A bilateral, immune-mediated gut-lung interaction shaping the respective microbiomes and influencing the health/disease balance in each organ is therefore plausible, but remains to be demonstrated in human neonates [124].

Bacterial metabolites and lung immune homeostasis: Gut microbiota generate metabolites during food assimilation that have direct effects on lung immune homeostasis (for review, see [125]). Among these, short chain fatty acids (SCFAs), in particular acetate, propionate and butyrate, reach the systemic circulation from the intestinal lymphatic system and modulate the lung immune balance. SCFAs promote regulatory T-cell generation and function through free fatty acid receptor 2 and 3 (FFAR 2/3) binding and histone deacetylase (HDAc) inhibition [126]. Mice with vancomycin-induced intestinal dysbiosis showing exacerbated Th-2 responses leading to allergic lung inflammation have been rescued by dietary SCFAs through attenuation of dendritic cell activation via programmed death ligand 1 (PD-L1) and decreased Immunoglobulin E (IgE) and interleukin 4 production [127]. Tryptophan metabolites generated by the intestinal microbiome, especially the lactobacillus genus, are natural ligands for the aryl hydrocarbon receptor (AhR), which in turn promotes regulatory T-cell development via interleukin 22 production [86]. In a human RCT of adults with emphysema, azithromycin treatment decreased intestinal microbiome diversity leading to increased bacterial metabolites such as glycolic acid, indol-3-acetate and linoleic acid, and reduced chemokine (C-X-C) ligand 1 (CXCL1), TNF)α, interleukin 13 and IL-12p40 in bronchoalveolar lavage fluid [128]. The role of these recently identified bioactive bacterial metabolites in neonatal lung disease are still to be unveiled.

6.3. Impact of Antibiotic Exposure

The wide exposure of infants to broad-spectrum antibiotics in the perinatal and neonatal periods has profound effects on microbiota. In a mouse BPD model, perinatal maternal antibiotic exposure increased pulmonary fibrosis, vascular remodeling, alveolar inflammation and mortality in offspring through disruption of commensal intestinal colonization, demonstrating a key role of the gut-lung axis [129]. Antenatal exposure to antibiotics can also influence a mother's gut microbiota [130]. In a similar way, maternal chorioamnionitis can negatively influence neonatal gut microbiota and outcome. Puri at al. studied the fecal microbiome of 106 preterm infants ≤28 weeks [131]. Neonates born to mothers with chorioamnionitis had a higher abundance of *Bacteroides* and *Fusobacteria* in fecal samples, and were at higher risk of sepsis or death. Recently, a large meta-analysis showed that BPD, not RDS, is strongly associated with maternal chorioamnionitis [132]. Considering that women with chorioamnionitis almost invariably receive broad-spectrum antibiotics, the majority of their fetuses are exposed. Therefore, we can speculate that not only inflammation but also dysbiosis contributes to the higher risk of BPD associated with chorioamnionitis. The Canadian Healthy Infant Longitudinal Development CHILD study, a prospective cohort study of Canadian infants followed up over a period of two years, found that that an infant's gut microbiota is persistently altered after intrapartum antibiotic prophylaxis exposure [133]. Does the dysbiosis induced postnatally by broad-spectrum antibiotics have an impact on the course of late-onset infectious disease? A retrospective paired cohort study comparing clinical courses in preterm infants with NEC suggests it's not the case, showing no difference between those receiving probiotics vs those not [19]. Antibiotic-induced alterations of physiological gut microflora have been shown to last into adulthood [134]. A recent RCT on peripartum maternal antibiotics prophylaxis, demonstrating that azithromycin in addition to the standard cephalosporin regimen for women undergoing non-elective cesarean section decreased the risk of post-operative wound infections and other infectious complications, led to a broader fetal exposure to macrolides in the USA, but failed to address short-term pulmonary effects and long-term respiratory outcomes in newborns [135]. Some studies suggest that macrolides have beneficial short-term effects on lung disease of prematurity. Given the prevalence of *ureaplasma* species in chorioamnionitis and its suspected role in BPD, adding azithromycin to the standard antibiotic regimen in women with PPROM <28 weeks of gestation improves perinatal respiratory outcomes and the BPD risk [136]. However, the lasting impact of the microbiome is still poorly understood, and potentially significant. In a large Finnish cohort study, penicillin in early life had only a transient effect on intestinal microbiota, whereas macrolides correlated with substantial, long-standing shifts from normally dominant Gram-positive phyla to Gram-negative species [137]. This alteration was associated with asthma and obesity in children aged two to seven years. Therefore, the benefits and risks of perinatal broad-spectrum antibiotics, including macrolides, should be carefully investigated and weighed in future strategies.

The use of postnatal antibiotics reportedly modifies the existing flora, and reduced microbiome diversity is associated to BPD predisposition. In fact, antibiotic exposure in the first two weeks of life is associated with increased BPD rate and severity [138]. Broad-spectrum antibiotics increase the risk of multi-resistant bacterial infection, which in turn is associated with a twofold increase in BPD [139]. Furthermore, preterm infants with negative cultures exposed to more than five days of antibiotics have shown an increased BPD rate [140,141]. The Surveillance and Correction Of Unnecessary antibiotic

Therapy SCOUT study, a multicenter observational study on antibiotic use in NICUs, showed that the majority of antibiotics are administered empirically and without clear evidence of infection [142].

Beyond antibiotics, other medications such as postnatal steroids influence the taxonomy and longitudinal development of microbiomes after birth. Grier et al. showed that steroids used for BPD prevention or treatment significantly altered the abundance of *bifidobacterium*, a beneficial intestinal genus, in a cohort of preterm infants followed longitudinally over the neonatal period [143]. The same authors showed that the lung and gut microbioma have distinct compositions, but develop in a tightly interdependent manner [144].

6.4. Acting on the Airway Microbiome

Conversely, would restoring a beneficial airway microbiome be a valid strategy for BPD prevention and treatment? Since the major source of microorganisms is the intestine, it is intuitive that the intestinal microbiome should translate into the lung microbiome, a hypothesis supported by some animal data [145]. Probiotics are live micro-organisms that, when administered in adequate amounts, confer a health benefit to the host. They exert a beneficial effect mostly by decreasing colonization and invasion by pathogenic organisms and by modifying the host immunity. Probiotic supplementation has proven to be effective for NEC prevention [22]. Animal studies have shown that enteral administration of probiotics impacts the respiratory microbiome [146], but no human studies have examined the effect of probiotic supplementation on the development of BPD as a primary outcome. Villamor-Martinez et al. conducted a systematic meta-analysis of 15 randomized trials on probiotics for NEC prevention and analyzed whether BPD incidence was affected in these studies [23]. While the meta-analysis confirmed a significant reduction of NEC (risk ratio (RR) 0.52, 95% confidence interval (CI) 0.33 to 0.81, $p = 0.004$), no significant effect on BPD could be demonstrated. In fact, every organ has a particular microbiome, and a probiotic beneficial for one system may not be for another. It is now accepted that differential bacterial strains of the same genus and species can have different effects on the host depending on the site of action. Therefore, every probiotic must be studied in order to act in a particular milieu [147]. The question whether intratracheal probiotic administration would improve respiratory outcomes in adults hospitalized in intensive care units is currently the object of a large RCT in Canada, the Prevention Of Severe Pneumonia and Endotracheal Colonization PROSPECT Trial [148]. If positive, this could represent an innovative approach for BPD prevention. In brief, modeling the lung microbiome is a potential alley for preventing BPD, but the modalities still have to be determined and properly tested.

7. Human Milk

Human milk plays a protective role towards the immature lung through various mechanisms including specific nutrients and factors, and through its influence on microbiota. A recent meta-analysis including 22 studies (17 cohort plus 5 RCTs) and 8661 infants [149] showed a trend towards a protective effect of human milk against BPD, calling for larger RCTs the determine a definite answer, which would undoubtedly raise ethical questions given its proven benefits in other diseases of prematurity such as necrotizing enterocolitis. In addition, differences exist between fresh maternal breast milk (MBM) and pasteurized human donor milk (DBM). In the largest meta-analysis to date based on 4984 infants, with 1416 BPD cases [150], there was a significant reduction of BPD incidence in exclusively MBM-fed infants compared with exclusive formula-fed (RR 0.74; 95% CI 0.57–0.96). Conversely, the same authors showed a trend but failed to formally demonstrate the same benefit comparing exclusive DBM and formula for BPD prevention (RR 0.89; CI 0.60–1.32), but suggested a protective effect of MBM vs. DBM (RR 0.77; 95% CI 0.62–0.96), even though the quality of evidence is low [18].

Many factors contribute to direct protective effects of MBM against prematurity co-morbidities, including specific macronutrients such as whey proteins, milk fat globules (MFG) and their specific lipids and membranes (MGFM), phosphoproteins and glycosylated proteins, oligosaccharides and many others [151]. In addition, antimicrobial factors such as lactoferrin, leucocytes, secretory IgA, complement factors, cytokines, lactoferrin and lysozyme play a fundamental immunomodulating role [152]. As recently discovered, human milk exosomes containing microRNA and other epigenetic factors interact with gene transcription and exert longstanding effects on gut homeostasis [153]. Pasteurization, which is considered a standard for DBM out of concerns for the transmission of infectious agents such as cytomegalovirus, Human Immunodeficiency Virus and Herpes Simplex Virus, inactivates many microcomponents and compromises its bactericidal and immunomodulating properties [152]. Alternative methods are currently under development, but have not reached prime time in the NICUs and DBM banks so far [154].

After birth, MBM promotes the colonization of the infant digestive tract and the development of the early microbiome [104] through various mechanisms. Bacteria are specific to the mother–infant dyad and the term of the pregnancy. In a 16S rRNA sequencing prospective study in healthy neonates, stable airway microbiomes characterized by predominant *moraxella* and *corynebacterium* species were associated with early breastfeeding and lower rates of infections in infancy [155]. Specific human milk oligosaccharides (HMOs), non-digestible prebiotics, act by promoting the development of *bifidobacteria* and *bacteroidetes*, which may have a beneficial effect on respiration and immunity. Indeed, HMO addition in formula provides protection against bronchiolitis in term infants [20]. However, HMO composition and concentration are significantly different in preterm compared to term breastmilk [156], and the effects of HMO on gut maturation and prevention of necrotizing enterocolitis appear to be age-dependent and uncertain in premature infants [21]. Up to now, evidence has been lacking indicating that early HMO supplementation has any beneficial effects in the preterm infant lung [21]. The influence of human milk nutrition on the airway microbiome in preterm infants and its potential effects in BPD prevention is still an open question.

8. Conclusions

Macro- and micronutrients have a profound influence on premature lung health and disease, raising the question of whether nutrition experts should be involved more systematically in neonatal intensive care teams. As bronchopulmonary dysplasia is a heterogeneous and multifactorial disease, single-bullet approaches have mostly failed to achieve significant progress. From this perspective, it is not surprising that a "simple" nutritional approach such as exclusive human milk feeding has shown an efficacy comparable to single-target drugs. The evidence of a neonatal lung microbiome playing a key role in RDS and BPD establishes new directions for prevention and therapeutic interventions, yet its origin, the dynamics of its establishment, its evolution and its interactions with the environment and its relationship with health maintenance and disease are still under intense investigation. The emerging concept of a placenta-gut-lung triangle should govern future research efforts, with the goal of preventing and potentially reversing the course of chronic lung disease of prematurity and preventing its lifelong consequences.

Author Contributions: F.P. and O.D. conceptualized and drafted the manuscript. B.V.G. contributed on microbiome-related studies review and discussion, C.H. contributed on effects on lung diseases. F.P. and O.D. finalized the manuscript and its revisions. All authors have read and agreed to the published version of the manuscript.

Acknowledgments: Karin Spijker made the illustration.

Abbreviations

LCPUFA	long chain polyinsaturatyed fatty acid
HMO	human milk oligosaccharide
BPD	bronchopulmonary dysplasia
RTI	respiratory tract infection
DHA	docosahexenoic acid
AA	arachidonic acid
NEC	necrotizing enterocolitis
LOS	late-onset sepsis
META	meta-analysis
MBM	maternal breast milk
DBM	donor breast milk
RCT	randomized controlled trial
RDS	respiratory distress syndrome
R	recommended
NR	not recommended

References

1. Hamvas, A.; Feng, R.; Bi, Y.; Wang, F.; Bhattacharya, S.; Mereness, J.; Kaushal, M.; Cotten, C.M.; Ballard, P.L.; Mariani, T.J.; et al. Exome sequencing identifies gene variants and networks associated with extreme respiratory outcomes following preterm birth. *BMC Genet.* **2018**, *19*, 94. [CrossRef] [PubMed]
2. Tyson, J.E.; Wright, L.L.; Oh, W.; Kennedy, K.A.; Mele, L.; Ehrenkranz, R.A.; Stoll, B.J.; Lemons, J.A.; Stevenson, D.K.; Bauer, C.R.; et al. Vitamin A supplementation for extremely-low-birth-weight infants. National Institute of Child Health and Human Development Neonatal Research Network. *N. E. J. Med.* **1999**, *340*, 1962–1968. [CrossRef] [PubMed]
3. Checkley, W.; West, K.P., Jr.; Wise, R.A.; Baldwin, M.R.; Wu, L.; LeClerq, S.C.; Christian, P.; Katz, J.; Tielsch, J.M.; Khatry, S.; et al. Maternal vitamin A supplementation and lung function in offspring. *N. E. J. Med.* **2010**, *362*, 1784–1794. [CrossRef] [PubMed]
4. Araki, S.; Kato, S.; Namba, F.; Ota, E. Vitamin A to prevent bronchopulmonary dysplasia in extremely low birth weight infants: A systematic review and meta-analysis. *PLoS ONE* **2018**, *13*, e0207730. [CrossRef] [PubMed]
5. Fort, P.; Salas, A.A.; Nicola, T.; Craig, C.M.; Carlo, W.A.; Ambalavanan, N. A Comparison of 3 Vitamin D Dosing Regimens in Extremely Preterm Infants: A Randomized Controlled Trial. *J. Pediatrics* **2016**, *174*. [CrossRef]
6. Hibbs, A.M.; Ross, K.; Kerns, L.A.; Wagner, C.; Fuloria, M.; Groh-Wargo, S.; Zimmerman, T.; Minich, N.; Tatsuoka, C. Effect of Vitamin D Supplementation on Recurrent Wheezing in Black Infants Who Were Born Preterm: The D-Wheeze Randomized Clinical Trial. *JAMA* **2018**, *319*, 2086–2094. [CrossRef]
7. Brion, L.P.; Bell, E.F.; Raghuveer, T.S. Vitamin E supplementation for prevention of morbidity and mortality in preterm infants. *Cochrane Database Syst. Rev.* **2003**, CD003665. [CrossRef]
8. Martin, C.R.; Dasilva, D.A.; Cluette-Brown, J.E.; Dimonda, C.; Hamill, A.; Bhutta, A.Q.; Coronel, E.; Wilschanski, M.; Stephens, A.J.; Driscoll, D.F.; et al. Decreased postnatal docosahexaenoic and arachidonic acid blood levels in premature infants are associated with neonatal morbidities. *J. Pediatrics* **2011**, *159*. [CrossRef]
9. Wang, Q.; Zhou, B.; Cui, Q.; Chen, C. Omega-3 Long-chain Polyunsaturated Fatty Acids for Bronchopulmonary Dysplasia: A Meta-analysis. *Pediatrics* **2019**, *144*. [CrossRef]
10. Martin, C.R. Fatty acid requirements in preterm infants and their role in health and disease. *Clin. Perinatol.* **2014**, *41*, 363–382. [CrossRef]

11. Ozkan, H.; Koksal, N.; Dorum, B.A.; Kocael, F.; Ozarda, Y.; Bozyigit, C.; Dogan, P.; Guney Varal, I.; Bagci, O. New-generation fish oil and olive oil lipid for prevention of oxidative damage in preterm infants: Single center clinical trial at university hospital in Turkey. *Pediatrics Int.* **2019**, *61*, 388–392. [CrossRef] [PubMed]
12. Najm, S.; Lofqvist, C.; Hellgren, G.; Engstrom, E.; Lundgren, P.; Hard, A.L.; Lapillonne, A.; Savman, K.; Nilsson, A.K.; Andersson, M.X.; et al. Effects of a lipid emulsion containing fish oil on polyunsaturated fatty acid profiles, growth and morbidities in extremely premature infants: A randomized controlled trial. *Clin. Nutr. ESPEN* **2017**, *20*, 17–23. [CrossRef] [PubMed]
13. Kapoor, V.; Malviya, M.N.; Soll, R. Lipid emulsions for parenterally fed preterm infants. *Cochrane Database Syst. Rev.* **2019**, *6*, CD013163. [CrossRef] [PubMed]
14. Hallman, M.; Bry, K.; Hoppu, K.; Lappi, M.; Pohjavuori, M. Inositol supplementation in premature infants with respiratory distress syndrome. *N. E. J. Med.* **1992**, *326*, 1233–1239. [CrossRef] [PubMed]
15. Howlett, A.; Ohlsson, A.; Plakkal, N. Inositol in preterm infants at risk for or having respiratory distress syndrome. *Cochrane Database Syst. Rev.* **2019**, *7*, CD000366. [CrossRef] [PubMed]
16. Pammi, M.; Suresh, G. Enteral lactoferrin supplementation for prevention of sepsis and necrotizing enterocolitis in preterm infants. *Cochrane Database Syst. Rev.* **2017**, *6*, CD007137. [CrossRef]
17. Griffiths, J.; Jenkins, P.; Vargova, M.; Bowler, U.; Juszczak, E.; King, A.; Linsell, L.; Murray, D.; Partlett, C.; Patel, M.; et al. Enteral lactoferrin supplementation for very preterm infants: A randomised placebo-controlled trial. *Lancet* **2019**, *393*, 423–433. [CrossRef]
18. Villamor-Martinez, E.; Pierro, M.; Cavallaro, G.; Mosca, F.; Kramer, B.W.; Villamor, E. Donor Human Milk Protects against Bronchopulmonary Dysplasia: A Systematic Review and Meta-Analysis. *Nutrients* **2018**, *10*, 238. [CrossRef]
19. Wang, Z.L.; Liu, L.; Hu, X.Y.; Guo, L.; Li, Q.Y.; An, Y.; Jiang, Y.J.; Chen, S.; Wang, X.Q.; He, Y.; et al. Probiotics may not prevent the deterioration of necrotizing enterocolitis from stage I to II/III. *BMC Pediatrics* **2019**, *19*, 185. [CrossRef]
20. Puccio, G.; Alliet, P.; Cajozzo, C.; Janssens, E.; Corsello, G.; Sprenger, N.; Wernimont, S.; Egli, D.; Gosoniu, L.; Steenhout, P. Effects of Infant Formula With Human Milk Oligosaccharides on Growth and Morbidity: A Randomized Multicenter Trial. *J. Pediatric Gastroenterol. Nutr.* **2017**, *64*, 624–631. [CrossRef]
21. Bering, S.B. Human Milk Oligosaccharides to Prevent Gut Dysfunction and Necrotizing Enterocolitis in Preterm Neonates. *Nutrients* **2018**, *10*, 1461. [CrossRef] [PubMed]
22. AlFaleh, K.; Anabrees, J. Probiotics for prevention of necrotizing enterocolitis in preterm infants. *Cochrane Database Syst. Rev.* **2014**, CD005496. [CrossRef]
23. Villamor-Martinez, E.; Pierro, M.; Cavallaro, G.; Mosca, F.; Kramer, B.; Villamor, E. Probiotic Supplementation in Preterm Infants Does Not Affect the Risk of Bronchopulmonary Dysplasia: A Meta-Analysis of Randomized Controlled Trials. *Nutrients* **2017**, *9*, 1197. [CrossRef] [PubMed]
24. Chen, H.J.; Gur, T.L. Intrauterine Microbiota: Missing, or the Missing Link? *Trends Neurosci.* **2019**, *42*, 402–413. [CrossRef] [PubMed]
25. Lal, C.V.; Travers, C.; Aghai, Z.H.; Eipers, P.; Jilling, T.; Halloran, B.; Carlo, W.A.; Keeley, J.; Rezonzew, G.; Kumar, R.; et al. The Airway Microbiome at Birth. *Sci. Rep.* **2016**, *6*, 31023. [CrossRef] [PubMed]
26. Pammi, M.; Lal, C.V.; Wagner, B.D.; Mourani, P.M.; Lohmann, P.; Luna, R.A.; Sisson, A.; Shivanna, B.; Hollister, E.B.; Abman, S.H.; et al. Airway Microbiome and Development of Bronchopulmonary Dysplasia in Preterm Infants: A Systematic Review. *J. Pediatrics* **2019**, *204*, 126–133. [CrossRef]
27. Arigliani, M.; Spinelli, A.M.; Liguoro, I.; Cogo, P. Nutrition and Lung Growth. *Nutrients* **2018**, *10*, 919. [CrossRef]
28. Lio, A.; Rosati, P.; Pastorino, R.; Cota, F.; Tana, M.; Tirone, C.; Aurilia, C.; Ricci, C.; Gambacorta, A.; Paladini, A.; et al. Fetal Doppler velocimetry and bronchopulmonary dysplasia risk among growth-restricted preterm infants: An observational study. *BMJ Open* **2017**, *7*, e015232. [CrossRef]
29. DeRegnier, R.A.; Guilbert, T.W.; Mills, M.M.; Georgieff, M.K. Growth failure and altered body composition are established by one month of age in infants with bronchopulmonary dysplasia. *J. Nutr.* **1996**, *126*, 168–175. [CrossRef]
30. Ehrenkranz, R.A.; Dusick, A.M.; Vohr, B.R.; Wright, L.L.; Wrage, L.A.; Poole, W.K. Growth in the neonatal intensive care unit influences neurodevelopmental and growth outcomes of extremely low birth weight infants. *Pediatrics* **2006**, *117*, 1253–1261. [CrossRef]

31. Agostoni, C.; Buonocore, G.; Carnielli, V.P.; De Curtis, M.; Darmaun, D.; Decsi, T.; Domellof, M.; Embleton, N.D.; Fusch, C.; Genzel-Boroviczeny, O.; et al. Enteral nutrient supply for preterm infants: Commentary from the European Society of Paediatric Gastroenterology, Hepatology and Nutrition Committee on Nutrition. *J. Pediatric Gastroenterol. Nutr.* **2010**, *50*, 85–91. [CrossRef] [PubMed]
32. Mihatsch, W.A.; Braegger, C.; Bronsky, J.; Cai, W.; Campoy, C.; Carnielli, V.; Darmaun, D.; Desci, T.; Domellof, M.; Embleton, N.; et al. ESPGHAN/ESPEN/ESPR/CSPEN guidelines on pediatric parenteral nutrition. *Clin. Nutr.* **2018**, *37*, 2303–2305. [CrossRef]
33. Becquet, O.; El Khabbaz, F.; Alberti, C.; Mohamed, D.; Blachier, A.; Biran, V.; Sibony, O.; Baud, O. Insulin treatment of maternal diabetes mellitus and respiratory outcome in late-preterm and term singletons. *BMJ Open* **2015**, *5*, e008192. [CrossRef] [PubMed]
34. McGillick, E.V.; Lock, M.C.; Orgeig, S.; Morrison, J.L. Maternal obesity mediated predisposition to respiratory complications at birth and in later life: Understanding the implications of the obesogenic intrauterine environment. *Paediatr. Respir. Rev.* **2017**, *21*, 11–18. [CrossRef] [PubMed]
35. Wemhoner, A.; Ortner, D.; Tschirch, E.; Strasak, A.; Rudiger, M. Nutrition of preterm infants in relation to bronchopulmonary dysplasia. *BMC Pulm. Med.* **2011**, *11*, 7. [CrossRef] [PubMed]
36. Cogo, P.E.; Ori, C.; Simonato, M.; Verlato, G.; Isak, I.; Hamvas, A.; Carnielli, V.P. Metabolic precursors of surfactant disaturated-phosphatidylcholine in preterms with respiratory distress. *J. Lipid Res.* **2009**, *50*, 2324–2331. [CrossRef]
37. Cogo, P.E.; Zimmermann, L.J.; Pesavento, R.; Sacchetto, E.; Burighel, A.; Rosso, F.; Badon, T.; Verlato, G.; Carnielli, V.P. Surfactant kinetics in preterm infants on mechanical ventilation who did and did not develop bronchopulmonary dysplasia. *Crit. Care Med.* **2003**, *31*, 1532–1538. [CrossRef]
38. Faucett, A.M.; Metz, T.D.; DeWitt, P.E.; Gibbs, R.S. Effect of obesity on neonatal outcomes in pregnancies with preterm premature rupture of membranes. *Am. J. Obstet. Gynecol.* **2016**, *214*. [CrossRef]
39. Mayor, R.S.; Finch, K.E.; Zehr, J.; Morselli, E.; Neinast, M.D.; Frank, A.P.; Hahner, L.D.; Wang, J.; Rakheja, D.; Palmer, B.F.; et al. Maternal high-fat diet is associated with impaired fetal lung development. *Am. J. Physiol. Lung Cell. Mol. Physiol.* **2015**, *309*, L360–L368. [CrossRef]
40. Wolfe, R.R.; Martini, W.Z.; Irtun, O.; Hawkins, H.K.; Barrow, R.E. Dietary fat composition alters pulmonary function in pigs. *Nutrition* **2002**, *18*, 647–653. [CrossRef]
41. Ma, L.; Li, N.; Liu, X.; Shaw, L.; Li Calzi, S.; Grant, M.B.; Neu, J. Arginyl-glutamine dipeptide or docosahexaenoic acid attenuate hyperoxia-induced lung injury in neonatal mice. *Nutrition* **2012**, *28*, 1186–1191. [CrossRef] [PubMed]
42. Lapillonne, A.; Jensen, C.L. Reevaluation of the DHA requirement for the premature infant. *Prostaglandins Leukot Essent Fatty Acids* **2009**, *81*, 143–150. [CrossRef] [PubMed]
43. Collins, C.T.; Makrides, M.; McPhee, A.J.; Sullivan, T.R.; Davis, P.G.; Thio, M.; Simmer, K.; Rajadurai, V.S.; Travadi, J.; Berry, M.J.; et al. Docosahexaenoic Acid and Bronchopulmonary Dysplasia in Preterm Infants. *N. E. J. Med.* **2017**, *376*, 1245–1255. [CrossRef] [PubMed]
44. Choudhary, N.; Tan, K.; Malhotra, A. Inpatient outcomes of preterm infants receiving omega-3 enriched lipid emulsion (SMOFlipid): An observational study. *Eur. J. Pediatrics* **2018**, *177*, 723–731. [CrossRef] [PubMed]
45. Huang, L.T.; Chou, H.C.; Lin, C.M.; Chen, C.M. Uteroplacental Insufficiency Alters the Retinoid Pathway and Lung Development in Newborn Rats. *Pediatrics Neonatol.* **2016**, *57*, 508–514. [CrossRef]
46. Darlow, B.A.; Graham, P.J. Vitamin A supplementation to prevent mortality and short- and long-term morbidity in very low birthweight infants. *Cochrane Database Syst. Rev.* **2011**, CD000501. [CrossRef]
47. Couroucli, X.I.; Placencia, J.L.; Cates, L.A.; Suresh, G.K. Should we still use vitamin A to prevent bronchopulmonary dysplasia? *J. Perinatol.* **2016**, *36*, 581–585. [CrossRef]
48. Wat, M.J.; Veenma, D.; Hogue, J.; Holder, A.M.; Yu, Z.; Wat, J.J.; Hanchard, N.; Shchelochkov, O.A.; Fernandes, C.J.; Johnson, A.; et al. Genomic alterations that contribute to the development of isolated and non-isolated congenital diaphragmatic hernia. *J. Med. Genet.* **2011**, *48*, 299–307. [CrossRef]
49. Coste, K.; Beurskens, L.W.; Blanc, P.; Gallot, D.; Delabaere, A.; Blanchon, L.; Tibboel, D.; Labbe, A.; Rottier, R.J.; Sapin, V. Metabolic disturbances of the vitamin A pathway in human diaphragmatic hernia. *Am. J. Physiol. Lung Cell. Mol. Physiol.* **2015**, *308*, L147–L157. [CrossRef]

50. Michikawa, T.; Yamazaki, S.; Sekiyama, M.; Kuroda, T.; Nakayama, S.F.; Isobe, T.; Kobayashi, Y.; Iwai-Shimada, M.; Suda, E.; Kawamoto, T.; et al. Maternal dietary intake of vitamin A during pregnancy was inversely associated with congenital diaphragmatic hernia: The Japan Environment and Children's Study. *Br. J. Nutr.* **2019**, 1–8. [CrossRef]
51. Lykkedegn, S.; Sorensen, G.L.; Beck-Nielsen, S.S.; Christesen, H.T. The impact of vitamin D on fetal and neonatal lung maturation. A systematic review. *Am. J. Physiol. Lung Cell. Mol. Physiol.* **2015**, *308*, L587–L602. [CrossRef] [PubMed]
52. Burris, H.H.; Van Marter, L.J.; McElrath, T.F.; Tabatabai, P.; Litonjua, A.A.; Weiss, S.T.; Christou, H. Vitamin D status among preterm and full-term infants at birth. *Pediatric Res.* **2014**, *75*, 75–80. [CrossRef] [PubMed]
53. Ataseven, F.; Aygun, C.; Okuyucu, A.; Bedir, A.; Kucuk, Y.; Kucukoduk, S. Is vitamin d deficiency a risk factor for respiratory distress syndrome? *Int. J. Vitam. Nutr. Res.* **2013**, *83*, 232–237. [CrossRef] [PubMed]
54. Backstrom, M.C.; Maki, R.; Kuusela, A.L.; Sievanen, H.; Koivisto, A.M.; Ikonen, R.S.; Kouri, T.; Maki, M. Randomised controlled trial of vitamin D supplementation on bone density and biochemical indices in preterm infants. *Arch. Dis. Child. Fetal Neonatal Ed.* **1999**, *80*, F161–F166. [CrossRef]
55. Camargo, C.A., Jr.; Ingham, T.; Wickens, K.; Thadhani, R.; Silvers, K.M.; Epton, M.J.; Town, G.I.; Pattemore, P.K.; Espinola, J.A.; Crane, J.; et al. Cord-blood 25-hydroxyvitamin D levels and risk of respiratory infection, wheezing, and asthma. *Pediatrics* **2011**, *127*, e180–e187. [CrossRef]
56. Joung, K.E.; Burris, H.H.; Van Marter, L.J.; McElrath, T.F.; Michael, Z.; Tabatabai, P.; Litonjua, A.A.; Weiss, S.T.; Christou, H. Vitamin D and bronchopulmonary dysplasia in preterm infants. *J. Perinatol.* **2016**, *36*, 878–882. [CrossRef]
57. Cetinkaya, M.; Cekmez, F.; Erener-Ercan, T.; Buyukkale, G.; Demirhan, A.; Aydemir, G.; Aydin, F.N. Maternal/neonatal vitamin D deficiency: A risk factor for bronchopulmonary dysplasia in preterms? *J. Perinatol.* **2015**, *35*, 813–817. [CrossRef]
58. Turner, S.W.; Campbell, D.; Smith, N.; Craig, L.C.; McNeill, G.; Forbes, S.H.; Harbour, P.J.; Seaton, A.; Helms, P.J.; Devereux, G.S. Associations between fetal size, maternal {alpha}-tocopherol and childhood asthma. *Thorax* **2010**, *65*, 391–397. [CrossRef]
59. Islam, S.; Narra, V.; Cote, G.M.; Manganaro, T.F.; Donahoe, P.K.; Schnitzer, J.J. Prenatal vitamin E treatment improves lung growth in fetal rats with congenital diaphragmatic hernia. *J. Pediatric Surg.* **1999**, *34*, 172–176. [CrossRef]
60. Falciglia, H.S.; Ginn-Pease, M.E.; Falciglia, G.A.; Lubin, A.H.; Frank, D.J.; Chang, W. Vitamin E and selenium levels of premature infants with severe respiratory distress syndrome and bronchopulmonary dysplasia. *J. Pediatr. Perinat. Nutr.* **1988**, *2*, 35–49. [CrossRef]
61. Stone, C.A., Jr.; McEvoy, C.T.; Aschner, J.L.; Kirk, A.; Rosas-Salazar, C.; Cook-Mills, J.M.; Moore, P.E.; Walsh, W.F.; Hartert, T.V. Update on Vitamin E and Its Potential Role in Preventing or Treating Bronchopulmonary Dysplasia. *Neonatology* **2018**, *113*, 366–378. [CrossRef] [PubMed]
62. Reiss, I.; Landmann, E.; Heckmann, M.; Misselwitz, B.; Gortner, L. Increased risk of bronchopulmonary dysplasia and increased mortality in very preterm infants being small for gestational age. *Arch. Gynecol. Obstet.* **2003**, *269*, 40–44. [CrossRef] [PubMed]
63. Thebaud, B.; Abman, S.H. Bronchopulmonary dysplasia: Where have all the vessels gone? Roles of angiogenic growth factors in chronic lung disease. *Am. J. Respir. Crit. Care Med.* **2007**, *175*, 978–985. [CrossRef]
64. Laughon, M.; Allred, E.N.; Bose, C.; O'Shea, T.M.; Van Marter, L.J.; Ehrenkranz, R.A.; Leviton, A.; Investigators, E.S. Patterns of respiratory disease during the first 2 postnatal weeks in extremely premature infants. *Pediatrics* **2009**, *123*, 1124–1131. [CrossRef] [PubMed]
65. Brett, K.E.; Ferraro, Z.M.; Yockell-Lelievre, J.; Gruslin, A.; Adamo, K.B. Maternal-fetal nutrient transport in pregnancy pathologies: The role of the placenta. *Int. J. Mol. Sci.* **2014**, *15*, 16153–16185. [CrossRef]
66. Lai, P.Y.; Jing, X.; Michalkiewicz, T.; Entringer, B.; Ke, X.; Majnik, A.; Kriegel, A.J.; Liu, P.; Lane, R.H.; Konduri, G.G. Adverse early-life environment impairs postnatal lung development in mice. *Physiol. Genom.* **2019**, *51*, 462–470. [CrossRef]
67. Carnielli, V.P.; Giorgetti, C.; Simonato, M.; Vedovelli, L.; Cogo, P. Neonatal Respiratory Diseases in the Newborn Infant: Novel Insights from Stable Isotope Tracer Studies. *Neonatology* **2016**, *109*, 325–333. [CrossRef]

68. Batenburg, J.J. Surfactant phospholipids: Synthesis and storage. *Am. J. Physiol.* **1992**, *262*, L367–L385. [CrossRef]
69. De Luca, D.; van Kaam, A.H.; Tingay, D.G.; Courtney, S.E.; Danhaive, O.; Carnielli, V.P.; Zimmermann, L.J.; Kneyber, M.C.J.; Tissieres, P.; Brierley, J.; et al. The Montreux definition of neonatal ARDS: Biological and clinical background behind the description of a new entity. *Lancet Respir. Med.* **2017**, *5*, 657–666. [CrossRef]
70. Merrill, J.D.; Ballard, R.A.; Cnaan, A.; Hibbs, A.M.; Godinez, R.I.; Godinez, M.H.; Truog, W.E.; Ballard, P.L. Dysfunction of pulmonary surfactant in chronically ventilated premature infants. *Pediatric Res.* **2004**, *56*, 918–926. [CrossRef]
71. Orgeig, S.; Crittenden, T.A.; Marchant, C.; McMillen, I.C.; Morrison, J.L. Intrauterine growth restriction delays surfactant protein maturation in the sheep fetus. *Am. J. Physiol. Lung Cell. Mol. Physiol.* **2010**, *298*, L575–L583. [CrossRef] [PubMed]
72. Chen, C.M.; Wang, L.F.; Su, B. Effects of maternal undernutrition during late gestation on the lung surfactant system and morphometry in rats. *Pediatric Res.* **2004**, *56*, 329–335. [CrossRef] [PubMed]
73. Khazaee, R.; McCaig, L.A.; Yamashita, C.; Hardy, D.B.; Veldhuizen, R.A.W. Maternal protein restriction during perinatal life affects lung mechanics and the surfactant system during early postnatal life in female rats. *PLoS ONE* **2019**, *14*, e0215611. [CrossRef] [PubMed]
74. Zhang, Q.; Chai, X.; Deng, F.; Ouyang, W.; Song, T. The reduction in FOXA2 activity during lung development in fetuses from diabetic rat mothers is reversed by Akt inhibition. *FEBS Open Bio.* **2018**, *8*, 1594–1604. [CrossRef] [PubMed]
75. Chao, A.C.; Ziadeh, B.I.; Diau, G.Y.; Wijendran, V.; Sarkadi-Nagy, E.; Hsieh, A.T.; Nathanielsz, P.W.; Brenna, J.T. Influence of dietary long-chain PUFA on premature baboon lung FA and dipalmitoyl PC composition. *Lipids* **2003**, *38*, 425–429. [CrossRef]
76. Kohri, T.; Sakai, K.; Mizunuma, T.; Kishino, Y. Levels of pulmonary surfactant protein A in fetal lung and amniotic fluid from protein-malnourished pregnant rats. *J. Nutr. Sci. Vitaminol. (Tokyo)* **1996**, *42*, 209–218. [CrossRef]
77. Briana, D.D.; Gourgiotis, D.; Baka, S.; Boutsikou, M.; Vraila, V.M.; Boutsikou, T.; Hassiakos, D.; Malamitsi-Puchner, A. The effect of intrauterine growth restriction on circulating surfactant protein D concentrations in the perinatal period. *Reprod. Sci.* **2010**, *17*, 653–658. [CrossRef]
78. Mourani, P.M.; Sontag, M.K.; Younoszai, A.; Miller, J.I.; Kinsella, J.P.; Baker, C.D.; Poindexter, B.B.; Ingram, D.A.; Abman, S.H. Early pulmonary vascular disease in preterm infants at risk for bronchopulmonary dysplasia. *Am. J. Respir. Crit. Care Med.* **2015**, *191*, 87–95. [CrossRef]
79. Lusk, L.A.; Wai, K.C.; Moon-Grady, A.J.; Steurer, M.A.; Keller, R.L. Persistence of pulmonary hypertension by echocardiography predicts short-term outcomes in congenital diaphragmatic hernia. *J. Pediatrics* **2015**, *166*. [CrossRef]
80. Wedgwood, S.; Warford, C.; Agvateesiri, S.C.; Thai, P.; Berkelhamer, S.K.; Perez, M.; Underwood, M.A.; Steinhorn, R.H. Postnatal growth restriction augments oxygen-induced pulmonary hypertension in a neonatal rat model of bronchopulmonary dysplasia. *Pediatric Res.* **2016**, *80*, 894–902. [CrossRef]
81. Wedgwood, S.; Warford, C.; Agvatisiri, S.R.; Thai, P.N.; Chiamvimonvat, N.; Kalanetra, K.M.; Lakshminrusimha, S.; Steinhorn, R.H.; Mills, D.A.; Underwood, M.A. The developing gut-lung axis: Postnatal growth restriction, intestinal dysbiosis, and pulmonary hypertension in a rodent model. *Pediatric Res.* **2019**. [CrossRef] [PubMed]
82. Zhong, Y.; Catheline, D.; Houeijeh, A.; Sharma, D.; Du, L.; Besengez, C.; Deruelle, P.; Legrand, P.; Storme, L. Maternal omega-3 PUFA supplementation prevents hyperoxia-induced pulmonary hypertension in the offspring. *Am. J. Physiol. Lung Cell. Mol. Physiol.* **2018**, *315*, L116–L132. [CrossRef] [PubMed]
83. Check, J.; Gotteiner, N.; Liu, X.; Su, E.; Porta, N.; Steinhorn, R.; Mestan, K.K. Fetal growth restriction and pulmonary hypertension in premature infants with bronchopulmonary dysplasia. *J. Perinatol.* **2013**, *33*, 553–557. [CrossRef] [PubMed]
84. Thebaud, B.; Goss, K.N.; Laughon, M.; Whitsett, J.A.; Abman, S.H.; Steinhorn, R.H.; Aschner, J.L.; Davis, P.G.; McGrath-Morrow, S.A.; Soll, R.F.; et al. Bronchopulmonary dysplasia. *Nat. Rev. Dis. Primers* **2019**, *5*, 78. [CrossRef] [PubMed]
85. Jackson, K.H.; Harris, W.S. A Prenatal DHA Test to Help Identify Women at Increased Risk for Early Preterm Birth: A Proposal. *Nutrients* **2018**, *10*, 1933. [CrossRef]

86. Collins, J.J.P.; Tibboel, D.; de Kleer, I.M.; Reiss, I.K.M.; Rottier, R.J. The Future of Bronchopulmonary Dysplasia: Emerging Pathophysiological Concepts and Potential New Avenues of Treatment. *Front. Med. (Lausanne)* **2017**, *4*, 61. [CrossRef]
87. Smithers, L.G.; Collins, C.T.; Simmonds, L.A.; Gibson, R.A.; McPhee, A.; Makrides, M. Feeding preterm infants milk with a higher dose of docosahexaenoic acid than that used in current practice does not influence language or behavior in early childhood: A follow-up study of a randomized controlled trial. *Am. J. Clin. Nutr.* **2010**, *91*, 628–634. [CrossRef]
88. Manley, B.J.; Makrides, M.; Collins, C.T.; McPhee, A.J.; Gibson, R.A.; Ryan, P.; Sullivan, T.R.; Davis, P.G.; Committee, D.S. High-dose docosahexaenoic acid supplementation of preterm infants: Respiratory and allergy outcomes. *Pediatrics* **2011**, *128*, e71–e77. [CrossRef]
89. Legrand, D. Overview of Lactoferrin as a Natural Immune Modulator. *J. Pediatrics* **2016**, *173* (Suppl. S10–S15). [CrossRef]
90. Manzoni, P.; Rinaldi, M.; Cattani, S.; Pugni, L.; Romeo, M.G.; Messner, H.; Stolfi, I.; Decembrino, L.; Laforgia, N.; Vagnarelli, F.; et al. Bovine lactoferrin supplementation for prevention of late-onset sepsis in very low-birth-weight neonates: A randomized trial. *JAMA* **2009**, *302*, 1421–1428. [CrossRef]
91. Group, N.H.W.; Peterson, J.; Garges, S.; Giovanni, M.; McInnes, P.; Wang, L.; Schloss, J.A.; Bonazzi, V.; McEwen, J.E.; Wetterstrand, K.A.; et al. The NIH Human Microbiome Project. *Genome Res.* **2009**, *19*, 2317–2323. [CrossRef] [PubMed]
92. Neu, J.; Pammi, M. Necrotizing enterocolitis: The intestinal microbiome, metabolome and inflammatory mediators. *Semin. Fetal Neonatal Med.* **2018**, *23*, 400–405. [CrossRef] [PubMed]
93. Morrow, A.L.; Lagomarcino, A.J.; Schibler, K.R.; Taft, D.H.; Yu, Z.; Wang, B.; Altaye, M.; Wagner, M.; Gevers, D.; Ward, D.V.; et al. Early microbial and metabolomic signatures predict later onset of necrotizing enterocolitis in preterm infants. *Microbiome* **2013**, *1*, 13. [CrossRef] [PubMed]
94. Whelan, F.J.; Waddell, B.; Syed, S.A.; Shekarriz, S.; Rabin, H.R.; Parkins, M.D.; Surette, M.G. Culture-enriched metagenomic sequencing enables in-depth profiling of the cystic fibrosis lung microbiota. *Nat. Microbiol.* **2020**. [CrossRef]
95. Dominguez-Bello, M.G.; Costello, E.K.; Contreras, M.; Magris, M.; Hidalgo, G.; Fierer, N.; Knight, R. Delivery mode shapes the acquisition and structure of the initial microbiota across multiple body habitats in newborns. *Proc. Natl. Acad. Sci. USA* **2010**, *107*, 11971–11975. [CrossRef]
96. Aagaard, K.; Ma, J.; Antony, K.M.; Ganu, R.; Petrosino, J.; Versalovic, J. The placenta harbors a unique microbiome. *Sci. Transl. Med.* **2014**, *6*, 237ra265. [CrossRef]
97. Prince, A.L.; Ma, J.; Kannan, P.S.; Alvarez, M.; Gisslen, T.; Harris, R.A.; Sweeney, E.L.; Knox, C.L.; Lambers, D.S.; Jobe, A.H.; et al. The placental membrane microbiome is altered among subjects with spontaneous preterm birth with and without chorioamnionitis. *Am. J. Obstet. Gynecol.* **2016**, *214*. [CrossRef]
98. Martinez, K.A., 2nd; Romano-Keeler, J.; Zackular, J.P.; Moore, D.J.; Brucker, R.M.; Hooper, C.; Meng, S.; Brown, N.; Mallal, S.; Reese, J.; et al. Bacterial DNA is present in the fetal intestine and overlaps with that in the placenta in mice. *PLoS ONE* **2018**, *13*, e0197439. [CrossRef]
99. Satokari, R.; Gronroos, T.; Laitinen, K.; Salminen, S.; Isolauri, E. Bifidobacterium and Lactobacillus DNA in the human placenta. *Lett. Appl. Microbiol.* **2009**, *48*, 8–12. [CrossRef]
100. Al Alam, D.; Danopoulos, S.; Grubbs, B.; Ali, N.; MacAogain, M.; Chotirmall, S.H.; Warburton, D.; Gaggar, A.; Ambalavanan, N.; Lal, C.V. Human Fetal Lungs Harbor a Microbiome Signature. *Am. J. Respir. Crit. Care Med.* **2020**. [CrossRef] [PubMed]
101. De Goffau, M.C.; Lager, S.; Sovio, U.; Gaccioli, F.; Cook, E.; Peacock, S.J.; Parkhill, J.; Charnock-Jones, D.S.; Smith, G.C.S. Human placenta has no microbiome but can contain potential pathogens. *Nature* **2019**, *572*, 329–334. [CrossRef] [PubMed]
102. Bushman, F.D. De-Discovery of the Placenta Microbiome. *Am. J. Obstet. Gynecol.* **2019**, *220*, 213–214. [CrossRef] [PubMed]
103. Perez-Munoz, M.E.; Arrieta, M.C.; Ramer-Tait, A.E.; Walter, J. A critical assessment of the "sterile womb" and "in utero colonization" hypotheses: Implications for research on the pioneer infant microbiome. *Microbiome* **2017**, *5*, 48. [CrossRef] [PubMed]
104. Mueller, N.T.; Bakacs, E.; Combellick, J.; Grigoryan, Z.; Dominguez-Bello, M.G. The infant microbiome development: Mom matters. *Trends Mol. Med.* **2015**, *21*, 109–117. [CrossRef]

105. Balany, J.; Bhandari, V. Understanding the Impact of Infection, Inflammation, and Their Persistence in the Pathogenesis of Bronchopulmonary Dysplasia. *Front. Med. (Lausanne)* **2015**, *2*, 90. [CrossRef]
106. Viscardi, R.M.; Hasday, J.D. Role of Ureaplasma species in neonatal chronic lung disease: Epidemiologic and experimental evidence. *Pediatric Res.* **2009**, *65*, 84R–90R. [CrossRef]
107. Nair, V.; Loganathan, P.; Soraisham, A.S. Azithromycin and other macrolides for prevention of bronchopulmonary dysplasia: A systematic review and meta-analysis. *Neonatology* **2014**, *106*, 337–347. [CrossRef]
108. Lohmann, P.; Luna, R.A.; Hollister, E.B.; Devaraj, S.; Mistretta, T.A.; Welty, S.E.; Versalovic, J. The airway microbiome of intubated premature infants: Characteristics and changes that predict the development of bronchopulmonary dysplasia. *Pediatric Res.* **2014**, *76*, 294–301. [CrossRef]
109. Sagar, S.; Morgan, M.E.; Chen, S.; Vos, A.P.; Garssen, J.; van Bergenhenegouwen, J.; Boon, L.; Georgiou, N.A.; Kraneveld, A.D.; Folkerts, G. Bifidobacterium breve and Lactobacillus rhamnosus treatment is as effective as budesonide at reducing inflammation in a murine model for chronic asthma. *Respir. Res.* **2014**, *15*, 46. [CrossRef]
110. Beck, T.F.; Campeau, P.M.; Jhangiani, S.N.; Gambin, T.; Li, A.H.; Abo-Zahrah, R.; Jordan, V.K.; Hernandez-Garcia, A.; Wiszniewski, W.K.; Muzny, D.; et al. FBN1 contributing to familial congenital diaphragmatic hernia. *Am. J. Med. Genet. A* **2015**, *167A*, 831–836. [CrossRef]
111. Ryan, F.J.; Drew, D.P.; Douglas, C.; Leong, L.E.X.; Moldovan, M.; Lynn, M.; Fink, N.; Sribnaia, A.; Penttila, I.; McPhee, A.J.; et al. Changes in the Composition of the Gut Microbiota and the Blood Transcriptome in Preterm Infants at Less than 29 Weeks Gestation Diagnosed with Bronchopulmonary Dysplasia. *mSystems* **2019**, *4*. [CrossRef]
112. Lal, C.V.; Kandasamy, J.; Dolma, K.; Ramani, M.; Kumar, R.; Wilson, L.; Aghai, Z.; Barnes, S.; Blalock, J.E.; Gaggar, A.; et al. Early airway microbial metagenomic and metabolomic signatures are associated with development of severe bronchopulmonary dysplasia. *Am. J. Physiol. Lung Cell. Mol. Physiol.* **2018**, *315*, L810–L815. [CrossRef]
113. Resch, B.; Gutmann, C.; Reiterer, F.; Luxner, J.; Urlesberger, B. Neonatal Ureaplasma urealyticum colonization increases pulmonary and cerebral morbidity despite treatment with macrolide antibiotics. *Infection* **2016**, *44*, 323–327. [CrossRef]
114. Goodrich, J.K.; Davenport, E.R.; Beaumont, M.; Jackson, M.A.; Knight, R.; Ober, C.; Spector, T.D.; Bell, J.T.; Clark, A.G.; Ley, R.E. Genetic Determinants of the Gut Microbiome in UK Twins. *Cell Host Microbe* **2016**, *19*, 731–743. [CrossRef]
115. Spor, A.; Koren, O.; Ley, R. Unravelling the effects of the environment and host genotype on the gut microbiome. *Nat. Rev. Microbiol.* **2011**, *9*, 279–290. [CrossRef]
116. Awany, D.; Allali, I.; Dalvie, S.; Hemmings, S.; Mwaikono, K.S.; Thomford, N.E.; Gomez, A.; Mulder, N.; Chimusa, E.R. Host and Microbiome Genome-Wide Association Studies: Current State and Challenges. *Front. Genet.* **2018**, *9*, 637. [CrossRef]
117. Mei, C.; Yang, W.; Wei, X.; Wu, K.; Huang, D. The Unique Microbiome and Innate Immunity During Pregnancy. *Front. Immunol.* **2019**, *10*, 2886. [CrossRef]
118. Ithier, M.C.; Parobchak, N.; Yadava, S.; Cheng, J.; Wang, B.; Rosen, T. Fetal lung C4BPA induces p100 processing in human placenta. *Sci. Rep.* **2019**, *9*, 5519. [CrossRef]
119. Gao, L.; Rabbitt, E.H.; Condon, J.C.; Renthal, N.E.; Johnston, J.M.; Mitsche, M.A.; Chambon, P.; Xu, J.; O'Malley, B.W.; Mendelson, C.R. Steroid receptor coactivators 1 and 2 mediate fetal-to-maternal signaling that initiates parturition. *J. Clin. Investig* **2015**, *125*, 2808–2824. [CrossRef]
120. Ho, T.T.B.; Groer, M.W.; Kane, B.; Yee, A.L.; Torres, B.A.; Gilbert, J.A.; Maheshwari, A. Dichotomous development of the gut microbiome in preterm infants. *Microbiome* **2018**, *6*, 157. [CrossRef]
121. Gill, N.; Wlodarska, M.; Finlay, B.B. The future of mucosal immunology: Studying an integrated system-wide organ. *Nat. Immunol.* **2010**, *11*, 558–560. [CrossRef]
122. Debock, I.; Flamand, V. Unbalanced Neonatal CD4(+) T-Cell Immunity. *Front. Immunol.* **2014**, *5*, 393. [CrossRef]
123. Rawls, J.F.; Mahowald, M.A.; Ley, R.E.; Gordon, J.I. Reciprocal gut microbiota transplants from zebrafish and mice to germ-free recipients reveal host habitat selection. *Cell* **2006**, *127*, 423–433. [CrossRef]

124. Tirone, C.; Pezza, L.; Paladini, A.; Tana, M.; Aurilia, C.; Lio, A.; D'Ippolito, S.; Tersigni, C.; Posteraro, B.; Sanguinetti, M.; et al. Gut and Lung Microbiota in Preterm Infants: Immunological Modulation and Implication in Neonatal Outcomes. *Front. Immunol.* **2019**, *10*, 2910. [CrossRef]
125. Anand, S.; Mande, S.S. Diet, Microbiota and Gut-Lung Connection. *Front. Microbiol.* **2018**, *9*, 2147. [CrossRef]
126. Morrison, D.J.; Preston, T. Formation of short chain fatty acids by the gut microbiota and their impact on human metabolism. *Gut Microbes* **2016**, *7*, 189–200. [CrossRef]
127. Gollwitzer, E.S.; Saglani, S.; Trompette, A.; Yadava, K.; Sherburn, R.; McCoy, K.D.; Nicod, L.P.; Lloyd, C.M.; Marsland, B.J. Lung microbiota promotes tolerance to allergens in neonates via PD-L1. *Nat. Med.* **2014**, *20*, 642–647. [CrossRef]
128. Segal, L.N.; Clemente, J.C.; Wu, B.G.; Wikoff, W.R.; Gao, Z.; Li, Y.; Ko, J.P.; Rom, W.N.; Blaser, M.J.; Weiden, M.D. Randomised, double-blind, placebo-controlled trial with azithromycin selects for anti-inflammatory microbial metabolites in the emphysematous lung. *Thorax* **2017**, *72*, 13–22. [CrossRef]
129. Willis, K.A.; Siefker, D.T.; Aziz, M.M.; White, C.T.; Mussarat, N.; Gomes, C.K.; Bajwa, A.; Pierre, J.F.; Cormier, S.A.; Talati, A.J. Perinatal maternal antibiotic exposure augments lung injury in offspring in experimental bronchopulmonary dysplasia. *Am. J. Physiol. Lung Cell. Mol. Physiol.* **2019**. [CrossRef]
130. Zou, Z.H.; Liu, D.; Li, H.D.; Zhu, D.P.; He, Y.; Hou, T.; Yu, J.L. Prenatal and postnatal antibiotic exposure influences the gut microbiota of preterm infants in neonatal intensive care units. *Ann. Clin. Microbiol. Antimicrob.* **2018**, *17*, 9. [CrossRef]
131. Puri, K.; Taft, D.H.; Ambalavanan, N.; Schibler, K.R.; Morrow, A.L.; Kallapur, S.G. Association of Chorioamnionitis with Aberrant Neonatal Gut Colonization and Adverse Clinical Outcomes. *PLoS ONE* **2016**, *11*, e0162734. [CrossRef]
132. Villamor-Martinez, E.; Alvarez-Fuente, M.; Ghazi, A.M.T.; Degraeuwe, P.; Zimmermann, L.J.I.; Kramer, B.W.; Villamor, E. Association of Chorioamnionitis With Bronchopulmonary Dysplasia Among Preterm Infants: A Systematic Review, Meta-analysis, and Metaregression. *JAMA Netw. Open* **2019**, *2*, e1914611. [CrossRef]
133. Azad, M.B.; Konya, T.; Persaud, R.R.; Guttman, D.S.; Chari, R.S.; Field, C.J.; Sears, M.R.; Mandhane, P.J.; Turvey, S.E.; Subbarao, P.; et al. Impact of maternal intrapartum antibiotics, method of birth and breastfeeding on gut microbiota during the first year of life: A prospective cohort study. *BJOG* **2016**, *123*, 983–993. [CrossRef]
134. Willing, B.P.; Russell, S.L.; Finlay, B.B. Shifting the balance: Antibiotic effects on host-microbiota mutualism. *Nat. Rev. Microbiol.* **2011**, *9*, 233–243. [CrossRef] [PubMed]
135. Mei, J.; Harter, K.; Danhaive, O.; Seidman, D.; Vargas, J. Implications of intrapartum azithromycin on neonatal microbiota. *Lancet Infect. Dis.* **2017**, *17*, 253–254. [CrossRef]
136. Tanaka, S.; Tsumura, K.; Nakura, Y.; Tokuda, T.; Nakahashi, H.; Yamamoto, T.; Ono, T.; Yanagihara, I.; Nomiyama, M. New antibiotic regimen for preterm premature rupture of membrane reduces the incidence of bronchopulmonary dysplasia. *J. Obstet. Gynaecol. Res.* **2019**, *45*, 967–973. [CrossRef] [PubMed]
137. Korpela, K.; Salonen, A.; Virta, L.J.; Kekkonen, R.A.; Forslund, K.; Bork, P.; de Vos, W.M. Intestinal microbiome is related to lifetime antibiotic use in Finnish pre-school children. *Nat. Commun.* **2016**, *7*, 10410. [CrossRef] [PubMed]
138. Cantey, J.B.; Huffman, L.W.; Subramanian, A.; Marshall, A.S.; Ballard, A.R.; Lefevre, C.; Sagar, M.; Pruszynski, J.E.; Mallett, L.H. Antibiotic Exposure and Risk for Death or Bronchopulmonary Dysplasia in Very Low Birth Weight Infants. *J. Pediatrics* **2017**, *181*. [CrossRef]
139. Alonso-Ojembarrena, A.; Martinez-Diaz, J.V.; Lechuga-Sancho, A.M.; Galan-Sanchez, F.; Lubian-Lopez, S.P. Broad spectrum antibiotics in newborns increase multi-drug resistant infections. *J. Chemother.* **2019**, *31*, 81–85. [CrossRef]
140. Fajardo, C.; Alshaikh, B.; Harabor, A. Prolonged use of antibiotics after birth is associated with increased morbidity in preterm infants with negative cultures. *J. Mater. Fetal Neonatal Med.* **2018**, 1–7. [CrossRef]
141. Ting, J.Y.; Synnes, A.; Roberts, A.; Deshpandey, A.C.; Dow, K.; Yang, J.; Lee, K.S.; Lee, S.K.; Shah, P.S.; Canadian Neonatal, N.; et al. Association of Antibiotic Utilization and Neurodevelopmental Outcomes among Extremely Low Gestational Age Neonates without Proven Sepsis or Necrotizing Enterocolitis. *Am. J. Perinatol.* **2018**, *35*, 972–978. [CrossRef] [PubMed]
142. Cantey, J.B.; Wozniak, P.S.; Sanchez, P.J. Prospective surveillance of antibiotic use in the neonatal intensive care unit: Results from the SCOUT study. *Pediatric Infect. Dis. J.* **2015**, *34*, 267–272. [CrossRef] [PubMed]

143. Grier, A.; Qiu, X.; Bandyopadhyay, S.; Holden-Wiltse, J.; Kessler, H.A.; Gill, A.L.; Hamilton, B.; Huyck, H.; Misra, S.; Mariani, T.J.; et al. Impact of prematurity and nutrition on the developing gut microbiome and preterm infant growth. *Microbiome* **2017**, *5*, 158. [CrossRef] [PubMed]
144. Grier, A.; McDavid, A.; Wang, B.; Qiu, X.; Java, J.; Bandyopadhyay, S.; Yang, H.; Holden-Wiltse, J.; Kessler, H.A.; Gill, A.L.; et al. Neonatal gut and respiratory microbiota: Coordinated development through time and space. *Microbiome* **2018**, *6*, 193. [CrossRef]
145. Vientos-Plotts, A.I.; Ericsson, A.C.; Rindt, H.; Grobman, M.E.; Graham, A.; Bishop, K.; Cohn, L.A.; Reinero, C.R. Dynamic changes of the respiratory microbiota and its relationship to fecal and blood microbiota in healthy young cats. *PLoS ONE* **2017**, *12*, e0173818. [CrossRef]
146. Vientos-Plotts, A.I.; Ericsson, A.C.; Rindt, H.; Reinero, C.R. Oral Probiotics Alter Healthy Feline Respiratory Microbiota. *Front. Microbiol.* **2017**, *8*, 1287. [CrossRef]
147. Abrahamsson, T.R. Not all probiotic strains prevent necrotising enterocolitis in premature infants. *Lancet* **2016**, *387*, 624–625. [CrossRef]
148. Johnstone, J.; Heels-Ansdell, D.; Thabane, L.; Meade, M.; Marshall, J.; Lauzier, F.; Duan, E.H.; Zytaruk, N.; Lamarche, D.; Surette, M.; et al. Evaluating probiotics for the prevention of ventilator-associated pneumonia: A randomised placebo-controlled multicentre trial protocol and statistical analysis plan for PROSPECT. *BMJ Open* **2019**, *9*, e025228. [CrossRef]
149. Huang, J.; Zhang, L.; Tang, J.; Shi, J.; Qu, Y.; Xiong, T.; Mu, D. Human milk as a protective factor for bronchopulmonary dysplasia: A systematic review and meta-analysis. *Arch. Dis. Child. Fetal Neonatal Ed.* **2019**, *104*, F128–F136. [CrossRef]
150. Villamor-Martinez, E.; Pierro, M.; Cavallaro, G.; Mosca, F.; Villamor, E. Mother's Own Milk and Bronchopulmonary Dysplasia: A Systematic Review and Meta-Analysis. *Front. Pediatrics* **2019**, *7*, 224. [CrossRef]
151. Casado, B.; Affolter, M.; Kussmann, M. OMICS-rooted studies of milk proteins, oligosaccharides and lipids. *J. Proteom.* **2009**, *73*, 196–208. [CrossRef] [PubMed]
152. Van Gysel, M.; Cossey, V.; Fieuws, S.; Schuermans, A. Impact of pasteurization on the antibacterial properties of human milk. *Eur. J. Pediatrics* **2012**, *171*, 1231–1237. [CrossRef] [PubMed]
153. De la Torre Gomez, C.; Goreham, R.V.; Bech Serra, J.J.; Nann, T.; Kussmann, M. "Exosomics"-A Review of Biophysics, Biology and Biochemistry of Exosomes With a Focus on Human Breast Milk. *Front. Genet.* **2018**, *9*, 92. [CrossRef] [PubMed]
154. Wesolowska, A.; Sinkiewicz-Darol, E.; Barbarska, O.; Bernatowicz-Lojko, U.; Borszewska-Kornacka, M.K.; van Goudoever, J.B. Innovative Techniques of Processing Human Milk to Preserve Key Components. *Nutrients* **2019**, *11*, 1169. [CrossRef] [PubMed]
155. Biesbroek, G.; Tsivtsivadze, E.; Sanders, E.A.; Montijn, R.; Veenhoven, R.H.; Keijser, B.J.; Bogaert, D. Early respiratory microbiota composition determines bacterial succession patterns and respiratory health in children. *Am. J. Respir. Crit. Care Med.* **2014**, *190*, 1283–1292. [CrossRef] [PubMed]
156. Austin, S.; De Castro, C.A.; Sprenger, N.; Binia, A.; Affolter, M.; Garcia-Rodenas, C.L.; Beauport, L.; Tolsa, J.F.; Fischer Fumeaux, C.J. Human Milk Oligosaccharides in the Milk of Mothers Delivering Term versus Preterm Infants. *Nutrients* **2019**, *11*, 1282. [CrossRef] [PubMed]

8

Characterising a Weight Loss Intervention in Obese Asthmatic Children

Shaun Eslick [1], Megan E. Jensen [2], Clare E. Collins [3], Peter G. Gibson [1], Jodi Hilton [4] and Lisa G. Wood [1,*]

[1] Priority Research Centre for Healthy Lungs, Hunter Medical Research Institute, The University of Newcastle, New Lambton Heights, NSW 2305, Australia; shaun.eslick@uon.edu.au (S.E.); peter.gibson@newcastle.edu.au (P.G.G.)

[2] Priority Research Centre Grow Up Well, Hunter Medical Research Institute, School of Medicine and Public Health, The University of Newcastle, New Lambton Heights, NSW 2305, Australia; megan.jensen@newcastle.edu.au

[3] Priority Research Centre in Physical Activity and Nutrition, Faculty of Health and Medicine, The University of Newcastle, Callaghan, NSW 2308, Australia; clare.collins@newcastle.edu.au

[4] Pediatric Respiratory and Sleep Medicine, John Hunter Children's Hospital, New Lambton Heights, NSW 2305, Australia; jodi.hilton@health.nsw.gov.au

[*] Correspondence: Lisa.Wood@newcastle.edu.au

Abstract: The prevalence of obesity in asthmatic children is high and is associated with worse clinical outcomes. We have previously reported that weight loss leads to improvements in lung function and asthma control in obese asthmatic children. The objectives of this secondary analysis were to examine: (1) changes in diet quality and (2) associations between the baseline subject characteristics and the degree of weight loss following the intervention. Twenty-eight obese asthmatic children, aged 8–17 years, completed a 10-week diet-induced weight loss intervention. Dietary intake, nutritional biomarkers, anthropometry, lung function, asthma control, and clinical outcomes were analysed before and after the intervention. Following the intervention, the body mass index (BMI) z-score decreased ($\Delta = 0.18 \pm 0.04$; $p < 0.001$), %energy from protein increased ($\Delta = 4.3 \pm 0.9\%$; $p = 0.002$), and sugar intake decreased ($\Delta = 23.2 \pm 9.3$ g; $p = 0.025$). Baseline lung function and physical activity level were inversely associated with Δ% fat mass. The ΔBMI z-score was negatively associated with physical activity duration at baseline. Dietary intervention is effective in achieving acute weight loss in obese asthmatic children, with significant improvements in diet quality and body composition. Lower lung function and physical engagement at baseline were associated with lesser weight loss, highlighting that subjects with these attributes may require greater support to achieve weight loss goals.

Keywords: weight loss; asthma; children; diet; nutritional biomarkers

---

1. Introduction

Over the past few decades, the prevalence of both obesity and asthma has increased significantly worldwide in children [1]. Asthma is the most common chronic childhood disease and was estimated in 2007–2008 to affect 10.4% of children aged 0–15 years in Australia [2,3]. Obesity is a worldwide epidemic, with a study of 188 countries reporting 23.8% of boys and 22.6% of girls aged 2–19 years are overweight or obese in developed countries [4]. Australian data from 2014–2015 found that 27% of children aged 5–14 years were overweight and an additional 7% were obese [5].

Childhood obesity has been identified as a strong predictor of obesity in adulthood, with 6.4% of males and 12.6% of females carrying obesity from childhood to adulthood [6]. Of concern are a myriad of obesity-related respiratory problems and, in adults, these include mechanical lung compression, resistance to steroid treatment, increased systemic inflammation, and altered airway inflammation [7–10]. In children, excess weight is associated with poorer asthma control, increased risk of exacerbations, reduced effectiveness of steroids, and decreased static lung function, implicating the need for obesity management in paediatrics [10–12]. Therefore, addressing obesity in children with asthma is of high importance, not only to improve short-term health, but also long-term health.

To date, few weight loss studies utilising a dietary intervention alone have been conducted in obese children with asthma. The present study is a secondary analysis of a trial by Jensen et al. [13], a randomised controlled trial of a short-term dietary intervention in obese asthmatic children, which achieved improvements in lung function and asthma control as a result of an average weight loss of 3.4 kg. Subsequently, there have been three weight loss studies undertaken in asthmatic children that have demonstrated improvements in asthma control and severity, quality of life, static lung function, and fewer acute asthma exacerbations and nocturnal symptoms following weight loss of 2.6–13% [13–16]. Considering the reported benefits of weight loss in childhood asthma, studies examining the various strategies used are warranted.

Therefore, the aims of the current study were: (1) To examine changes in diet quality in obese asthmatic children during a weight loss intervention, and (2) To examine the association between the baseline subject characteristics and degree of weight loss following the intervention.

2. Materials and Methods

2.1. Study Design

This is a secondary analysis of a group of obese children with physician-diagnosed asthma who participated in a 10-week dietary intervention trial, which has been previously described [13]. Briefly, obese children (body mass index (BMI) z-score ≥ 1.64 standard deviation score (SDS)), aged between 8–17 years, with stable asthma (defined as no exacerbation, respiratory tract infection, oral corticosteroid use, or change in asthma medications in the past 4 weeks) were recruited from the John Hunter Children's Hospital (JHCH) outpatient clinics, local medical centres, and the general community in Newcastle, Australia. Exclusion criteria for this study included: unexplained weight change during the past 3 months, inflammatory or endocrine disorders, and respiratory disorders other than asthma. Participants were randomised to either the dietary intervention group (DIG) or the wait-list control group (WLC), who received the same intervention as the DIG group after an initial 10 week waiting period. As the degree of weight loss was similar in the DIG and WLC groups, these were combined for this secondary analysis. Participant approval and guardian consent were acquired prior to enrolment. The study was registered with the Australian New Zealand Clinical Trials Registry (ACTRN12610000955011) and was approved by the Hunter New England and University of Newcastle Human Research Ethics Committees (09/05/20/5.08).

2.2. Intervention

The 10-week dietary intervention pursued a 2000-kilojoule/day (KJ/day) energy reduction from individually calculated age- and gender-appropriate energy requirements (Schofield equation to estimate basal metabolic rate using activity factor of 1.55) [17]. Participants attended face-to-face counselling sessions with an Accredited Practising Dietitian in weeks 0, 1, 2, 4, 6, 8, and 10 with telephone contact in alternate weeks. Counselling sessions involved theoretical and practical education on food selection as well as appropriate serving sizes to optimize macronutrient and micronutrient intakes within an energy-restricted diet, identification and resolution of barriers to dietary change, and goal-setting. Materials included individually adapted meal plans and a commercial calorie counter. Meal plans routinely encouraged participants to increase intake of wholegrain breads and cereals, fruit and vegetables, and low-fat dairy products and lean meats. Additionally, intake of foods high in excess energy, fat, sugar, and salt such as chips, pizza, sausage rolls, cakes, soft drinks, and fried foods such as chicken nuggets and hot chips, were discouraged. Participants and their guardians were instructed to self-monitor energy intake using a food diary throughout the study period.

2.3. Clinical Assessment

At baseline and post-intervention, participants attended John Hunter Children's Hospital after an overnight fast (≥12 h) and withholding antihistamines and asthma medications (≥24 h). Baseline clinical asthma pattern (Global Initiative for Asthma (GINA) guidelines) and atopy (skin prick test) were assessed as described previously [18]. The following data were assessed at baseline and post-intervention: asthma control (Juniper Asthma Control Questionnaire (ACQ)), quality of life (Paediatric Asthma Quality of Life Questionnaire (standardized) (PAQLQ(s))), dynamic and static lung function via spirometry (Windows KoKo PFT System Version 4.9 2005, PDS Inc., Louisville, KY, USA), and plethysmography (MedGraphics Elite Series Plethysmograph, St. Paul, MN, USA; Breeze Suite 6.4.1.14 Version 510 2008, MedGraphics Corp., St. Paul, MN, USA) [19,20]. Forced expiratory volume in one second (FEV1), forced vital capacity (FVC), and expiratory reserve volume (ERV) values were expressed as a percentage of the predicted values [21,22].

2.4. Anthropometry

Height and weight were measured at baseline and post-intervention using 150 kg max scales (EB8271 NuWeigh, Newcastle Weighing Services, Newcastle, NSW, Australia) and a 2 m wall-suspended measuring tape with wall stop (Surgical and Medical Supplies Pty Ltd., Rose Park, SA, Australia). Waist circumference measurement was collected using a tape measure (Lufkin Executive Thin line 2 m W606 PM tape measure). BMI was calculated (weight (kg)/height (m^2)) and converted to BMI z-scores [23]. Body composition, including total body fat and lean mass, was measured as a percentage (%) of total body weight by dual energy X-ray absorptiometry (DEXA) (GE Lunar Prodigy, Medtel, Madison, WI, USA; GE Healthcare encore 2007 software Version 11.40.004, Madison, WI, USA) at baseline and post-intervention.

2.5. Diet Quality

2.5.1. Dietary Intake

Dietary intake was estimated pre- and post- intervention using a 4-day food record completed by participants using household measures. Records were analysed using the AUSNUT 2010 database available on nutrient analysis software Foodworks (Foodworks version 7.0.3016, Xyris Software, Brisbane, QLD, Australia) to quantify macronutrient and micronutrient intake. Nutrient intake was compared to the age and gender specific Nutrient Reference Values (NRVs) for Australians [24].

2.5.2. Nutritional Biomarkers

Plasma Carotenoid and Tocopherol Analysis

High performance liquid chromatography (HPLC) methodology was used to determine β-carotene, lycopene, α-carotene, β-cryptoxanthin, lutein/zeaxanthin, α-tocopherol, and γ-tocopherol concentrations in plasma, as described previously [25,26].

Plasma and Red Blood Cell Fatty Acid Analysis

Gas chromatography (GC) was used to determine red blood cell (RBC) fatty acid (FA) proportions and plasma FA concentrations of saturated fatty acids (SFA), polyunsaturated fatty acids (PUFA), monounsaturated fatty acids (MUFA), and omega 3 and 6. RBC membrane and plasma FAs were methylated, and the total FAs were determined using the validated method established by Lepage and Roy as described previously [27,28].

2.6. *Physical Activity*

Baseline physical activity measurements, including the amount of exercise (duration) undertaken and the intensity of physical activity as measured by metabolic equivalent (METs) for subjects, was obtained via the Adolescent Physical Activity and Recall Questionnaire (APARQ).

2.7. *Statistical Analysis*

Data are presented as mean (standard deviation, SD), median (interquartile range, IQR), or proportion (n, (%)). Continuous data were assessed using a paired mean-comparison *t*-test or Wilcoxon sign-rank test for within-group comparisons. Correlation analysis was conducted using Pearson's correlation coefficient or Spearman's Rank correlation coefficient to identify variables that correlated with weight loss, indicated by change in (Δ) BMI z-score and %fat mass. Results were considered statistically significant at $p < 0.05$. Statistical analysis was performed using Statistical Software for the Social Sciences Version 24.0 (SPSS Release 24.0; IBM Corp., Armonk, NY, USA). No adjustments were made for multiple testing.

3. Results

3.1. *Participant Characteristics*

Baseline characteristics for the 28 participants are presented in Table 1. Participants were predominantly mild asthmatics, with normal lung function between 80–120% predicted values. Baseline characteristics revealed that participants were predominantly male and atopic.

Table 1. Subject characteristics at baseline.

Characteristics	Baseline
Subjects; n	28
Gender (%females)	11 (39.3)
Age (years)	12.1 ± 2.3
Height (cm)	156.6 ± 12.2
Weight (kg)	73.3 ± 3.9
BMI z-score	2.1 ± 0.3
Waist Circumference (cm)	98.1 ± 10.6
Total body fat mass (%)	45.1 ± 6.8
Total lean mass (%)	53.3 ± 6.4
ACQ score	1.0 (0.4, 1.4)
PAQLQ score	6.1 (5.2, 6.5)
FEV1 %predicted	92.8 ± 2.4
FVC %predicted	100.5 (93.7, 108.4)
FEV1/FVC %	94.2 (88.1, 96.5)
ERV %predicted	94.6 (66.2, 147.9)
Atopic; n (%)	19 (67.9)
Metabolic Equivalent (METs)	5.2 (3.9, 5.8)
Activity Duration (mins)	436.3 (285.0, 702.5)
Short-acting Beta-antagonist; n (%)	24 (84.7)
Inhaled Corticosteroid; n (%)	10 (35.7)

Data are presented as mean ± SD or median (interquartile range, IQR) unless stated. BMI z-score: Body Mass Index z-score; ACQ: Asthma Control Questionnaire; PAQLQ: Paediatric Asthma Quality of Life Questionnaire; FEV1: Forced Expiratory Volume in 1 s; FVC: Forced Vital Capacity; ERV1: Expiratory Reserve Volume; METs: Metabolic Equivalent of Task; SABA: Short acting β-agonist; ICS: Inhaled Corticosteroids.

3.2. *Changes Following The Intervention*

3.2.1. Lung Function and Medication Use

No significant change in lung function or medication use were observed following the intervention [13].

3.2.2. Anthropometric and Body Composition

Complete pre- and post-intervention anthropometric and body composition data were available for 27 participants. Following the intervention, a significant reduction in various anthropometric and body composition measurements (p-value ≤ 0.001) were observed. Furthermore, a significant increase in lean mass (1.9%) was observed following the intervention (Table 2).

Table 2. Change in anthropometric variables in obese asthmatic children following a 10-week dietary intervention.

Anthropometry and Body Composition	Pre-Intervention	Post-Intervention	*p*-Value
Weight (kg)	73.3 ± 20.71	70.8 ± 19.35	0.001
BMI z-score	2.13 ± 0.30	1.95 ± 0.31	<0.001
Waist circumference (cm)	98.1 ± 9.72	94.4 ± 9.05	<0.001
Total body fat mass (%)	45.1 ± 6.74	42.9 ± 7.38	<0.001
Lean mass (%)	53.1 ± 6.3	55.0 ± 7.2	<0.001

Data are presented as mean ± SD or median (QR) unless stated.

3.2.3. Diet Quality

Dietary Change

Complete pre- and post-intervention diet quality data were available for 16 participants. A significant increase in mean % energy derived from protein (16.2 ± 3.1 versus 20.5 ± 3.7, $p < 0.001$) and a significant decrease in absolute sugar intake (g) (115.3 ± 34.6 versus 92.2 ± 29.4, $p = 0.025$) were detected post intervention (Figure 1). A trend towards decreased intake of energy and % energy from fat was observed (Table 3). At baseline, the mean intake of fibre, Vitamin A, potassium, and calcium were below age and gender specific recommendations. Post-intervention, the mean intake of fibre, Vitamin A, potassium, and calcium intake remained inadequate. The intake of saturated fat as % total fat intake was relatively high, approximately 38%, and remained unchanged post-intervention.

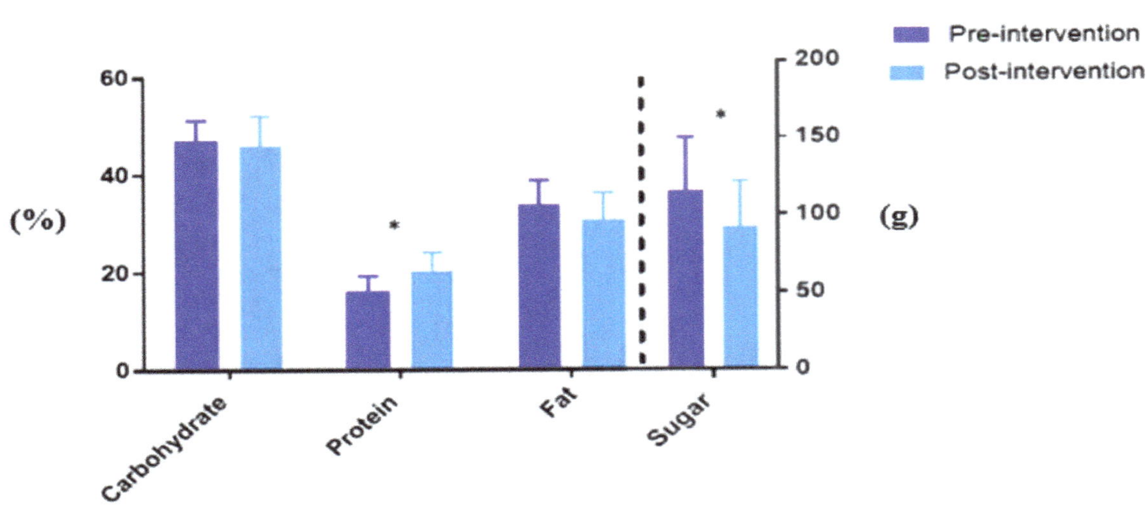

Figure 1. The % Energy intake from carbohydrate, protein, and fat as well as absolute sugar intake (g) pre- and post-intervention. * $p < 0.05$ for pre- versus post-intervention values.

Table 3. Change in dietary intakes in obese asthmatic children following a 10-week dietary intervention.

Energy and Macronutrients	Pre-Intervention	RDI/AI (%)	Post-Intervention	RDI/AI (%)	*p*-Value
Energy (kJ)	8678.6 ± 2089.9	-	7548.3 ± 866.6	-	0.123
%Protein	16.2 ± 3.1	-	20.5 ± 3.7	-	<0.001
%Fat	33.8 ± 5.0	-	30.7 ± 5.6	-	0.147
%SFA	38.4 ± 2.8	-	38.7 ± 3.9	-	0.794
%MUFA	12.7 (11.0, 18.0)	-	16.5 (12.7, 18.9)	-	0.109
%PUFA	48.6 (44.8, 51.4)	-	45.1 (40.9, 49.0)	-	0.121
%Carbohydrate	47.2 ± 4.1	-	45.9 ± 6.3	-	0.493
Sugar (g)	115.3 ± 34.6	-	92.2 ± 29.4	-	0.025
Fibre (g)	19.8 (16.5, 23.2)	89.5 (76.3, 113.4)	21.9 (15.7, 28.2)	99.4 (73.1, 122.2)	0.438
β-Carotene (μg)	2066.1 (836.2, 4436.1)	53.5 (23.2, 102.3)	2116.1 (1442.9, 3210.3)	52.9 (36.9, 94.5)	0.717
Thiamine (mg)	2.2 (1.7, 3.4)	229.6 (176.4, 318.7)	2.2 (1.6, 3.0)	214.9 (174.3, 338.9)	0.717
Riboflavin (mg)	2.7 (1.7, 3.2)	275.2 (190.1, 323.5)	2.5 (1.8, 3.0)	279.8 (194.1, 334.0)	0.959
Niacin (mg)	43.3 ± 12.4	361.6 ± 26.2	45.8 ± 16.0	395.1 ± 42.7	0.649
Vitamin C (mg)	95.9 (70.2, 117.8)	239.6 (175.4, 294.5)	61.2 (29.9, 91.3)	153.1 (74.6, 228.1)	0.179
Vitamin E (mg)	8.8 ± 5.3	102.1 ± 13.0	6.9 ± 2.2	81.8 ± 6.8	0.197
Potassium (mg)	2409.0 ± 509.1	78.0 ± 4.2	2570.2 ± 706.6	84.7 ± 7.2	0.497
Calcium (mg)	754.2 ± 245.3	66.6 ± 6.4	802.2 ± 385.7	72.1 ± 10.2	0.477
Iron (mg)	11.2 ± 3.6	127.6 ± 11.1	11.8 ± 5.2	134.9 ± 15.6	0.661
Zinc (mg)	9.3 (8.0, 13.0)	155.4 (127.2, 216.5)	12.2 (8.3, 14.5)	184.6 (116.2, 236.7)	0.756

Data are presented as mean ± SD or median (IQR) unless stated. kJ: kilojoules; RDI: Recommended Daily Intake; AI: Adequate Intake; - not applicable.

Nutritional Biomarkers

No significant change in plasma carotenoid and tocopherol concentrations was detected following the intervention (Table 4). No significant differences in total red blood cell membrane fatty acids or individual fatty acids was seen in participants following the intervention (Table 5).

Table 4. Change in plasma carotenoids and tocopherols in obese asthmatic children following a 10-week dietary intervention.

Nutritional Biomarker	Pre-Intervention	Post-Intervention	p-Value
	Carotenoids (mg/mL)		
Lutein	171.0 (152.5, 250.8)	207.5 (138.5, 268.8)	0.349
β-Cryptoxanthin	220.5 (78.0, 543.0)	254.5 (146.8, 346.8)	0.896
Lycopene	64.5 (42.3, 168.5)	53.0 (36.3, 97.5)	0.653
α-carotene	21.0 (0.00, 35.3)	21.0 (10.8, 31.8)	0.463
β-carotene	311.0 (114.0, 568.8)	304.5 (114.0, 711.8)	0.352
Total Carotenoids	995.5 (528.5, 1504.3)	946.0 (494.3, 1494.3)	0.472
	Tocopherols (mg/mL)		
γ-tocopherol	1.56 (0.93, 2.26)	1.95 (1.18, 2.41)	0.396
α-tocopherol	19.17 ± 2.41	23.56 ± 2.82	0.157
Total Tocopherols	20.88 (9.69, 29.46)	26.22 (18.23, 29.28)	0.157

Data are presented as mean ± SD or median [IQR] unless stated.

Table 5. Change in red blood cell membrane fatty acids in obese asthmatic children following a 10-week dietary intervention.

Nutritional Biomarker	Pre-Intervention	Post-Intervention	p-Value
SFA %	44.0 (43.8, 45.3)	43.9 (43.8, 45.2)	0.326
PUFA %	38.0 ± 1.6	37.9 ± 1.1	0.366
MUFA %	17.6 ± 0.8	17.9 ± 0.7	0.205
Omega 3 %	5.4 (4.0, 7.2)	6.7 (5.0, 7.7)	0.281
Omega 6 %	43.9 (36.8, 49.0)	42.0 (37.0, 47.6)	0.379

Data are presented as mean ± SD or median (IQR) unless stated.

3.3. Correlations

The Δ% fat mass was negatively associated with baseline % predicted FEV1 ($r = -0.429$, $p = 0.026$) (Figure 2 a) and baseline METs ($r = -0.454$, $p = 0.023$) (Figure 2b). Baseline duration of physical activity (mins/week) was negatively associated with ΔBMI z-score ($r = -0.445$, $p = 0.023$) (Figure 3).

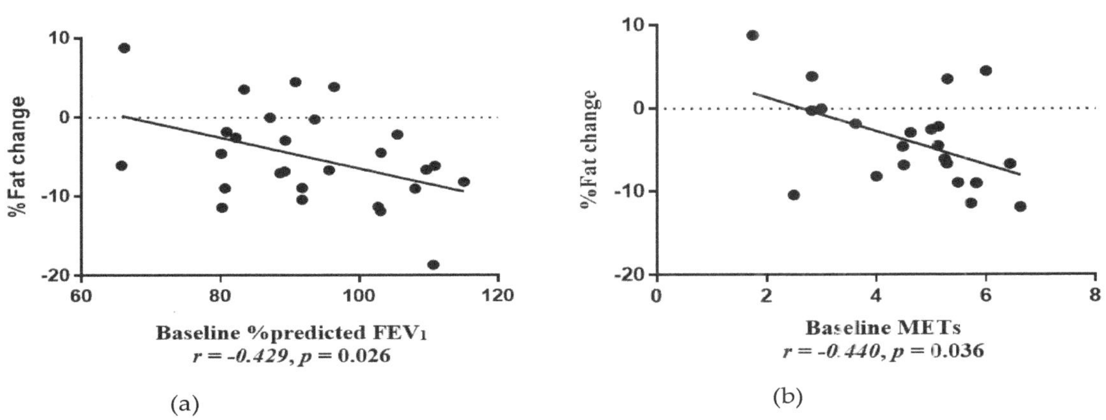

Figure 2. (**a**) Correlation between % fat mass change and baseline %predicted forced expiratory volume in 1 s (FEV_1) ($r = -0.429$, $p = 0.026$). (**b**) Correlation between % fat mass change and baseline Metabolic Equivalents (METs) ($r = -0.440$, $p = 0.036$).

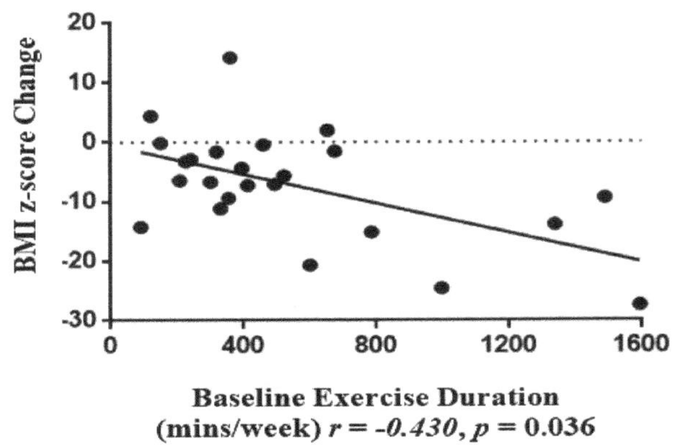

Figure 3. Correlations between BMI z-score change and baseline physical activity duration (mins/week) ($r = -0.430$, $p = 0.036$).

4. Discussion

In this secondary analysis of a cohort of obese asthmatic children who participated in a 10-week diet-induced weight loss intervention, we evaluated diet quality, which was assessed by dietary intake and key nutritional biomarkers, and examined the association between baseline subject characteristics with degree of weight loss following the intervention [13]. Following the intervention, improvements in diet quality were observed, notably a significant increase in protein intake and a significant decrease in sugar consumption. No significant changes in micronutrient intake, plasma carotenoids, or fatty acids were observed. Interestingly, children who had better baseline lung function (%predicted FEV1), or who undertook higher intensity physical activity at baseline, had a greater loss of % body fat. Additionally, children who engaged in a longer duration of physical activity at baseline had a greater decrease in BMI z-score.

The dietary intervention was successful in inducing acute weight loss in this group of obese asthmatic children, with a mean 3.4% weight loss and a 0.18 SDS reduction in the BMI z-score over 10 weeks. This is comparable to previous work reporting a 2.6% weight loss and a 0.2 SDS reduction in the BMI z-score in overweight/obese asthmatic children who undertook a dietary intervention over 6 weeks [15]. Of recent weight loss studies in non-asthmatic children that included a dietary component, BMI z-score reductions of 0.1–0.4 have been reported in interventions conducted over longer periods of time, lasting 4–9 months, whilst other studies found no significant change in BMI z-score [29,30]. Our results also show a significant decrease in the mean waist circumference of 3.7 cm compared to a 6 cm reduction in waist circumference in non-asthmatic overweight children involved in a multi-faceted lifestyle intervention conducted over a much longer 6-month period by Reinehr et al. [31]. Lastly, significant reductions in fat mass were also observed in our study, with a mean fat loss of 2.2% and significant reductions in segmental fat. A multicomponent lifestyle intervention study by da Silva et al. in asthmatic adolescents also reported significant fat loss with a reduction of 6%, albeit over a longer period of 6 months [14]. The lean mass of participants in our study significantly increased by 1.9% compared to a non-significant improvement in lean mass between control and intervention groups following the 6-month intervention carried out by Reinehr et al. [31]. This is a notable finding in the absence of a structured exercise component. Improvement seen in lean mass may have been attributable to the main dietary findings of increased protein and decreased sugar intake following the intervention. Therefore, the study outcomes suggest the efficacy of this short-term dietary intervention in reducing weight loss, BMI z-score, waist circumference, and fat mass in obese asthmatic children.

Participants had a significant increase of 4.3% in energy derived from protein and a 20% reduction in absolute sugar intake. Additionally, a trend of decreased % energy from total fat (−3.1%) was observed; however, this did not reach statistical significance. The observed dietary changes as a result of the intervention are likely attributable to the nutrition strategies employed in the intervention, such as meal plans and portion size education, which discouraged large intakes of foods high in excess energy, fat, sugar, and salt. Similarly, studies by Davis et al. [32,33] in non-asthmatic overweight adolescent females that focused on inducing weight loss through energy restriction achieved significant decreases in sugar intake and trended towards increased % energy intake from protein, mainly achieved by reducing the intake of processed foods. Therefore, our data demonstrate that an intervention spanning 10 weeks can induce important dietary changes; however, it is unknown if these changes can be maintained long term, and longer-term studies in this population are warranted. Additionally, the use of electronic data collection, such as a mobile phone application to record dietary intake, may reduce the burden of completing a 4-day record and increase compliance, particularly in this age group [34,35].

Dietary records revealed that baseline consumption of various micronutrients: vitamin A, fibre, calcium, and potassium, was inadequate when compared to the NRVs, and remained inadequate following the intervention. Interestingly, when compared to the 2011–2012 Australian health survey, inadequate intakes of calcium and Vitamin A were common in the average Australian child [36]. Approximately 70% of males and 87% of females aged 12–18 years were reported to have inadequate intakes of calcium [36]. Inadequate intake of vitamin A was seen in 33% of males and 27% of females aged 14–18 years [36]. Adequate intakes of these nutrients are particularly important in children for a range of essential body functions such as the use of Vitamin A to promote normal vision and a strong immunity to infectious disease, fibre to promote good bowel health, and calcium to support adequate growth and development. Therefore, it is concerning that intakes of these nutrients within this cohort are inadequate [24]. The study intervention did not specifically target these micronutrients; the focus was on dietary energy reduction and improving overall diet quality. Furthermore, the relatively short time frame of the intervention limited the amount of dietary change achievable. Studies inducing sustained increased intakes of fruit and vegetables in children have been conducted over 6–12 months, indicating that improving micronutrient intakes is possible in studies of longer duration [37,38]. Notably, intake of saturated fatty acids remained relatively high (38% of total fat intake) pre- and post-intervention. In dietary interventions of longer duration, this may be an important area to target as high saturated fat intake is associated with increased risk of cardiovascular disease [39,40]. Interestingly, vitamin E intake reduced following the intervention. A large number of polyunsaturated oils and processed foods are fortified with or contain vitamin E; therefore, a decreased intake of these foods as a result of dietary strategies may explain a decrease in the dietary intake of vitamin E [41].

Significant changes in plasma carotenoids, tocopherols, and fatty acid biomarkers were not detected following the 10-week weight loss intervention, despite improvements in dietary intake. To our knowledge, this is the first study in children with asthma that was conducted to examine the change in nutritional biomarkers following a weight loss intervention. Findings from nutritional biomarker analysis are consistent with the findings from 4-day food records, indicating that fruit, vegetable, and fat intake of participants did not significantly change as a result of the dietary intervention in this small sample. Future studies including longer dietary interventions, to promote micronutrient improvements as well as energy restrictions, are required in obese asthmatic children. Adequate nutrient intake in childhood, including fibre and vitamins A and E, is not only essential for optimal growth and development, but could also potentially provide beneficial anti-inflammatory and antioxidant effects in the asthmatic population [42–44].

An investigation of the baseline characteristics that were associated with the degree of weight loss in our study found that children who presented with better lung function at baseline achieved greater fat loss. This opposes results from a dietary intervention trial in obese asthmatic adults, whereby having poorer lung function was a positive predictor of weight loss [45]. Our results, which suggest that poorer asthma status is a barrier to lifestyle change in children, may be due to factors such as exercise avoidance and increased corticosteroid use in children with more severe disease [46,47]. Indeed, we found that more intense physical activity at baseline (METs) was correlated with greater % fat loss, and longer participation in physical activity at baseline was correlated with a greater reduction in the BMI z-score. Our data suggest that those with better lung function or physical engagement would be a good target for future interventions as they are more likely to achieve weight loss goals. In contrast, these findings suggest that children who do not have these attributes experience a barrier to weight loss and may benefit from a different type of intervention. Such an intervention may require extra assistance to achieve weight loss goals through asthma education on approaches to exercising safely.

There are a few limitations that should be acknowledged. Firstly, the small sample size potentially limited our ability to detect significant changes in some outcomes; nonetheless, we had adequate power to detect key changes in weight status and diet quality, which provided novel and important data to stimulate research in this area of childhood obesity and asthma. Secondly, we do not have follow up data on participants; therefore, long-term diet quality, weight loss, or maintenance could not be examined. Lastly, due to a low response rate, analysis of 4-day food records was limited and reporting bias may have affected results. However, the assessment of diet quality was strengthened by the use of gold standard objective measurement tools such as high performance liquid chromatography and gas chromatography to analyse nutritional biomarkers in the majority of subjects.

Analysis of diet quality revealed that a short term, diet-induced weight loss intervention was successful in reducing overall energy intake and intake of sugary foods; however, dietary data and nutritional biomarker analysis indicated no change in fruit and vegetable or fatty acid intake, perhaps due to a delay in the adoption of these positive practices. The study indicated that partaking in more regular or intense exercise at baseline was correlated with greater weight loss success, whilst those children with poorer lung function at baseline achieved less weight loss, so may require greater support to achieve their weight loss goals. The findings from this study support the need for future larger trials to further investigate the efficacy of weight loss interventions in obese asthmatic children. Future trials should include a longer intervention period to allow the implementation and adoption of more comprehensive dietary strategies targeting a reduction in dietary energy and improvements in diet quality, including an increase in fruit and vegetable intake and a reduction in saturated fatty acid intake. Importantly, this study has highlighted subgroups of obese asthmatic children, specifically those with low lung function or low physical activity levels, that may require additional support in order to succeed in weight loss interventions.

Author Contributions: S.E. was responsible for the analysis of data and writing of the article. M.E.J. was responsible for formulating the research question, designing the primary study, data collection and reviewing the manuscript. C.E.C. was responsible for designing the primary study, and reviewing the manuscript. P.G.G. was responsible for designing the primary study and the supervision of data collection and data interpretation. J.H. was responsible for designing the primary study. L.G.W. was responsible for formulating the research question, designing the study, data collection and reviewing the manuscript. All authors have read and agreed to the published version of the manuscript.

Acknowledgments: The authors thank Respiratory Research (Hunter Medical Research Institute) laboratory and clinical staff members for assistance with sample collection and processing and Majella Maher (John Hunter Children's Hospital) for performing lung plethysmography.

References

1. Lv, N.; Xiao, L.; Ma, J. Weight Management Interventions in Adult and Pediatric Asthma Populations: A Systematic Review. *J. Pulm. Respir. Med.* **2015**, *5*, 1000232. [CrossRef] [PubMed]
2. Lang, J.E. Obesity, Nutrition, and Asthma in Children. *Pediatri. Allergy Immunol. Pulmonol.* **2012**, *25*, 64–75. [CrossRef] [PubMed]
3. Marks, G.; Reddel, H.; Copper, S.; Poulos, L.; Ampon, R.; Waters, A.M. *Asthma in Australia 2011: with a Focus Chapter on Chronic Obstructive Pulmonary Disease*; Australian Centre for Asthma Monitoring; Series No.4; Australian Institute of Health and Welfare: Canberra, Australia, 2011.
4. Ng, M.; Fleming, T.; Robinson, M.; Thomson, B.; Graetz, N.; Margono, C.; Mullany, E.C.; Biryukov, S.; Abbafati, C.; Abera, S.F.; et al. Global, regional, and national prevalence of overweight and obesity in children and adults during 1980–2013: A systematic analysis for the Global Burden of Disease Study 2013. *Lancet* **2014**, *384*, 766–781. [CrossRef]

5. *A picture of overweight and obesity in Australia 2017*; Australian Institute of Health and Welfare: Canberra, Australia, 2017.
6. Venn, A.J.; Thomson, R.J.; Schmidt, M.D.; Cleland, V.J.; Curry, B.A.; Gennat, H.C.; Dwyer, T. Overweight and obesity from childhood to adulthood: A follow-up of participants in the 1985 Australian Schools Health and Fitness Survey. *Med. J. Aust.* **2007**, *186*, 458–460. [CrossRef]
7. Haldar, P.; Pavord, I.D.; Shaw, D.E.; Berry, M.A.; Thomas, M.; Brightling, C.E.; Wardlaw, A.J.; Green, R.H. Cluster analysis and clinical asthma phenotypes. *Am. J. Respir. Crit. Care Med.* **2008**, *178*, 218–224. [CrossRef]
8. Scott, H.A.; Gibson, P.G.; Garg, M.L.; Wood, L.G. Airway inflammation is augmented by obesity and fatty acids in asthma. *Eur. Respir. J.* **2011**, *38*, 594–602. [CrossRef]
9. Sood, A. Obesity, adipokines, and lung disease. *J. Appl. Physiol.* **2010**, *108*, 744–753. [CrossRef]
10. Sutherland, E.R. Linking obesity and asthma. *Ann. N. Y. Acad. Sci.* **2014**, *1311*, 31–41. [CrossRef]
11. Forno, E.; Lescher, R.; Strunk, R.; Weiss, S.; Fuhlbrigge, A.; Celedón, J.C. Decreased response to inhaled steroids in overweight and obese asthmatic children. *J. Allergy Clin. Immunol.* **2011**, *127*, 741–749. [CrossRef]
12. Li, A.; Chan, D.; Wong, E.; Yin, J.; Nelson, E.; Fok, T. The effects of obesity on pulmonary function. *Arch. Dis. Child.* **2003**, *88*, 361–363. [CrossRef]
13. Jensen, M.E.; Gibson, P.G.; Collins, C.E.; Hilton, J.M.; Wood, L.G. Diet-induced weight loss in obese children with asthma: A randomized controlled trial. *Clin. Exp. Allergy* **2013**, *43*, 775–784. [CrossRef] [PubMed]
14. da Silva, P.L.; de Mello, M.T.; Cheik, N.C.; Sanches, P.L.; Correia, F.A.; de Piano, A.; Corgosinho, F.C.; da Silveira Campos, R.M.; do Nascimento, C.M.; Oyama, L.M.; et al. Interdisciplinary therapy improves biomarkers profile and lung function in asthmatic obese adolescents. *Pediatr. Pulmonol.* **2012**, *47*, 8–17. [CrossRef] [PubMed]
15. van Leeuwen, J.C.; Hoogstrate, M.; Duiverman, E.J.; Thio, B.J. Effects of dietary induced weight loss on exercise-induced bronchoconstriction in overweight and obese children. *Pediatr. Pulmonol.* **2014**, *49*, 1155–1161. [CrossRef] [PubMed]
16. Abd El-Kader, M.S.; Al-Jiffri, O.; Ashmawy, E.M. Impact of weight loss on markers of systemic inflammation in obese Saudi children with asthma. *Afr. Health Sci.* **2013**, *13*, 682–688. [CrossRef] [PubMed]
17. Mahut, B.; Beydon, N.; Delclaux, C. Overweight is not a comorbidity factor during childhood asthma: The GrowthOb study. *Eur. Respir. J.* **2012**, *39*, 1120–1126. [CrossRef]
18. Global Initiative for Asthma. *Pocket Guide for Asthma Management and Prevention in Children*; National Institute of Health: USA, 2005; Contract No.:02-3659.
19. Juniper, E.; Guyatt, G.; Ferrie, P.; King, D. Development and validation of a questionnaire to measure asthma control. *Eur. Respi. J.* **1999**, *14*, 902–907. [CrossRef]
20. Seid, M.; Limbers, C.A.; Driscoll, K.A.; Opipari-Arrigan, L.A.; Gelhard, L.R.; Varni, J.W. Reliability, validity, and responsiveness of the Pediatric Quality of Life Inventory™(PedsQL™) Generic Core Scales and Asthma Symptoms Scale in vulnerable children with asthma. *J. Asthma* **2010**, *47*, 170–177. [CrossRef]
21. Hankinson, J.L.; Odencrantz, J.R.; Fedan, K.B. Spirometric reference values from a sample of the general US population. *Am. J. Respir. Crit. Care Medi.* **1999**, *159*, 179–187. [CrossRef]
22. Ruppel, G.L.; Enright, P.L. Pulmonary function testing. *Respir. Care* **2012**, *57*, 165–175. [CrossRef]
23. Division of Nutritional Physical Activity and Obesity. National Center for Chronic Disease Prevention and Health Promotion. A SAS Program for the CDC Growth Charts; Center for Disease Control and Prevention. Available online: https://www.cdc.gov/nccdphp/dnpao/growthcharts/resources/sas-who.htm (accessed on 22 November 2017).
24. *Nutrient Reference Values for Australia and New Zealand: Including Recommended Dietary Intakes*; Australian Government Department of Health and Ageing; National Health and Medical Research Council (Eds.) Version 1.2; National Health and Medical Research Council: Canberra, Australia, 2006.
25. Barua, A.B.; Kostic, D.; Olsen, J.A. New simplified procedures for the extraction and simultaneous high-performance liquid chromatographic analysis of retinol, tocopherols, and carotenoids in human serum. *J. Chromatogr. B* **1993**, *617*, 257–264. [CrossRef]
26. Wood, L.G.; Garg, M.L.; Blake, R.J.; Garcia-Caraballo, S.; Gibson, P.G. Airway and circulating levels of carotenoids in asthma and healthy controls. *J. Am. Coll. Nutr.* **2005**, *24*, 448–455. [CrossRef] [PubMed]

27. Wood, L.G.; Fitzgerald, D.A.; Lee, A.K.; Garg, M.L. Improved antioxidant and fatty acid status of patients with cystic fibrosis after antioxidant supplementation is linked to improved lung function. *Am. Clin. Nutr.* **2003**, *77*, 150–159. [CrossRef] [PubMed]
28. Lepage, G.; Roy, C.C. Direct transesterification of all classes of lipids in a one-step reaction. *J. Lipid Res.* **1986**, *27*, 114–120. [PubMed]
29. Ho, M.; Garnett, S.P.; Baur, L.; Burrows, T.; Stewart, L.; Neve, M.; Collins, C. Effectiveness of lifestyle interventions in child obesity: Systematic review with meta-analysis. *Pediatrics* **2012**, *130*, e1647–e1671. [CrossRef] [PubMed]
30. McCallum, Z.; Wake, M.; Gerner, B.; Baur, L.; Gibbons, K.; Gold, L.; Gunn, J.; Harris, C.; Naughton, G.; Riess, C.; et al. Outcome data from the LEAP (Live, Eat and Play) trial: A randomized controlled trial of a primary care intervention for childhood overweight/mild obesity. *Int. J. Obes.* **2007**, *31*, 630–636. [CrossRef]
31. Reinehr, T.; Schaefer, A.; Winkel, K.; Finne, E.; Toschke, A.; Kolip, P. An effective lifestyle intervention in overweight children: Findings from a randomized controlled trial on "Obeldicks light". *Clin. Nutr.* **2010**, *29*, 331–336. [CrossRef]
32. Davis, J.N.; Tung, A.M.Y.; Chak, S.S.; Ventura, E.E.; Byrd-Williams, C.E.; Alexander, K.E.; Lane, C.J.; Weigensberg, M.J.; Spruijt-Metz, D.; Goran, M.I. Aerobic and Strength Training Reduces Adiposity in Overweight Latina Adolescents. *Med. Sci. Sports Exerc.* **2009**, *41*, 1494–1503. [CrossRef]
33. Davis, J.N.; Ventura, E.E.; Shaibi, G.Q.; Weigensberg, M.J.; Spruijt-Metz, D.; Watanabe, R.M.; Goran, M.I. Reduction in Added Sugar Intake and Improvement in Insulin Secretion in Overweight Latina Adolescents. *Metab. Syndr. Relat. D.* **2007**, *5*, 183–193. [CrossRef]
34. Casperson, S.L.; Sieling, J.; Moon, J.; Johnson, L.; Roemmich, J.N.; Whigham, L. A Mobile Phone Food Record App to Digitally Capture Dietary Intake for Adolescents in a Free-Living Environment: Usability Study. *JMIR MHealth UHealth* **2015**, *3*, e30. [CrossRef]
35. Daugherty, B.L.; Schap, T.E.; Ettienne-Gittens, R.; Zhu, F.M.; Bosch, M.; Delp, E.J.; Ebert, D.S.; Kerr, D.A.; Boushey, C.J. Novel Technologies for Assessing Dietary Intake: Evaluating the Usability of a Mobile Telephone Food Record Among Adults and Adolescents. *J. Med. Internet Res.* **2012**, *14*, e58. [CrossRef]
36. Australian Bureau of Statistics and Food Standards Australia and New Zealand. *4364.0.55.008—Australian Health Survey: Usual Nutrient Intakes, 2011–2012*; Australian Bureau of Statistics: Canberra, Australia, 2015.
37. Raynor, H.A.; Osterholt, K.M.; Hart, C.N.; Jelalian, E.; Vivier, P.; Wing, R.R. Efficacy of U.S. Pediatric Obesity Primary Care Guidelines: Two Randomized Trials. *Pediatr. Obes.* **2012**, *7*, 28–38. [CrossRef]
38. Wright, K.; Norris, K.; Newman Giger, J.; Suro, Z. Improving healthy dietary behaviors, nutrition knowledge, and self-efficacy among underserved school children with parent and community involvement. *Child. Obes.* **2012**, *8*, 347–356. [CrossRef]
39. Siri-Tarino, P.W.; Sun, Q.; Hu, F.B.; Krauss, R.M. Saturated fatty acids and risk of coronary heart disease: Modulation by replacement nutrients. *Curr. Atheroscler. Rep.* **2010**, *12*, 384–390. [CrossRef] [PubMed]
40. Zong, G.; Li, Y.; Wanders, A.J.; Alssema, M.; Zock, P.L.; Willett, W.C.; Hu, F.B.; Sun, Q. Intake of individual saturated fatty acids and risk of coronary heart disease in US men and women: Two prospective longitudinal cohort studies. *BMJ* **2016**, *355*, i5796. [CrossRef] [PubMed]
41. Reboul, E.; Richelle, M.; Perrot, E.; Desmoulins-Malezet, C.; Pirisi, V.; Borel, P. Bioaccessibility of carotenoids and vitamin E from their main dietary sources. *J. Agric. Food Chem.* **2006**, *54*, 8749–8755. [CrossRef] [PubMed]
42. Wood, L.G.; Gibson, P.G. Dietary factors lead to innate immune activation in asthma. *Pharmacol. Ther.* **2009**, *123*, 37–53. [CrossRef] [PubMed]
43. Romieu, I.; Sienra-Monge, J.J.; Ramírez-Aguilar, M.; Téllez-Rojo, M.M.; Moreno-Macías, H.; Reyes-Ruiz, N.I.; del Río-Navarro, B.E.; Ruiz-Navarro, M.X.; Hatch, G.; Slade, R.; et al. Antioxidant supplementation and lung functions among children with asthma exposed to high levels of air pollutants. *Am. J. Respir. Crit. Care Med.* **2002**, *166*, 703–709. [CrossRef]
44. Chatzi, L.; Apostolaki, G.; Bibakis, I.; Skypala, I.; Bibaki-Liakou, V.; Tzanakis, N.; Kogevinas, M.; Cullinan, P. Protective effect of fruits, vegetables and the Mediterranean diet on asthma and allergies among children in Crete. *Thorax.* **2007**, *62*, 677–683. [CrossRef]
45. Scott, H.A.; Gibson, P.G.; Garg, M.L.; Pretto, J.J.; Morgan, P.J.; Callister, R.; Wood, L.G. Determinants of weight loss success utilizing a meal replacement plan and/or exercise, in overweight and obese adults with asthma. *Respirology* **2015**, *20*, 243–250. [CrossRef]

46. Glazebrook, C.; McPherson, A.C.; Macdonald, I.A.; Swift, J.A.; Ramsay, C.; Newbould, R.; Smyth, A. Asthma as a barrier to children's physical activity: Implications for body mass index and mental health. *Pediatrics* **2006**, *118*, 2443–2449. [CrossRef] [PubMed]
47. Lang, D.M.; Butz, A.M.; Duggan, A.K.; Serwint, J.R. Physical activity in urban school-aged children with asthma. *Pediatrics* **2004**, *113*, e341–e346. [CrossRef] [PubMed]

9

Higher Omega-3 Index is Associated with Better Asthma Control and Lower Medication Dose

Isobel Stoodley [1,2], Manohar Garg [3], Hayley Scott [1,3], Lesley Macdonald-Wicks [2], Bronwyn Berthon [1,3] and Lisa Wood [1,3,*]

1 Priority Research Centre for Healthy Lungs, Hunter Medical Research Institute, Newcastle, NSW 2305, Australia; Isobel.Stoodley@uon.edu.au (I.S.); Hayley.Scott@newcastle.edu.au (H.S.); Bronwyn.Berthon@newcastle.edu.au (B.B.)
2 School of Health Sciences, University of Newcastle, Callaghan, NSW 2308, Australia; Lesley.Wicks@newcastle.edu.au
3 School of Biomedical Science and Pharmacy, University of Newcastle, Callaghan, NSW 2308, Australia; Manohar.Garg@newcastle.edu.au
* Correspondence: Lisa.Wood@newcastle.edu.au

Abstract: Asthma is a chronic inflammatory airway disease, associated with systemic inflammation. Omega-3 polyunsaturated fatty acids (n-3 PUFA) have established anti-inflammatory effects, thus having potential as an adjunct therapy in asthma. This study aimed to compare erythrocyte n-3 PUFA in adults with (n = 255) and without (n = 137) asthma and determine the relationship between erythrocyte n-3 PUFA and clinical asthma outcomes. Subjects had blood collected, lung function measured and Juniper Asthma Control Questionnaire (ACQ) score calculated. Fatty acids were measured in erythrocyte membranes by gas chromatography, and the omega-3 index (O3I) was calculated (% eicosapentaenoic acid + % docosahexaenoic acid). O3I was similar in subjects with and without asthma ($p = 0.089$). A higher O3I was observed in subjects with controlled or partially controlled asthma (ACQ < 1.5) compared to subjects with uncontrolled asthma (ACQ ≥ 1.5) (6.0% (5.4–7.2) versus 5.6% (4.6–6.4) $p = 0.033$). Subjects with a high O3I (≥8%) had a lower maintenance dose of inhaled corticosteroids (ICS) compared to those with a low O3I (<8%) (1000 µg (400–1000) versus 1000 µg (500–2000) $p = 0.019$). This study demonstrates that a higher O3I is associated with better asthma control and with lower ICS dose, suggesting that a higher erythrocyte n-3 PUFA level may have a role in asthma management.

Keywords: omega-3 index; asthma; inflammation; fatty acids; nutritional biomarkers

---

1. Introduction

Asthma is a chronic inflammatory disease of the airways, affecting 2.5 million Australians in 2014–2015 [1]. Globally, it is estimated that 334 million people have asthma [2]. Airway inflammation in asthma is triggered by exposures such as allergens and viruses, and causes airway hyper-responsiveness (AHR), airway smooth muscle contraction and excess mucous production [3,4]. This results in the hallmark symptoms of asthma including breathlessness, wheezing, chest tightness and persistent cough [2]. Systemic inflammation is also a feature of asthma, with circulating C-reactive protein (CRP) levels shown to be elevated in people with asthma [4–6], which is associated with poorer lung function and more severe airway inflammation [6].

Current treatment for asthma predominantly involves inhaled corticosteroid (ICS) medication, which helps to control symptoms and exacerbations and to improve lung function and quality of life by reducing airway inflammation [7,8]. However, dietary patterns are also being investigated for their potential preventative or therapeutic role. It has been suggested that a Western dietary pattern, high in energy, saturated fats, sugars and salt, may increase the prevalence and severity of asthma, independent of socioeconomic and lifestyle factors [9]. Additionally, a Mediterranean dietary pattern, which is nutrient dense and high in fish, fruit and vegetables, could be protective, reducing the incidence and the severity of asthma symptoms [9].

One such way that the Mediterranean diet might be effective in reducing asthma symptoms is due to the high intake of omega-3 polyunsaturated fatty acids (n-3 PUFA). n-3 PUFA include eicosapentaenoic acid (EPA, C20:5n-3), docosapentaenoic acid (DPA, C22:5n-3) and docosahexaenoic acid (DHA, C22:6n-3) and are commonly found in significant amounts in marine sources such as salmon, herring and sardines [10]. These fatty acids have been found to inhibit inflammatory processes within the body, with benefits in cardiovascular disease well established [10]. These include suppression of transcription factors that control the production of circulating inflammatory cytokines CRP, tumour necrosis factor alpha (TNF-α), interleukin (IL)-1β and IL-6 [11,12]. n-3 PUFA also compete with omega-6 polyunsaturated fatty acids (n-6 PUFA), resulting in the downregulation of arachidonic acid-derived immune and inflammatory mediators including 3- and 5-series prostaglandins, thromboxanes, leukotrienes and lipoxins [3,13]. These same pathways and inflammatory mediators are involved in AHR in people with asthma [11,12]. Hence, it is possible that n-3 PUFA could play a role in the prevention or treatment of asthma.

Various studies have investigated n-3 PUFA in asthma. Mouse models have shown that increased DHA intake is associated with reduced eosinophil infiltration into the lungs [13] and that by increasing the ratio of n-3:n-6 in lung tissue, interleukins can be downregulated [14]. In humans, research is conflicting. Some studies have found that supplementation with n-3 PUFA can decrease inflammatory markers and improve asthma symptoms [15,16], while others found no changes to AHR or airway inflammation [17]. A Cochrane meta-analysis conducted in 2000, and updated in 2011 with nil changes, including 9 randomised control trials (RCTs) of both adults and children, concluded that there was no benefit or risk for the use of dietary marine fatty acids in people with asthma [18,19]. Furthermore the European Academy of Allergy and Clinical Immunology have released a position statement emphasizing that until more standardized trials with assessment of pre-intervention fatty acid levels have been conducted, there is no recommendation for n-3 PUFA in asthma and other allergic diseases [20].

The conflicting evidence highlights a need for more research in this area. Hence, this study aimed to examine the relationship between n-3 PUFA status and clinical outcomes in Australian adults with asthma. Firstly, it is unclear whether n-3 PUFA status is impaired in Australian subjects with asthma compared to health controls, thus an aim of this project was to investigate and describe the differences between these two groups. We hypothesized that individuals with asthma would have poorer n-3 PUFA status compared to those without asthma. Furthermore we hypothesized that subjects with asthma and a high n-3 PUFA status would have better clinical outcomes than those with low n-3 PUFA status. These aims were examined using the omega-3 index (O3I), which has been validated as a reliable measure of dietary n-3 PUFA intake and reflects long-term n-3 PUFA status [21,22]. O3I is the sum of erythrocyte EPA and DHA, expressed as a percentage of total erythrocyte membrane fatty acids [23]. A secondary aim of this project was to examine the effects of obesity on O3I in adults with asthma. Obesity in asthma is associated with poorer asthma control, greater severity, higher medication doses and more frequent exacerbations than healthy weight individuals [24]. One mechanism suggested to underpin this relationship is the chronic low-grade inflammation associated with obesity [25,26]. Considering the anti-inflammatory properties attributed to n-3 PUFA, it is possible that n-3 PUFA may attenuate this inflammation. Whether these interactions exist in obese asthmatic subjects is unknown. Therefore, we hypothesized that in an obese asthmatic population, those with a lower O3I would have poorer clinical and biochemical outcomes compared to those with a higher O3I.

2. Materials and Methods

2.1. Subjects

Subjects were pooled from seven previously published research studies [25,27–31]. Subjects were adults (≥18 years of age) with (n = 255) and without (n = 137) asthma, recruited at the Hunter Medical Research Institute (HMRI), NSW Australia, from existing research volunteer databases or by media release. Subjects were nonsmoking (never smoked, or ceased at least 6 months prior). Asthma was defined as a doctor's diagnosis of asthma with documented history of AHR. All asthmatic subjects were classified as stable with no asthma exacerbation, respiratory tract infection or oral corticosteroid use in the preceding four weeks. Exclusions included current smokers, use of systemic anti-inflammatory or immunosuppressant medications or current cancer diagnosis. All studies were conducted at the Hunter Medical Research Institute, Newcastle, Australia between 2006–2015. All procedures involving human subjects were approved by the Hunter New England Human Research Ethics Committee (Ethics approval numbers: 11/06/15/3.03; 14/02/19/3.01; 13/07/17/4.03; 08/10/15/5.07; 09/03/18/5.05; 05/03/09/3.09; 09/05/20/5.07). All subjects provided written informed consent.

Clinical assessment and blood collection were performed during a single clinic visit. Subjects underwent spirometry including forced expiratory volume in one second (FEV_1) and forced vital capacity (FVC) (Koko, nSpire Health, Longmont, CO, USA or Medgraphics, PFS/D and BreezeSuite software; Medgraphics, Saint Paul, MN, USA) in accordance with American Thoracic Society and European Respiratory Society guidelines [32,33]. All asthmatic subjects completed the six-item Juniper Asthma Control Questionnaire (ACQ6) [34]. Partially or well controlled asthma was defined as ACQ < 1.5, while uncontrolled asthma was defined as ≥1.5 [34]. Clinical asthma pattern was determined according to Global Initiative for Asthma (GINA) recommendations [8]. Maintenance ICS doses were recorded and converted to beclomethasone equivalents. Body weight was measured in 0.1 kg increments using calibrated electronic scales (Nuweigh EB8271; Newcastle Weighing Services, Wickham, Australia). Height was calculated to the nearest millimetre using a wall-mounted stadiometer (Seca 220; Seca, Hamburg, Germany). Body mass index (BMI) was calculated as body weight (kg)/height $(m)^2$.

2.2. Sputum Induction and Analysis

Sputum induction and bronchial provocation were performed using 4.5% hypertonic saline over 15.5-min nebuliser time [35]. Lower respiratory sputum portions were selected and dispersed using dithiothreitol. Total cell counts and cell viability (trypan blue exclusion) were determined from cytospins.

2.3. Plasma Inflammatory Markers

Venous blood was collected after a 12 h overnight fast. Commercial ELISAs were used to determine plasma high sensitivity CRP (MP-Biomedicals, Orangeburg, NY, USA), IL-6 and TNF-α (R&D Systems, Minneapolic, MN, USA), according to manufacturer's instructions.

2.4. Erythrocyte Membrane Fatty Acid Preparation

Whole blood was collected in EDTA tubes and centrifuged at 3000× g at 4 °C for 10 min. Red blood cells were separated and stored at −70 °C before analysis.

After thawing, the erythrocytes were lysed, and their membranes solubilised and purified using the method described by Tomoda et al. [36]. Then, 12 mL of hypotonic tris buffer (10 mM tris hydroxymethyamino methane/5 mM ascorbate buffer, pH 7.4) was added to approximately 500 µL of erythrocytes and vortexed. After standing on ice for five minutes, 12 mL of 0.25 M glucose solution was added. The sample was vortexed, stood on ice for another five minutes, then centrifuged at 10,000 rpm at 4 °C for 10 min. The supernatant was discarded and the procedure repeated twice more (resuspending the pellet by vortexing) using the same quantities of tris and glucose solutions above, but centrifuging at 12,000 rpm at 4 °C for 10 min and then 15,000 rpm at 4 °C for 20 min. The pellet was then resuspended in approximately 250 μL each of tris and glucose solutions and stored at −20 °C prior to analysing for fatty acid content.

2.5. Fatty Acid Determination

Total erythrocyte fatty acids were determined using the method established by Lepage and Roy [37]. Here, 2 mL of a methanol/toluene mixture (4:1 *v*/*v*), containing C21:0 (0.02 g/L) as internal standard and BHT (0.12 g/L), was added to 200 μL of erythrocyte membrane suspension. Fatty acids were methylated by adding 200 μL acetyl chloride dropwise while vortexing and heating to 100 °C for one hour. After cooling, the reaction was stopped by adding 5 mL 6% K_2CO_3. The sample was centrifuged at 3000 rpm at 4 °C for 10 min to facilitate separation of layers. The upper toluene layer was used for gas chromatography analysis of the fatty acid methyl esters, using a 30 m × 0.25 m (DB-225) fused carbon-silica column coated with cyanopropylphenyl (J & W Scientific, Folsom, CA, USA). Both injector and detector port temperatures were set at 250 °C. The oven temperature was 170 °C for two minutes, increased 10 °C/min to 190 °C, held for one minute, then increased 3 °C/min up to 220 °C and maintained to give a total run time of 30 min. A split ratio of 10:1 and an injection volume of 5 mL was used. The chromatograph was equipped with a flame ionisation detector, autosampler and autodetector. Sample fatty acid methyl ester peaks were identified by comparing their retention times with those of standard mixture of fatty acid methyl esters and quantified using a Hewlett Packard 6890 Series Gas Chromatograph with Chemstations Version A.04.02.

2.6. Fatty Acid Calculations

Saturated, monounsaturated, polyunsaturated, n-3 PUFA and n-6 PUFA are reported as a percentage of total fatty acids. Omega-3 Index is calculated as ((erythrocyte membrane EPA (mg) + erythrocyte membrane DHA (mg))/total erythrocyte fatty acids (mg)) × 100 [22]. Harris et al. [22] classify an O3I between 0–4% as undesirable, 4–8% as intermediate and ≥8% as desirable, for cardioprotective benefits. An O3I cutpoint of ≥8% was used for the current analysis to represent a high O3I. The omega-6:omega-3 ratio was determined by dividing total omega-6 fatty acids (%) by total omega-3 fatty acids (%).

2.7. Statistical Analysis

Data are reported as median (interquartile range (IQR)) for nonparametric data or mean ± standard deviation (SD) for parametric data. Data were analysed using GraphPad Prism 7.0 for Windows (GraphPad Software, La Jolla, California, USA) and STATA 15 (StataCorp, College Station, TX, USA). Comparisons for continuous data were performed using either the unpaired *t*-test or Mann–Whitney test for nonparametric variables. Logistic regression analysis was used, adjusted for age, BMI and sex, for comparisons between subjects with versus without asthma; subjects with asthma with well or partially controlled asthma versus poorly controlled asthma; and subjects with asthma with low versus high O3I. Age and gender adjusted two-factor ANOVA was used to analyse the interaction between obesity and O3I status on clinical and biochemical asthma outcomes. Chi-squared testing was used for categorical variables. In this study, p-values < 0.05 were considered statistically significant.

3. Results

3.1. Comparison of Nonasthmatic and Asthmatic Subjects

Table 1 shows the clinical characteristics of subjects with and without asthma. There was no significant difference in age between the groups, however the BMI was higher and there were fewer females in the nonasthmatic group. After adjusting for age, gender and BMI, lung function was lower in the asthmatic population. CRP was significantly higher in the asthma population, however there was no significant difference in the other systemic inflammatory markers. Subjects without asthma had a significantly lower percentage of eosinophils in sputum, higher percentage of macrophages in sputum, higher percentage of SFAs, a lower percentage of MUFAs and omega-3 PUFA and a higher ratio of n-6:n-3 fatty acids.

Table 1. Subject characteristics.

	No Asthma	Asthma	*p*-Value *	Odds Ratio (95% CI)
Subjects	137	255		
Age	53.5 (45.2–64.35)	57.1 (40.9–66.0)	0.8473 ^	
Gender (% female)	39.4 (n = 54)	50.6 (n = 129)	**0.0435 #**	
BMI (kg/m^2)	33.5 (28.9–41.45)	31.0 (26.9–36.2)	**0.0011 ^**	
Smokers (% Ex)	46.72 (n = 64)	43.14 (n = 110)	0.854	0.98 (0.79–1.22)
Smoking history (pack years)	4.0 (0.0–11.0)	5.5 (0.0–20.0)	**0.011**	1.03 (1.00–1.06)
ACQ6		0.7 (0.2–1.3) (n = 206)		
GINA Classification (%1/2/3/4)		25/20/39/16 (n = 243)		
FEV$_1$ (% predicted)	98.54 ± 13.04 (n = 71)	79.42 ± 18.77 (n = 235)	**<0.001**	0.93 (0.90–0.95)
FVC (% predicted)	102.8 ± 14.07 (n = 71)	91.46 ± 16.11 (n = 235)	**<0.001**	0.95 (0.93–0.97)
FEV$_1$/FVC (%)	77.0 (74.0–81.0) (n = 71)	70.0 (63.1–77.0) (n = 235)	**<0.001**	0.88 (0.84–0.92)
Airway markers				
Neutrophils (%)	30.5 (12.0–47.25) (n = 51)	34.75 (10.25–54.75) (n = 206)	0.782	1.00 (0.99–1.02)
Eosinophils (%)	0.75 (0.25–1.25) (n = 51)	2.5 (0.72–14.4) (n = 206)	**0.003**	1.25 (1.08–1.44)
Macrophages (%)	61.5 (46.0–74.0) (n = 51)	38.31 (18.9–61.31) (n = 206)	**<0.001**	0.97 (0.96–0.98)
Lymphocytes (%)	1.75 (0.75–3.0) (n = 51)	1.0 (0.25–3.25) (n = 206)	**0.032**	1.06 (1.01–1.11)
Systemic markers				
CRP (mg/L)	3.0 (1.5–5.5) (n = 135)	3.41 (1.2–8.18) (n = 196)	0.018	1.06 (1.01–1.11)
IL-6 (pg/mL)	1.45 (1.05–1.94) (n = 34)	1.51 (0.89–2.58) (n = 171)	0.289	1.19 (0.87–1.63)
TNF-a (pg/mL)	1.05 (0.88–1.34) (n = 44)	1.18 (0.64–1.77) (n = 143)	0.168	1.43 (0.86–2.38)
Erythrocyte fatty acids				
SFA (%)	43.29 (42.54–44.26) (n = 127)	41.92 (40.87–43.11) (n = 242)	**0.001**	0.89 (0.83–0.96)
MUFA (%)	18.27 (17.29–19.28) (n = 127)	19.06 (17.67–20.13) (n = 242)	0.526	1.02 (0.96–1.09)
PUFA (%)	29.13 (27.27–30.44) (n = 127)	28.77 (27.29–30.39) (n = 242)	0.995	1.00 (0.91–1.10)
n-3 PUFA (%)	8.91 (7.85–10.25) (n = 127)	10.03 (8.74–12.54) (n = 242)	**<0.001**	1.24 (1.12–1.37)
O3I (%)	6.1 (4.9–7.4) (n = 127)	6.2 (5.4–7.9) (n = 242)	0.089	1.10 (0.99–1.23)
n-6:n-3	3.31 (2.72–3.74) (n = 127)	2.82 (2.30–3.40) (n = 242)	**<0.001**	0.58 (0.44–0.78)

Data are presented as median (interquartile range) or mean ± standard deviation. Significant effects are highlighted in bold. BMI: Body mass index; FEV$_1$: Forced expiratory volume in 1 s; FVC: Forced vital capacity; ACQ: Asthma Control Questionnaire; GINA: Global Initiative for Asthma; CRP: C-reactive protein; IL-6: Interleukin-6; TNF-α: Tumour necrosis factor α; SFA: Saturated fatty acids; MUFA: Monounsaturated fatty acids; n-6 PUFA: Omega-6 polyunsaturated fatty acids; n-3 PUFA: Omega-3 polyunsaturated fatty acids; O3I: Omega-3 index. GINA classification: 1 = intermittent, 2 = mild persistent, 3 = moderate persistent, 4 = severe persistent. *: Logistic regression analysis performed, adjusting for age, gender and BMI unless otherwise stated. Reference population is nonasthmatic. ^: Mann–Whitney test, unadjusted. #: Chi-squared test, unadjusted.

3.2. Asthma Clinical Markers, Systemic Inflammation and O3I

While O3I did not differ between subjects with and without asthma, when comparing within the asthma group alone, subjects with partially controlled or well controlled asthma (ACQ6 < 1.5) had a significantly higher O3I compared to those with uncontrolled asthma (ACQ6 ≥ 1.5) (6.0% (5.4–7.2) versus 5.6% (4.6–6.4), respectively, $p = 0.033$) (Figure 1).

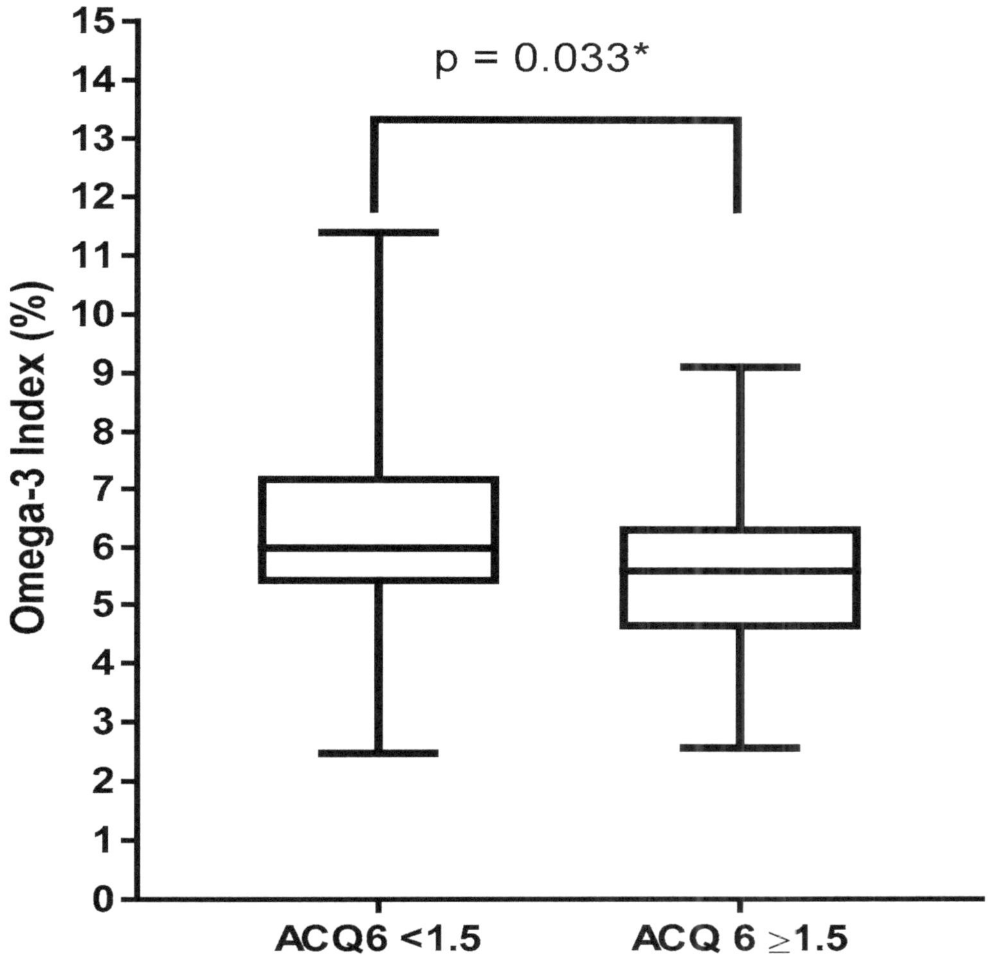

Figure 1. Omega-3 index classified by asthma control, ACQ < 1.5 $n = 150$, ACQ ≥ 1.5 $n = 44$. * Logistic regression adjusting for age, BMI and gender.

When analysing clinical asthma measures, there was no significant difference in lung function or asthma severity in subjects with a higher (≥8%) versus lower (<8%) O3I (Table 2). However subjects with higher O3I had a significantly lower range of maintenance ICS dose (beclomethasone equivalents) (Table 2, Figure 2). There were no significant differences in systemic inflammatory markers between higher and lower O3I after adjusting for age, gender and BMI (Table 2).

Table 2. Clinical asthma markers of subjects with asthma by O3I status.

	Asthma, Low O3I (<8%)	Asthma, High O3I (≥8%)	p-Value *	Odds Ratio (95% CI)
n	185	57		
Age	57.9 (42.8–66.4)	54.6 (36.5–65.6)	0.1938 ^	
BMI (kg/m^2)	30.6 (26.9–37.7)	31.7 (28.1–35.5)	0.9591 ^	
ICS (ug beclomethasone eq/d)	1000 (500–2000) (n = 120)	1000 (400–1000) (n = 51)	**0.019**	0.999 (0.9989–0.9999)
ACQ6	0.7 (0.2–1.3) (n = 170)	0.42 (0.2–1.11) (n = 24)	0.311	0.71 (0.37–1.37)
GINA Classification: 1/2/3/4 (%)	24/22/38/16 (n = 176)	19/25/41/15 (n = 54)	0.7638 #	
FEV_1 (% predicted)	79.11 ± 19.4 (n = 169)	78.93 ± 16.78 (n = 54)	0.610	1.00 (0.98–1.01)
FVC (% predicted)	91.01 ± 16.82 (n = 169)	91.71 ± 13.43 (n = 54)	0.760	1.00 (0.98–1.02)
FEV_1/FVC (%)	70 (63–77) (n = 169)	69.55 (59.78–75.33) (n = 54)	0.249	0.98 (0.95–1.01)
CRP (mg/mL)	3.8 (1.3–8.7) (n = 140)	2.9 (1.1–7.8) (n = 44)	0.124	0.94 (0.87–1.02)
IL-6 (pg/mL)	1.8 (1.3–8.7) (n = 41)	0.9 (0.1–1.7) (n = 41)	0.212	0.85 (0.65–1.10)
TNF (pg/mL)	1.3 (0.9–1.8) (n = 99)	0.4 (0.2–1.2) (n = 37)	0.944	1.01 (0.85–1.19)

Data are presented as median (interquartile range) or mean ± standard deviation unless stated. Significant effects are highlighted in bold. ICS: inhaled corticosteroid; ACQ: Asthma Control Questionnaire; GINA: Global Initiative for Asthma; FEV_1: Forced expiratory volume in 1 s; %; FVC: Forced vital capacity; CRP: C-reactive protein; IL-6: Interleukin-6; TNF-α: Tumour necrosis factor α. *: Logistic regression analysis performed, adjusting for age, gender and BMI unless otherwise stated. Reference population is low O3I. ^: Mann–Whitney test, unadjusted. #: Chi-squared test, unadjusted.

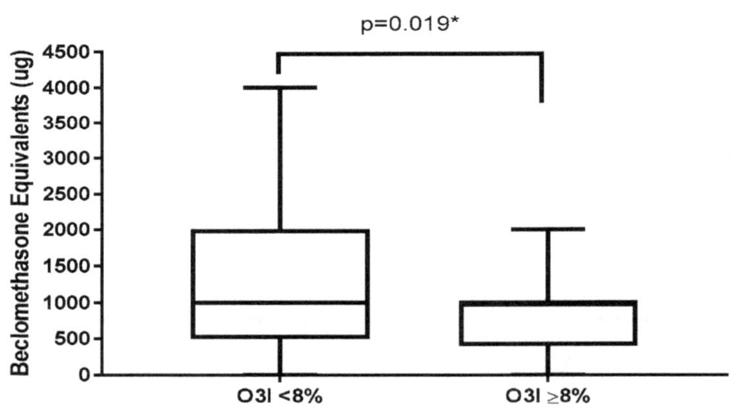

Figure 2. Inhaled corticosteroid dose classified by omega-3 index status. * Logistic regression adjusting for age, BMI and gender.

3.3. *Asthma, O3I and Obesity*

Due to the interesting nexus of asthma and obesity, we compared clinical asthma markers and systemic inflammation in subjects with asthma divided into obese (BMI ≥ 30 kg/m^2) and nonobese (BMI < 30 kg/m^2) groups with high (≥8%) and low (<8%) O3I (Table 3). The analysis was adjusted for gender and age. We found that subjects who were obese with a lower O3I had a significantly higher range of maintenance ICS medication dose compared with obese subjects with a higher O3I (p = 0.0002) (Table 3). While there was significance difference detected in all lung function measures, only FEV1/FVC ratio revealed an obesity interaction. Both obesity and O3I were significant predictors of CRP, but not for TNF-α or Il-6. Obesity and O3I were not significant predictors for ACQ.

Table 3. Clinical asthma markers and inflammatory markers of subjects with asthma, classified by weight and O3I.

	Obese Asthma		Nonobese Asthma					
Obese Asthma	**>8% O3I**	**<8% O3I**	**>8% O3I**	**<8% O3I**	***p*-Value ***	**Obesity × O3I Interaction**	**High vs. Low O3I**	**Obese vs. Nonobese**
n	37	98	20	87				
ICS (μg beclomethasone eq/d)	1000 (212.5–1000) (*n* = 36)	1000 (1000–2000) (*n* = 61)	1000 (500–1000) (*n* = 15)	500 (500–1000) (*n* = 59)	**0.0002**	0.1556	0.0104	0.0077
ACQ6	0.33 (0–1.8) (*n* = 7)	0.75 (0.3–1.5) (*n* = 86)	0.5 (0.3–1.0) (*n* = 17)	0.7 (0.2–1.3) (*n* = 84)	0.6981	0.8864	0.4235	0.4948
FEV_1 (% predicted)	82.49 ± 15.08 (*n* = 35)	80.18 ± 19.37 (*n* = 84)	72.37 ± 18.15 (*n* = 19)	78.05 ± 19.48 (*n* = 85)	**0.0001**	0.6616	0.4851	0.3445
FVC (% predicted)	94.04 ± 13.87 (*n* = 35)	88.61 ± 15.84 (*n* = 84)	87.42 ± 11.74 (*n* = 19)	93.38 ± 17 (*n* = 85)	**<0.0001**	0.2197	0.8011	0.3537
FEV_1/FVC (5)	71.5 (63.9–77.7) (*n* = 35)	74 (66.25–80) (*n* = 84)	66 (55–71.6) (*n* = 19)	68 (60–74) (*n* = 85)	**<0.0001**	0.6012	0.1146	0.0035
CRP (mg/mL)	3.1 (1.25–8) (*n* = 33)	5.59 (2.67–12.42) (*n* = 74)	1.57 (0.9–7.28) (*n* = 11)	1.77 (0.97–5) (*n* = 67)	**0.0003**	0.0475		
IL-6 (pg/mL)	0.30 (0.04–1.13) (*n* = 30)	2.35 (1.61–3.37) (*n* = 53)	1.77 (1.16–2.42) (*n* = 11)	1.38 (0.9–2.11) (*n* = 65)	**0.0326**	0.6909	0.1857	0.3207
TNF (pg/mL)	0.35 (0.18–0.9) (*n* = 27)	1.41 (0.96–1.92) (*n* = 50)	1 (0.46–1.54) (*n* = 10)	1.23 (0.82–1.75) (*n* = 49)	0.4769	0.3315	0.8142	0.2666

Data are presented as median (interquartile range) or mean ± standard deviation. Significant effects are highlighted in bold. ICS: inhaled corticosteroid; ACQ: Asthma Control Questionnaire; GINA: Global Initiative for Asthma; FEV1: Forced expiratory volume in 1 s; FVC: Forced vital capacity; CRP: C-reactive protein; IL-6: Interleukin-6; TNF-α: Tumour necrosis factor α. *: Two-factor ANOVA analysis performed, adjusted for age and gender, unless otherwise stated.

4. Discussion

To the best of our knowledge, this is the first study reporting that a lower omega-3 index is associated with poorer asthma control in adults with asthma. Additionally, a higher O3I was associated with a lower maintenance ICS dose. Interestingly, this was most significant in the subjects who were also obese, showing a similar dose range of maintenance ICS to nonobese subjects with asthma. Considering the high medication burden and reduced quality of life in people with asthma, our study suggests that higher levels of n-3 PUFA could be utilised as an adjunct therapy in the treatment of asthma.

Our first aim was to investigate the differences in erythrocyte fatty acid levels and O3I between subjects with and without asthma in an Australian population. Contrary to our hypothesis there was no difference in O3I, subjects with asthma had a better fatty acid profile, with lower saturated fatty acids, higher monounsaturated and n-3 fatty acids and a lower n-6 PUFA to n-3 PUFA ratio. This is in contrast to the results of Zhou et al. [38], who found that subjects in China with asthma had a fatty acid profile composed mostly of SFAs, while those without asthma contained more PUFAs. Similar to our study, supplement and dietary intake data were not available to determine whether these differences were reflective of different dietary or supplement patterns or an effect of asthma. In severe asthma, dysregulation of lipid metabolism pathways has been observed; in particular, n-3 PUFA pathways are impaired, while n-6 PUFA pathways remain unaffected [39]. This may explain the differences between the two studies, as our population had mild to moderate asthma while Zhou et al. did not present data on the severity in their population and potentially had more severe asthma phenotypes. Furthermore, the subjects with asthma were older than the control group (mean 58 years old versus 25 years old), and without adjusting for this may have been a confounder explaining the differences between the two groups.

This study demonstrated that a lower omega-3 index is associated with poorer asthma control in adults. Subjects with uncontrolled asthma had a significantly lower O3I than those with well controlled or partially controlled asthma. Our findings are supported by a cross-sectional study conducted in 2011, which observed a significant positive relationship between EPA and DHA consumption (measured using a Food Frequency Questionnaire (FFQ)) with asthma control and lung function (FEV_1) [40]. Our study reinforces this finding, using the objective and longer-term measure of O3I, which provides stronger evidence for this relationship.

Another significant finding was the relationship between O3I and maintenance ICS dose. Subjects with a higher O3I had a significantly lower range of maintenance ICS dose. A similar finding has been shown in a recent RCT by Papamichael et al. [41], where children with asthma were prescribed a Mediterranean diet supplemented with two meals of 150 g cooked fatty fish per week for 6 months, compared to a control group following their normal diet. They found that while there was no difference between lung function, asthma control and quality of life scores, there was a significant reduction in medication use for children in the intervention group [41]. In a study examining exercise-induced bronchoconstriction, n-3 PUFA supplementation (3200 mg EPA + 200 mg DHA for eight weeks) has also been demonstrated to reduce bronchodilator use in adults [42]. Given irregular reporting of respiratory outcomes such as ICS dose and asthma control in the available literature, systematic reviews on n-3 PUFA in asthma have highlighted the need for more high quality research in this area [19,43]. In particular, the relationship between n-3 PUFA and medication use would be of great interest for future research, given our results. Our findings suggest that achieving an O3I $\geq$ 8% could be a beneficial target for people with asthma in order to reduce maintenance ICS dose. This target also corresponds with cardioprotective recommendations [22]. Nutritionally, to achieve this O3I, it would equate to consuming $\geq$800 mg EPA and DHA per day, or 4–5 serves of mostly oily fish per week [44]. Intervention studies are required to confirm our observations, particularly to elucidate the ideal dose and duration needed to achieve this status in an asthmatic population, as well as the most effective pathway (supplementation versus whole foods).

As obesity is generally associated with increased asthma severity, poorer asthma control and more frequent exacerbations, it was important to analyse the relationship between O3I, obesity and asthma outcomes [24]. When we examined obese and nonobese asthmatics according to O3I, obese asthmatics with a higher O3I had a lower range of maintenance ICS doses compared with obese asthmatics with a lower O3I. This is particularly important, as obesity is associated with a reduced response to ICS medication, requiring higher doses to achieve protective effects [45]. Our findings suggest that omega-3 fatty acids could be a potential nonpharmacological approach to assist in the management of asthma, however our findings require confirmation by intervention studies. A recent study by Lang et al. found that supplementing with 4 g/day of fish oil over 24 weeks did not affect asthma control, lung function, exacerbations or have any impact on medication use in overweight and obese adolescents and young adults with asthma [46]. This study did not investigate inflammation. Rather, it reported fatty acid status within inflammatory cells such as monocytes and granulocytes, so without confirmation that the supplementation was reducing inflammatory pathways it may be possible that the dose or length of treatment was not sufficient to affect clinical changes in asthma.

Interestingly, we did not find any differences in systemic inflammatory markers between asthmatics with lower and higher O3I, after adjusting for age, gender and BMI. This has been confirmed in other studies investigating the association between n-3 PUFA and inflammatory markers in asthma [47–49]. However, one study used a semiquantitative FFQ rather than objectively measuring n-3 PUFA [47]. Another study trialed a fish oil supplement for eight weeks (800 mg or 3400 mg per day), with neither dose producing a reduction in CRP [48].

However, other studies have found positive effects of n-3 PUFA on systemic inflammatory markers in asthma. Farjadian et al. [15] studied children with asthma and demonstrated a reduction in TNF-α and IL-17A in 72% of subjects after n-3 PUFA supplementation (180 mg EPA and 120 mg DHA daily) for 3 months [15]. This study also demonstrated an improvement in asthma symptoms, while Mickleborough et al. [16] found that supplementing n-3 PUFA (3.2 g EPA and 2.2 g DHA) in elite athletes over three weeks suppressed exercise-induced bronchoconstriction and inflammatory markers such as TNF-α and IL-1β.

A review examining the impact of n-3 PUFA supplementation on inflammatory biomarkers across a variety of diseases found that, particularly in cardiac populations and the critically ill, omega-3 fatty acid supplementation can reduce a variety of inflammatory biomarkers including CRP, IL-6 and TNF-α [50]. However systematic inflammation is not reported in systematic reviews on n-3 PUFA and asthma due to irregularity in reporting [19,43]. Considering the heterogeneity between studies with pathway, dose and duration, further research is needed to further elucidate this relationship.

A recent review by Kumar et al. [51] highlighted a need for further research involving n-3 PUFA in specific asthma sub-populations, as there is a gap in knowledge for the use of n-3 PUFA in obese subjects with asthma. Considering our findings, which demonstrate that a higher O3I in obese asthmatics is associated with lower CRP and maintenance ICS dose, n-3 PUFA supplementation may provide a unique nonpharmacological approach to treating asthma in this population and demands further research.

As expected, subjects with asthma had poorer lung function and increased airway inflammation compared to those without asthma. Airway inflammation is a key feature of asthma and is characterised by increased levels of eosinophils, neutrophils, or both, in the airways [25,52]. While increased systemic inflammation has been reported in some studies of asthma, this was only significant in CRP between our two groups. This may be related to the higher erythrocyte percentage of n-3 fatty acids that we observed in asthma compared to controls. We are unsure why this occurred in our cohort, but we suspect this must be due to higher dietary intake or supplement use by the asthma group.

Strengths of our study include the use of O3I. O3I is an objective and validated measure of n-3 PUFA intake, as erythrocyte fatty acids represent habitual intake and individual bioavailability as opposed to plasma fatty acids, which reflect shorter term intake [12,22,23]. Erythrocyte fatty acids are more accurate than subjective measures such as FFQs, which rely on accurate recounting of dietary intake, as well as interpretation.

There were some limitations to the study. This was an older cohort, limiting our study's ability to be generalised to younger populations. In addition, subjects with and without asthma were not matched for sex or BMI. However, where differences existed, analyses have been adjusted for sex, age and BMI. Another limitation was that fish oil supplementation and dietary intake of fish were not recorded across the studies. It would be important to account for this in future research to determine which pathway more effectively changes n-3 PUFA status in this population. Dietary intake data would also be able to address possible confounding by other anti- or proinflammatory foods or nutrients, which we were not able to account for in this study. Lastly, socioeconomic status data for subjects were not available. Considering the established relationship between education and financial status with n-3 PUFA status [53,54] it would have been beneficial to investigate this relationship in a population with asthma, and would be important to assess in future studies. Furthermore, this cohort may be more representative of subjects with high socioeconomic advantage. The higher median O3I in our asthmatic and nonasthmatic subjects was higher than expected for average Australians. Previous research suggests that, on average, Australians consume 395 mg of n-3 PUFA per day [55], equivalent to an O3I of approximately 4–5%.

The cross-sectional study design cannot determine causality; as such, further intervention studies are needed. Nevertheless, our study adds important insight into the relationship between n-3 PUFA and asthma outcomes.

5. Conclusions

In conclusion, we have shown that a higher O3I is associated with better asthma control, lower inhaled corticosteroid medication dose and lower systemic inflammatory markers, suggesting that n-3 PUFA may have a role in asthma management. In particular, n-3 PUFA may be clinically relevant for an obese asthma population as our findings show lower ICS dose and CRP in this population with a higher O3I. Our findings suggest that achieving an O3I $\geq$ 8% may be an appropriate target for therapeutic benefit in both an asthma and an older population. However intervention studies are needed to confirm this hypothesis, particularly in specific subpopulations such as obese people with asthma who may benefit most from this type of dietary intervention.

Author Contributions: I.S., H.S., L.W. and B.B. conceived the study; I.S. and M.G. conducted the laboratory analysis; I.S., H.S and B.B. conducted formal analysis; I.S. wrote original draft; H.S., B.B., L.M.-W., M.G. and L.W.; reviewed and edited the draft. All authors have read and agreed to the published version of the manuscript.

Acknowledgments: The authors wish to thank Rebecca McLoughlin, Evan Williams and Sarah Hiles at the Hunter Medical Research Institute for their assistance with sample analysis and statistical analysis.

References

1. Australian Bureau of Statistics. *National Health Survey First Results 2014-15*; 4364.0.55.001; Australian Bureau of Statistics: Canberra, Australia, 2015.
2. Global Asthma Network. *The Global Asthma Report*; Global Asthma Network: Auckland, New Zealand, 2014.
3. Beermann, C.; Neumann, S.; Fussbroich, D.; Zielen, S.; Schubert, R. Combinations of distinct long-chain polyunsaturated fatty acid species for improved dietary treatment against allergic bronchial asthma. *Nutr. Burbank Los Angeles Cty. Calif.* **2016**, *32*, 1165–1170. [CrossRef] [PubMed]
4. Wood, L.G.; Baines, K.J.; Fu, J.; Scott, H.A.; Gibson, P.G. The neutrophilic inflammatory phenotype is associated with systemic inflammation in asthma. *Chest* **2012**, *142*, 86–93. [CrossRef] [PubMed]
5. Olafsdottir, I.S.; Gislason, T.; Thjodleifsson, B.; Olafsson, I.; Gislason, D.; Jogi, R.; Janson, C. C reactive protein levels are increased in non-allergic but not allergic asthma: A multicentre epidemiological study. *Thorax* **2005**, *60*, 451–454. [CrossRef] [PubMed]

6. Takemura, M.; Matsumoto, H.; Niimi, A.; Ueda, T.; Matsuoka, H.; Yamaguchi, M.; Jinnai, M.; Muro, S.; Hirai, T.; Ito, Y.; et al. High sensitivity C-reactive protein in asthma. *Eur. Respir. J.* **2006**, *27*, 908–912. [CrossRef] [PubMed]
7. Scott, H.A.; Jensen, M.E.; Wood, L.G. Dietary interventions in asthma. *Curr. Pharm. Des.* **2014**, *20*, 1003–1010. [CrossRef]
8. The Global Initiative for Asthma. GINA Report: Global Strategy for Asthma Management and Prevention. 2007. Available online: http://www.ginasthma.org (accessed on 8 October 2019).
9. Barros, R.; Moreira, A.; Padrao, P.; Teixeira, V.H.; Carvalho, P.; Delgado, L.; Lopes, C.; Severo, M.; Moreira, P. Dietary patterns and asthma prevalence, incidence and control. *Clin. Exp. Allergy J. Br. Soc. Allergy Clin. Immunol.* **2015**, *45*, 1673–1680. [CrossRef]
10. Calder, P.C. Marine omega-3 fatty acids and inflammatory processes: Effects, mechanisms and clinical relevance. *Biochim. Biophys. Acta* **2015**, *1851*, 469–484. [CrossRef]
11. Endo, J.; Arita, M. Cardioprotective mechanism of omega-3 polyunsaturated fatty acids. *J. Cardiol.* **2016**, *67*, 22–27. [CrossRef]
12. Olliver, M.; Veysey, M.; Lucock, M.; Niblett, S.; King, K.; MacDonald-Wicks, L.; Garg, M.L. Erythrocyte omega-3 polyunsaturated fatty acid levels are associated with biomarkers of inflammation in older Australians. *J. Nutr. Intermed. Metab.* **2016**, *5*, 61–69. [CrossRef]
13. Yokoyama, A.; Hamazaki, T.; Ohshita, A.; Kohno, N.; Sakai, K.; Zhao, G.D.; Katayama, H.; Hiwada, K. Effect of aerosolized docosahexaenoic acid in a mouse model of atopic asthma. *Int. Arch. Allergy Immunol.* **2000**, *123*, 327–332. [CrossRef]
14. Bilal, S.; Haworth, O.; Wu, L.; Weylandt, K.H.; Levy, B.D.; Kang, J.X. Fat-1 transgenic mice with elevated omega-3 fatty acids are protected from allergic airway responses. *Biochim. Biophys. Acta* **2011**, *1812*, 1164–1169. [CrossRef] [PubMed]
15. Farjadian, S.; Moghtaderi, M.; Kalani, M.; Gholami, T.; Hosseini Teshnizi, S. Effects of omega-3 fatty acids on serum levels of T-helper cytokines in children with asthma. *Cytokine* **2016**, *85*, 61–66. [CrossRef] [PubMed]
16. Mickleborough, T.D.; Murray, R.L.; Ionescu, A.A.; Lindley, M.R. Fish oil supplementation reduces severity of exercise-induced bronchoconstriction in elite athletes. *Am. J. Respir. Crit. Care Med.* **2003**, *168*, 1181–1189. [CrossRef] [PubMed]
17. Brannan, J.D.; Bood, J.; Alkhabaz, A.; Balgoma, D.; Otis, J.; Delin, I.; Dahlen, B.; Wheelock, C.E.; Nair, P.; Dahlen, S.E.; et al. The effect of omega-3 fatty acids on bronchial hyperresponsiveness, sputum eosinophilia, and mast cell mediators in asthma. *Chest* **2015**, *147*, 397–405. [CrossRef]
18. Woods, R.K.; Thien, F.C.; Abramson, M.J. Dietary marine fatty acids (fish oil) for asthma in adults and children. *Cochrane Database Syst. Rev.* **2002**. [CrossRef]
19. Thien, F.C.K.; De Luca, S.; Woods, R.K.; Abramson, M.J. Cochrane Review: Dietary marine fatty acids (fish oil) for asthma in adults and children. *Evid. Based Child Health Cochrane Rev. J.* **2011**, *6*, 984–1012. [CrossRef]
20. Venter, C.; Meyer, R.W.; Nwaru, B.I.; Roduit, C.; Untersmayr, E.; Adel-Patient, K.; Agache, I.; Agostoni, C.; Akdis, C.A.; Bischoff, S.C.; et al. EAACI position paper: Influence of dietary fatty acids on asthma, food allergy and atopic dermatitis. *Allergy* **2019**, *74*, 1429–1444. [CrossRef]
21. Harris, W.S.; Pottala, J.V.; Vasan, R.S.; Larson, M.G.; Robins, S.J. Changes in erythrocyte membrane trans and marine fatty acids between 1999 and 2006 in older Americans. *J. Nutr.* **2012**, *142*, 1297–1303. [CrossRef]
22. Harris, W.S.; Von Schacky, C. The Omega-3 Index: A new risk factor for death from coronary heart disease? *Prev. Med.* **2004**, *39*, 212–220. [CrossRef]
23. Ferguson, J.J.; Veysey, M.; Lucock, M.; Niblett, S.; King, K.; MacDonald-Wicks, L.; Garg, M.L. Association between omega-3 index and blood lipids in older Australians. *J. Nutr. Biochem.* **2016**, *27*, 233–240. [CrossRef]
24. Stoodley, I.; Williams, L.; Thompson, C.; Scott, H.; Wood, L. Evidence for lifestyle interventions in asthma. *Breathe* **2019**, *15*, e50. [CrossRef] [PubMed]
25. Scott, H.A.; Gibson, P.G.; Garg, M.L.; Wood, L.G. Airway inflammation is augmented by obesity and fatty acids in asthma. *Eur. Respir. J.* **2011**, *38*, 594–602. [CrossRef] [PubMed]
26. Wood, L.G. Diet, Obesity, and Asthma. *Ann. Am. Thorac. Soc.* **2017**, *14*, S332–S338. [CrossRef] [PubMed]
27. Berthon, B.S.; Gibson, P.G.; McElduff, P.; MacDonald-Wicks, L.K.; Wood, L.G. Effects of short-term oral corticosteroid intake on dietary intake, body weight and body composition in adults with asthma—A randomized controlled trial. *Clin. Exp. Allergy J. Br. Soc. Allergy Clin. Immunol.* **2015**, *45*, 908–919. [CrossRef] [PubMed]

28. Williams, E.J.; Baines, K.J.; Berthon, B.S.; Wood, L.G. Effects of an Encapsulated Fruit and Vegetable Juice Concentrate on Obesity-Induced Systemic Inflammation: A Randomised Controlled Trial. *Nutrients* **2017**, *9*, 116. [CrossRef] [PubMed]
29. Scott, H.A.; Gibson, P.G.; Garg, M.L.; Pretto, J.J.; Morgan, P.J.; Callister, R.; Wood, L.G. Dietary restriction and exercise improve airway inflammation and clinical outcomes in overweight and obese asthma: A randomized trial. *Clin. Exp. Allergy J. Br. Soc. Allergy Clin. Immunol.* **2013**, *43*, 36–49. [CrossRef]
30. Wood, L.G.; Garg, M.L.; Smart, J.M.; Scott, H.A.; Barker, D.; Gibson, P.G. Manipulating antioxidant intake in asthma: A randomized controlled trial. *Am. J. Clin. Nutr.* **2012**, *96*, 534–543. [CrossRef]
31. Periyalil, H.A.; Wood, L.G.; Wright, T.A.; Karihaloo, C.; Starkey, M.R.; Miu, A.S.; Baines, K.J.; Hansbro, P.M.; Gibson, P.G. Obese asthmatics are characterized by altered adipose tissue macrophage activation. *Clin. Exp. Allergy J. Br. Soc. Allergy Clin. Immunol.* **2018**, *48*, 641–649. [CrossRef]
32. Wanger, J.; Clausen, J.L.; Coates, A.; Pedersen, O.F.; Brusasco, V.; Burgos, F.; Casaburi, R.; Crapo, R.; Enright, P.; van der Grinten, C.P.; et al. Standardisation of the measurement of lung volumes. *Eur. Respir. J.* **2005**, *26*, 511–522. [CrossRef]
33. Miller, M.R.; Hankinson, J.; Brusasco, V.; Burgos, F.; Casaburi, R.; Coates, A.; Crapo, R.; Enright, P.; van der Grinten, C.P.; Gustafsson, P.; et al. Standardisation of spirometry. *Eur. Respir. J.* **2005**, *26*, 319–338. [CrossRef]
34. Juniper, E.F.; O'Byrne, P.M.; Guyatt, G.H.; Ferrie, P.J.; King, D.R. Development and validation of a questionnaire to measure asthma control. *Eur. Respir. J.* **1999**, *14*, 902–907. [CrossRef] [PubMed]
35. Gibson, P.G.; Wlodarczyk, J.W.; Hensley, M.J.; Gleeson, M.; Henry, R.L.; Cripps, A.W.; Clancy, R.L. Epidemiological association of airway inflammation with asthma symptoms and airway hyperresponsiveness in childhood. *Am. J. Respir. Crit. Care Med.* **1998**, *158*, 36–41. [CrossRef] [PubMed]
36. Tomoda, A.; Kodaira, K.; Taketo, A.; Tanimoto, K.; Yoneyama, Y. Isolation of human erythrocyte membranes in glucose solution. *Anal. Biochem.* **1984**, *140*, 386–390. [CrossRef]
37. Lepage, G.; Roy, C.C. Direct transesterification of all classes of lipids in a one-step reaction. *J. Lipid Res.* **1986**, *27*, 114–120. [PubMed]
38. Zhou, J.; Chen, L.; Liu, Z.; Sang, L.; Li, Y.; Yuan, D. Changes in erythrocyte polyunsaturated fatty acids and plasma eicosanoids level in patients with asthma. *Lipids Health Dis.* **2018**, *17*, 206. [CrossRef] [PubMed]
39. Miyata, J.; Arita, M. Role of omega-3 fatty acids and their metabolites in asthma and allergic diseases. *Allergol. Int.* **2015**, *64*, 27–34. [CrossRef]
40. Barros, R.; Moreira, A.; Fonseca, J.; Delgado, L.; Castel-Branco, M.G.; Haahtela, T.; Lopes, C.; Moreira, P. Dietary intake of alpha-linolenic acid and low ratio of n-6:n-3 PUFA are associated with decreased exhaled NO and improved asthma control. *Br. J. Nutr.* **2011**, *106*, 441–450. [CrossRef]
41. Papamichael, M.M.; Katsardis, C.; Lambert, K.; Tsoukalas, D.; Koutsilieris, M.; Erbas, B.; Itsiopoulos, C. Efficacy of a Mediterranean diet supplemented with fatty fish in ameliorating inflammation in paediatric asthma: A randomised controlled trial. *J. Hum. Nutr. Diet. Off. J. Br. Diet. Assoc.* **2019**, *32*, 185–197. [CrossRef]
42. Mickleborough, T.D.; Lindley, M.R.; Ionescu, A.A.; Fly, A.D. Protective effect of fish oil supplementation on exercise-induced bronchoconstriction in asthma. *Chest* **2006**, *129*, 39–49. [CrossRef]
43. Reisman, J.; Schachter, H.M.; Dales, R.E.; Tran, K.; Kourad, K.; Barnes, D.; Sampson, M.; Morrison, A.; Gaboury, I.; Blackman, J. Treating asthma with omega-3 fatty acids: Where is the evidence? A systematic review. *BMC Complementary Altern. Med.* **2006**, *6*, 26. [CrossRef]
44. *AUSNUT 2011–13–Australian Food Composition Database*; Food Standards Australia New Zealand: Canberra, Australia, 2014.
45. Peters, U.; Dixon, A.E.; Forno, E. Obesity and asthma. *J. Allergy Clin. Immunol.* **2018**, *141*, 1169–1179. [CrossRef] [PubMed]
46. Lang, J.E.; Mougey, E.B.; Hossain, M.J.; Livingston, F.; Balagopal, P.B.; Langdon, S.; Lima, J.J. Fish Oil Supplementation in Overweight/Obese Patients with Uncontrolled Asthma. A Randomized Trial. *Ann. Am. Thorac. Soc.* **2019**, *16*, 554–562. [CrossRef] [PubMed]
47. Haidari, F.; Mohammadshahi, M.; Borsi, S.H.; Haghighizadeh, M.H.; Malgard, S. Comparison of essential fatty acid intakes and serum levels of inflammatory factors between asthmatic and healthy adults: A case-control study. *Iran. J. Allergy Asthma Immunol.* **2014**, *13*, 335–342. [PubMed]

48. Skulas-Ray, A.C.; Kris-Etherton, P.M.; Harris, W.S.; Vanden Heuvel, J.P.; Wagner, P.R.; West, S.G. Dose-response effects of omega-3 fatty acids on triglycerides, inflammation, and endothelial function in healthy persons with moderate hypertriglyceridemia. *Am. J. Clin. Nutr.* **2011**, *93*, 243–252. [CrossRef]
49. Geelen, A.; Brouwer, I.A.; Schouten, E.G.; Kluft, C.; Katan, M.B.; Zock, P.L. Intake of n-3 fatty acids from fish does not lower serum concentrations of C-reactive protein in healthy subjects. *Eur. J. Clin. Nutr.* **2004**, *58*, 1440–1442. [CrossRef]
50. Khorsan, R.; Crawford, C.; Ives, J.A.; Walter, A.R.; Jonas, W.B. The effect of omega-3 fatty acids on biomarkers of inflammation: A rapid evidence assessment of the literature. *Mil. Med.* **2014**, *179*, 2–60. [CrossRef]
51. Kumar, A.; Mastana, S.S.; Lindley, M.R. n-3 Fatty acids and asthma. *Nutr. Res. Rev.* **2016**, *29*, 1–16. [CrossRef]
52. Wood, L.G.; Powell, H.; Gibson, P.G. Mannitol challenge for assessment of airway responsiveness, airway inflammation and inflammatory phenotype in asthma. *Clin. Exp. Allergy J. Br. Soc. Allergy Clin. Immunol.* **2010**, *40*, 232–241. [CrossRef]
53. Wagner, A.; Simon, C.; Morio, B.; Dallongeville, J.; Ruidavets, J.B.; Haas, B.; Laillet, B.; Cottel, D.; Ferrieres, J.; Arveiler, D. Omega-3 index levels and associated factors in a middle-aged French population: The MONA LISA-NUT Study. *Eur. J. Clin. Nutr.* **2015**, *69*, 436–441. [CrossRef]
54. Cohen, B.E.; Garg, S.K.; Ali, S.; Harris, W.S.; Whooley, M.A. Red Blood Cell Docosahexaenoic Acid and Eicosapentaenoic Acid Concentrations Are Positively Associated with Socioeconomic Status in Patients with Established Coronary Artery Disease: Data from the Heart and Soul Study. *J. Nutr.* **2008**, *138*, 1135–1140. [CrossRef]
55. Meyer, B.J. Australians are not Meeting the Recommended Intakes for Omega-3 Long Chain Polyunsaturated Fatty Acids: Results of an Analysis from the 2011-2012 National Nutrition and Physical Activity Survey. *Nutrients* **2016**, *8*, 111. [CrossRef] [PubMed]

10

Perinatal Undernutrition, Metabolic Hormones and Lung Development

Juan Fandiño, Laura Toba, Lucas C. González-Matías, Yolanda Diz-Chaves and Federico Mallo *

Laboratory of Endocrinology (LabEndo), The Biomedical Research Centre (CINBIO), University of Vigo, Campus Universitario de Vigo (CUVI), 36310 Vigo, Spain; jufandinogom@gmail.com (J.F.); lauratoba7@gmail.com (L.T.); lucascgm@uvigo.es (L.C.G.-M.); dizyolanda@gmail.com (Y.D.-C.)

* Correspondence: fmallo@uvigo.es3

Abstract: Maternal and perinatal undernutrition affects the lung development of litters and it may produce long-lasting alterations in respiratory health. This can be demonstrated using animal models and epidemiological studies. During pregnancy, maternal diet controls lung development by direct and indirect mechanisms. For sure, food intake and caloric restriction directly influence the whole body maturation and the lung. In addition, the maternal food intake during pregnancy controls mother, placenta, and fetal endocrine systems that regulate nutrient uptake and distribution to the fetus and pulmonary tissue development. There are several hormones involved in metabolic regulations, which may play an essential role in lung development during pregnancy. This review focuses on the effect of metabolic hormones in lung development and in how undernutrition alters the hormonal environment during pregnancy to disrupt normal lung maturation. We explore the role of GLP-1, ghrelin, and leptin, and also retinoids and cholecalciferol as hormones synthetized from diet precursors. Finally, we also address how metabolic hormones altered during pregnancy may affect lung pathophysiology in the adulthood.

Keywords: lung development; undernutrition; lung diseases; ghrelin; leptin; GLP-1; retinoids; cholecalciferol; fetal growth restriction; respiratory distress syndrome

---

1. Introduction

Maternal diet is an essential factor that controls fetal growth, both directly by providing nutrients to the embryo and indirectly by regulating the expression of endocrine mechanisms that control the uptake and use of nutrients by the fetus; it also contributes indirectly by changing epigenetic profile and so modulating the expression of genes. The reduction in caloric supply during pregnancy that usually comes accompanied by deficiency of macro and several oligonutrients is called maternal undernutrition. It is demonstrated that maternal undernutrition reduces fetal and placental growth in animals and humans [1]. The reduction in fetal growth is explained by the reduction in cell division [2], which is the result of the adaptation of the cells to the lack of nutrients and the alteration of growth factor and hormone supplies, especially insulin and growth hormone [3]. Fetal growth restriction (FGR) is defined as the fetal growth in lower rate than the normal growth potential, and is an important cause of fetal and neonatal morbidity and mortality [4].

Lung development is a complex process that initiates in utero and continues until early adulthood. In humans, lung development starts as soon as week 3 of gestation [5]. Lung organogenesis comprises five differentiated stages in humans [6]. In the embryonic stage (4 to 6 weeks of gestation, WG), the two lung buds and primary bronchi emerge from the primitive foregut. In the pseudoglandular stage (5 to 17 WG), there is an expansion of the conducting airways. Following this, in the canalicular stage (16 to 27 WG), the epithelia differentiates to separate conducting and respiratory airways and the pulmonary surfactant starts to be synthetized by alveolar type II cells (ATII). In the saccular stage (28 to 31 WG), there is a transition from branching morphogenesis to alveologenesis. In the final alveolar stage (32 WG until early postnatal life), alveoli form and grow.

Other mammal species used for the study of lung development show similar stages, but at different timing during gestation. Rodents have an immature lung at birth—they are in the saccular stage and the alveoli develop postnatally [7]. The deficit of nutrients may alter normal lung development, and promotes a long-lasting impact in the lung structure and function [8].

2. Effect of Metabolic Hormones in Lung Development

Hormones and growth factors lead lung morphogenesis. Some key hormones for metabolic control such as insulin, glucocorticoids, and thyroid hormones are at the core of regulatory management of organ development. However, there is extensive literature about their role in lung development and organogenesis that the interested reader might easily find, and thus they are not included in our review, despite their undoubted relevance.

Instead, new hormones modulating metabolism have been recently shown to have a key role in the maturation of several organs, including the lung. In the next paragraphs, we summarize the actions of some of the most relevant metabolic hormones, such as ghrelin, leptin, GLP-1, and gene-regulating hormones such as retinoids and cholecalciferols.

2.1. Ghrelin

Ghrelin is a 28 amino acid acylated peptide derived from preproghrelin, a 117 AA precursor. It was firstly identified in rat and human stomachs [9], but later, ghrelin expression was found in other adult organs such as the pituitary, hypothalamus, kidneys, heart, and placenta [10]. Ghrelin acts trough a G protein-coupled receptor known as growth hormone secretagogue receptor subtype 1a (GHS-R1a) [9], because it potently stimulates growth hormone (GH) release from the pituitary. In addition, ghrelin stimulates food intake, acting at hypothalamus, and it is involved in the regulation of metabolism, having an overall anabolic effect [11].

Ghrelin hormone is detected in cord blood in human fetuses from 20 weeks of gestation [12]. Interestingly, ghrelin is expressed in neuroendocrine cells of the bronchial wall in the pseudoglandular stage of fetal lung development (7–18 WG), but its levels decrease from 19 WG to the second year of postnatal life, and remains afterwards [13]. GHS-R1a is also widely expressed in fetal lung tissue [14,15]. It has been postulated that ghrelin acts as a regulator of fetal lung development in an autocrine/paracrine way, and when exogenously administered, it contributes to fetal lung branching in in vivo and in vitro studies [15,16].

It has been observed that in congenital diaphragmatic hernia (CDH), the ghrelin gene is overexpressed in humans and in an animal model of CDH induced by nitrofen administration. These data suggest a potential role of ghrelin in the mechanisms involved in attenuation of lung hypoplasia [16]. In addition, and very relevant, ghrelin administration sensitizes lung fetal tissue to the action of retinoic acid (RA) by upregulating RA receptors, what may be part of the underlying mechanism to explain the effect of ghrelin in lung growth and development [17]. Moreover, ghrelin administration improved pulmonary hypertension and attenuated pulmonary vascular remodeling in newborn pups from an animal model of persistent pulmonary hypertension [18].

2.2. Leptin

Leptin is a 164 AA peptide product of the *ob* gene [19]. Leptin is produced and secreted by the white adipose tissue, and so it is considered an adipokine. The circulating leptin levels seem to be related to the whole amount of fat stored in adipose tissues [20]. Interestingly, leptin has shown to have pleiotropic effects and it can modulate food intake and energy expenditure, immune response, reproduction, and blood pressure homeostasis [21].

Leptin acts through the leptin receptor (Ob-R), encoded by the *db* gene [22]. Ob-R is a member of the class I cytokine receptor family and it is composed for six different isoforms, all of them products of the alternative splicing of the Ob-R mRNA [23]. Leptin and Ob-R are expressed in many other tissues, like the placenta and lungs [24,25]. In lung adult tissue, leptin expression was identified in bronchial epithelial cells, ATII cells, which produce the surfactant, and in alveolar and interstitial macrophages [26]. Leptin receptor expression is detected in the distal lung both in the alveolar and bronchial epithelia [27].

In the fetal lung, leptin gene is expressed in lipofibroblasts, and its levels increases during alveolar differentiation, when pulmonary surfactant phospholipid synthesis is induced [28]. The lung is one of the few tissues that expresses the Ob-R leptin receptor during fetal development [29,30]. Ob-R is expressed specifically by fetal ATII cells [30] and it is enhanced in late gestation, which suggests a key role of leptin in lung maturity [31]. In FGR, the expression of leptin and Ob-R diminishes during the canalicular stage of lung development, being a relevant pathogenic event to explain the lung immaturity in that condition [32]. Moreover, leptin increases surfactant-associated protein (SFTP) expression in in vitro culture of fetal lung explants and in fetal ATII cells [32,33]. The stimulation of SFTP production by leptin is been postulated to be the result of a regulatory paracrine feedback loop between the lipofibroblasts inside the lung and the type II alveolar epithelial cells [28]. On the other hand, the administration of leptin to control animals in vivo produces contradictory findings. While leptin did not modify surfactant synthesis in sheep and mice fetal lungs [34], in more recent studies, it was able to increase the mRNA expression of surfactant-associated protein B (SFTPB) in fetal ewes [35]. In addition, leptin administration to pregnant rats between GD19 and GD20 prevented the alterations in fetal lung architecture and normalized the expression of surfactant-associated protein A (SFTPA) in a model of FGR [32].

Furthermore, the role of leptin in lung maturation may be clarified in *ob/ob* mice, which lack leptin expression [36]. These mice, which show a clear obese phenotype, also present an altered alveolar formation that may be observed from the second week of postnatal life onwards, with a clear decrease in lung volumes and reduced alveolar number and total alveolar surface area. The postnatal leptin replacement in *ob/ob* mice stimulates alveolar enlargement and increases lung volume and alveolar surface area [37].

On the other hand, the excessive leptin levels may also have deleterious effects. In rats, a maternal high fat diet increases offspring serum leptin levels, and increases inflammatory cell infiltration and interstitial remodeling, although in this case, it is not clear whether these effects might alternatively be secondary to obese phenotype and dysregulation of metabolism [38]. In fact, there is a negative correlation between leptin levels and forced expiratory volume in first second (FEV1), in obese children and adolescents [39].

Again, all of the little experimental data reported to date clearly indicate that leptin may play a relevant role in lung development, and in some way, this hormone might contribute to explain the functional and pathophysiological connections already observed between adipose tissue and lungs.

2.3. GLP-1

Glucagon-like peptide 1 (GLP-1) is an insulinotropic hormone produced by enteroendocrine L-cells of the ileum in response to food intake [40]. GLP-1 is the product of post-translational processing of proglucagon gene. GLP-1 acts by binding to GLP-1 receptor (GLP-1R), a G protein-coupled receptor that is widely expressed in many tissues, including a very high expression in fetal and adult lungs [41,42].

During fetal development, GLP-1 receptor is expressed in lung tissue, and its expression is greatly increased just immediately before birth, in coincidence with a period of high surfactant demand before alveolar expansion at first breath after birth [42]. GLP-1R activation increases in vitro phosphatidylcholine secretion in rodent and human ATII cell primary cultures [43,44]. GLP-1 analogue, exendin-4 also, increases perinatal SFTP expression and secretion in rats [42]. In the animal model of lung hypoplasia induced by nitrofen in pregnant rats, exendin-4 administration promotes the expression of SFTPA and SFTPB in similar amounts as dexamethasone, but it also improves the structural development of alveoli and the interstitial tissue, thus allowing the survival of a significant number of newborn rats [42], which never found in untreated animals. In addition, transplacental administration of the GLP-1R agonist liraglutide improved the morphology of the pulmonary vascular vessel in an animal model of congenital diaphragmatic hernia in rabbits [45]. Moreover, GLP-1R activation promoted a marked induction of the ACE2 expression, which enhanced the activity of the ACE2/Ang(1-7)/MasR branch of the renin–angiotensin system, with vasodilatory instead of vasoconstrictor properties, in an animal model of FGR by perinatal food restriction of the mothers [46]. This was also observed in diabetic rats, showing right ventricle hypertrophy, which is prevented by just one-week administration of liraglutide [47].

In summary, our group and others have shown that GLP-1 receptor agonists have very important effects in different aspects of lung physiology. These molecules stimulate the production of both components of surfactant, phospholipids, and SFTPs; they regulate the vascular tone of the pulmonary vessel, promoting vasorelaxation instead of vasoconstriction, thus preventing pulmonary hypertension by the modulation of the components of the renin-angiotensin system; and they improve the alveolar and interstitial histological structure of the lung tissue (Figure 1). GLP-1 receptor expression is also regulated in relation to key events in the lung physiology, and it is overexpressed immediately before birth. Altogether, GLP-1 receptor agonists show protective effects that improve lung function in different physiological and pathophysiological conditions, suggesting a very relevant role in this organ.

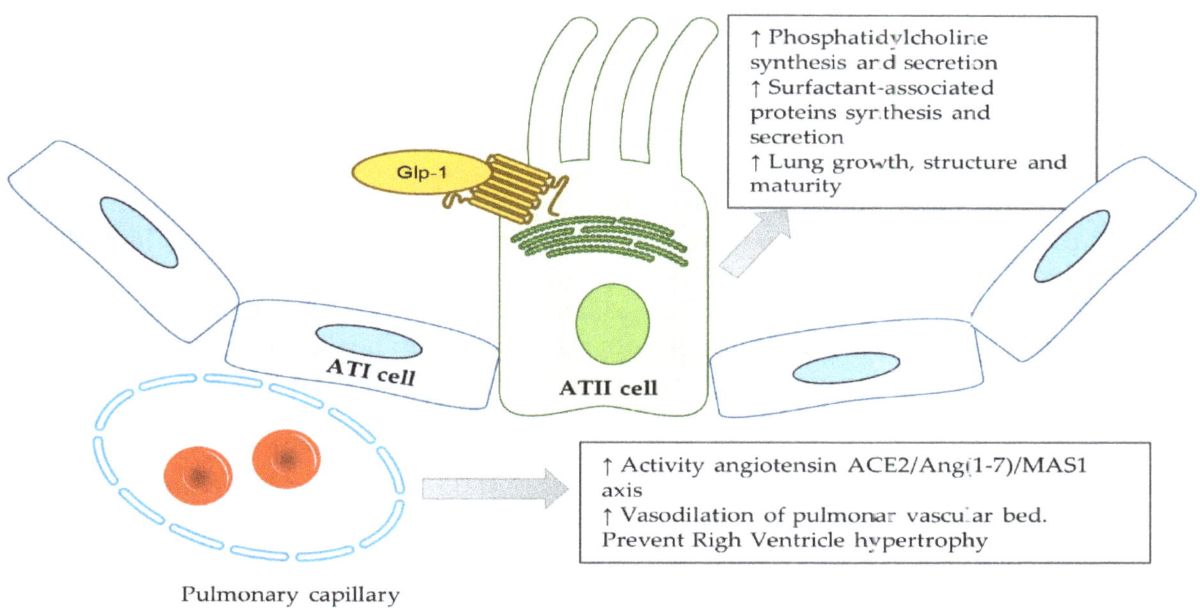

Figure 1. Schematic representation of the main effects of GLP-1R activation in fetal lung tissue. Abbreviations: ATI cell, alveolar type I cell; ATII cell, alveolar type II cell; Glp-1, glucagon-like peptide-1; ACE2, angiotensin-converting enzyme 2; Ang (1-7), angiotensin 1-7; MAS1, Mas proto-oncogene, G protein-coupled receptor.

2.4. *Retinoids*

Retinoic acid (RA) is a metabolite derived from diet that acts properly like a hormone regulating gene expression [48]. This hormone is obtained as a micronutrient, either as retinyl-esters, present in animal origin food, or as carotenoids, present in vegetables. The hepatocytes are the main reservoir of retinoids, where they accumulate up to 70% in the form of retinyl-esters [49]. When an extrahepatic tissue requires RA, retinyl-esters are cleaved to retinol, which is transported to target tissue bound to retinol-binding protein (RBP) [50]. In target tissues, retinol undergoes two successive oxidations to produce all-trans retinoic acid (ATRA), the biologically active hormone [49].

Retinoids exert their actions through two different families of nuclear receptors that are ligand-dependent transcription factors: Retinoid acid receptors (RARs) and retinoid X receptors

(RXRs) [51]. ATRA binds to an RAR, which then forms a heterodimer with an RXR molecule. This complex binds to specific retinoic acid response elements (RAREs) present in the genomic DNA upstream of the sequence of the gene promotor region. The RA receptors work as hormone-dependent transcription regulators of several genes, interacting with other hormonal families such as estrogens and thyroid hormones [51].

ATRA plays an essential role in fetal development and in tissue homeostasis by regulating cellular differentiation, tissue maturation, remodeling and apoptosis, and tissue repair [52]. It was shown that reduced levels of RA might promote fetal malformations of several organs [53], whereas very high levels may trigger teratogenesis [54]. Therefore, circulating RA levels must remain within normal ranges during pregnancy.

During fetal lung development, and since early embryonic stages, there is synthesis of RA and expression of RA receptors in the primordial lung buds [55,56]. In fact, RA regulates the formation of the bronchial tubules during the pseudoglandular phase [57]. This may be why the maternal deficiency of retinoid results in lung hypoplasia—and even lung agenesis in the most severe cases [53,58]. This effect was shown in fetuses of the RARα/RARβ2 double knockout mice, which had blunted the capacity to respond to RA [59].

In murine animal models, lung maturation is finished after birth. In that case, it can be observed that RA also plays a key role during perinatal lung maturation, when there is a relative depletion of retinyl-ester levels in lung tissue [60], but RAR expression is upregulated in alveoli with respect to mature lung, which suggests RA is involved in the genesis of alveoli [61]. Moreover, RA induces the proliferation and differentiation of fetal type II to type I alveolar epithelial cells in vitro [62], and it increases the expression of mRNA for surfactant-associated protein D [63].

Congenital diaphragmatic hernia (CDH) is a major life threatening disease, characterized by a failure in both alveolar and vascular pulmonary development [64]. There is evidence that a defective mechanism in the retinoid signaling pathway is involved in the etiology of CDH [65]. In classical studies, an incidence of 25–70% of CDH in the offspring of pregnant rats with a deficient intake of RA precursors was reported [66]. Whereas in humans, CDH-affected newborns present a 50% reduction of plasma levels of retinol and retinol binding protein with respect to healthy newborns [67].

ATRA has been shown to also be very effective in other animal models of lung diseases. For example, in bronchopulmonary dysplasia (BPD), the pups are exposed to hypoxia conditions from postnatal day 1, disrupting normal septation and lung alveolarization [68]. In this model, postnatal treatment with RA improves alveolar structure, reduces septal fibrosis, and increases survival [69–71].

In addition, RA contributes to ameliorate the status of the pups in experimental models of lung hypoplasia. In one of these models, the perinatal caloric restriction decreases the RARα expression, and the intraperitoneal administration of RA to the pups improves alveolar formation, likely overcoming the partial deficit of receptors but also stimulating the expression of RARα [72].

There are different strategies for modeling lung hypoplasia in laboratory animals. Nitrofen (2, 4-dichlorophenyl-p-nitro phenyl ether) is a molecule developed as a herbicide, without toxicological effects in adult rats. However, administration of nitrofen to pregnant rats on day 9 of gestation induces deep alterations in lung development, to the end that pups show lung hypoplasia, making them not viable for extra uterine life [73]. Nitrofen-induced lung hypoplasia might involve abnormalities in the synthesis, uptake, and signaling pathway of the retinoid system [74–76], since retinoid administration to lung explants of nitrofen-treated animals greatly improves the indicators of lung growth [77]. In addition, in vivo, the administration of retinoid precursors to the mothers during gestation reduces the incidence of CDH, and increases survival and lung maturity of the litters [78,79]. It was also shown that RA administration to mothers treated with nitrofen increases postnatal alveologenesis in the progenies [80], likely by promoting the proliferation of type I alveolar epithelial cells [81]. All these data suggest that an increase in the substrate supply for RA synthesis could counteract the decreased activity of the retinal dehydrogenase 2 (RALDH2), a key enzyme in retinol synthesis, as observed in nitrofen-treated fetal lungs [74].

2.5. Cholecalciferol

Cholecalciferol or vitamin D3 is a secosteroid that is obtained directly from food of animal origin, or indirectly by synthesis in the skin from 7-dehydrocholesterol after ultraviolet B exposure. This prohormone is inactive, and it experiences two sequential hydroxylation steps to produce 1,25-Hydroxyvitamin D (1,25$(OH)_2$D), the hormone active form [82]. 1,2(OH)$_2$D, also called calcitriol, interacts with this specific receptor, called vitamin D receptor (VDR), that is a ligand-dependent transcription factor [83]. After ligand binding, it requires the formation of a heterodimer with a retinoid X receptor (RXR) to interact with vitamin D response elements (VDRE) present in the DNA and to regulate gene expression [84].

As the action mechanism of calcitriol requires forming heterodimers with the promiscuous receptor for retinoids (RXR), it is not surprising that it may be involved in lung development, maturation, and functional regulation. In fact, the lung is likely one of the main target tissues for calcitriol during fetal development [85]. VDR receptor is expressed in fetal ATII cells, where its activation induces proliferation and the synthesis and secretion of surfactant of both the fractions proteins and phospholipids [86–89]. The incubation of human fetal and adult ATII cells with 1,25$(OH)_2$D in vitro culture increases VDR and the expression of SFTPB [90].

The maternal calcitriol deficiency during lung development in animal models modifies the expression of genes involved in organ development, branching morphogenesis, and regulation of inflammation process [91]. Therefore, several respiratory parameters may be affected, including the reduction in lung volume, vital capacity and oxygen saturation, and increases in airway smooth muscle mass and airway contractility [92–94]. All of these changes alter normal lung physiology and might compromise the survival of the litters. In this condition, the supplementation of mothers with calcitriol precursors completely prevents the negative effects of the deficiency. In addition, calcitriol supplementation during lactation in rodents with previous deficiency during gestation improves alveolar septation and lung function [95]. Even in pups from normal pregnant rats, the aerosol administration of calcitriol precursors contributes to lung maturity by increasing the expression of markers of epithelial, mesenchymal, and vascular differentiation that is followed by an increase in the synthesis of surfactant phospholipids [96]. In human studies, there is an association between a reduction of calcitriol levels in 18 WG and a reduced lung function in childhood [97]. It is also demonstrated that severe deficiency of 25(OH)D in preterm infants is related to the development of respiratory distress syndrome [98]. Thus, preterm supplementation with calcitriol precursors reduces the time of assisted ventilation and oxygen supplementation [99], which confirms the essential role of this hormone in lung maturation. In addition, it has been proposed that supplementation with calcitriol precursors during pregnancy may be an effective mean of preventing childhood asthma [100].

3. Effect of Undernutrition on Lung Development and Adult Lung Function

There are several different animal models for the study of FGR, including genetic manipulation models, but also mother food restriction during pregnancy [101]. The most frequently used animal species for modeling FGR are mice, rats, and lambs.

In a model of lamb FGR by the removal of endometrial caruncles, there is a reduction in fetal lung weight, lung liquid volume, and phospholipid concentration in liquid of alveolar lavage [102]. In this model, the lung weight is reduced by a similar rate to fetal body weight reduction, but carrying structural alterations that reveal a retarded maturation [103]. FGR reduces alveolar number and vascular density, but increases septal thickness [104,105]. These alterations become more pronounced during postnatal lung development [104], which leads to a smaller number of large alveoli, alveolar fenestrations, and increased number of mast cells in the lungs of adult animals, anticipating a premature lung aging [106]. At least part of these changes in lung architecture could be explained by a marked reduction in elastin synthesis and deposition [107]. FGR also promotes the reduction of the mRNA and protein expression of the SFTPs [108]. SFTP expression is higher after the delivery in FGR ewes due to the activation of the hypoxia-signaling pathway by increasing HIF-2α mRNA expression [109].

FGR alters normal structure of the lamellar bodies of ATII cells involved in surfactant synthesis and secretion, in the saccular stage before birth in rodents [110]. This alteration also reduces mRNA expression of SFTPs [111]. However, after birth, there is a reduction in lung surfactant lipid levels, just in the early postnatal period, without modifying the expression of surfactant-associated proteins in the remaining postnatal period [112]. As described in lambs, FGR also disrupts normal lung architecture in rodents, and it decreases alveolar number and increases septal thickness [113] from postnatal day 1 through adulthood. Moreover, this is accompanied by a decline in synthesis and secretion of elastin, and an increase in static lung compliance [114].

In humans, fetal undernutrition can be caused by at least five situations:

(1) Severe nausea and vomiting period that persists more than the first trimester [115];
(2) The "Maternal Depletion Syndrome," a product of a short inter-pregnancy interval, not allowing sufficient time to replenish energy reserves and recovery of mothers, which promotes a depletion of both macro- and micronutrients [116];
(3) Teenager pregnancy, where the mother, who may still be growing, competes with the fetus for resources [117];
(4) Use and abuse of tobacco [118]; and
(5) Alcohol/drugs [119], which may promote placenta under-function and reduced nutrient supply to fetus and/or maternal undernutrition.

There are few studies linking FGR, fetal lung development, and neonatal lung pathology in humans. In fact, there are some conflicting results about the effect of FGR over respiratory distress syndrome (RDS). Several studies have concluded that FGR reduces the incidence of RDS and increases the ratio of lecithin/sphingomyelin in amniotic fluid, a marker of lung maturation [120,121]. They explain this accelerated lung maturation as a consequence of the chronic intrauterine stress that increases fetal glucocorticoid levels. Nevertheless, other studies have concluded that FGR increases the risk of developing RDS and the risk of respiratory failure and death [122], and yet others did not find this relation [123]. On the other hand, there is an association between perinatal growth restriction and an increased risk of developing bronchopulmonary dysplasia in preterm infants [124]. Moreover, low birth weight, but not prematurity, decreases lung size and bronchial airflow, and conversely increases bronchial hyperreactivity in children [125].

In the mature lung, there is a clear relationship between the early fetal nutritional environment and adult pulmonary diseases—despite the mechanistic basis of this relationship being unknown [126]. In the adult lung, there is a suggestive, not fully consistent, association between FGR and pulmonary function in adulthood [127]. There are some evidences that FGR can decrease adult lung function [128], whereas other studies did not find any effect over lung function [129]. Another study shows that prenatal exposure to famine did not modify the lung function, but increased the prevalence of COPD [130]. This risk is greater when severe famine exposure occurs during infancy [131]. Asthma is another lung pathology that is related with FGR. There are some studies that link FGR with an increased risk of developing adult asthma [132], whereas other studies conclude that environmental factors during childhood rather than fetal undernutrition are responsible for the increased risk of developing asthma in adult life [133].

4. Undernutrition and Hormones in Lung Development

Undernutrition in pregnancy promotes several changes in metabolic control and hormone levels, which are needed to adapt the energy demands to reduced supplies. It is easy to link a caloric deficit with reduced availability of precursor for hormones that are obtained in diet, such as retinoids and carotenoids [134,135]. However, these precursors may be stored in some amounts in the liver and fat depots. In such a way, nutritional deficits of these hormones must be set up likely before pregnancy, for reducing the reserves enough to affect fetus development during gestation. In developed countries, the follow-up of every pregnant women and nutritional advice should be enough to prevent this kind of deficit. A large part of the population is in the lower range or outside the normal range for cholecalciferols (VitD), which may be especially critical in some susceptible populations: Low sun exposure, low intake of fish and dairy products, obesity, or undernutrition.

The effect in the modulation on gene transcription by the activation of the retinoid hormone system is so important that it might be a source of teratogeny when in elevated levels during pregnancy. In addition, on the other hand, a deficit of retinoids promotes alterations in reproduction, placentation, and organ development. However, there is not a recommendation to supplement nutrition with retinoid precursors in pregnancy apart from in known deficient populations. In some African countries, this deficit may be present in the 21–48% of all pregnant women [135]. On the other hand, some hormones are involved in the short-term availability of energy resources, and may eventually be relevant in the case of reduced food intake during pregnancy. In this context, and as described above, leptin seems to be a relevant hormone in lung development. This hormone is mainly secreted by adipose tissue in proportion to total fat storage. During starving, even partial, fat depots and, consequently, leptin circulating levels are reduced [136]. Leptin is also produced by the placenta, where it plays a local role in protein synthesis and proliferation of placental cells. It has been also postulated that leptin is very important for maternal–fetal exchanges, regulating the growth and development of many organs, including the lung. In fact, dysregulation of leptin mechanisms is link to several disorders occurring in pregnancy, such as gestational diabetes and intrauterine growth restriction [137]. In FGR neonates, there is a reduction in circulating leptin levels, due to a reduction in fetal fat mass and placental production [138,139] The fetal reduction in leptin levels may compromise correct lung development. The reduction in fetal circulating leptin levels is usually compensated by a postnatal increase when enough energy supply is set up, which explains the catch-up lung growth in FGR offspring [140]; however, it may also be related to the augmented incidence of childhood asthma in FGR offspring [141].

Another hormone that has a relevant role in metabolic and food intake control is ghrelin. Ghrelin is a peptide with orexigenic, adipogenic, and GH-releasing properties [142]. Regarding all described effects for ghrelin, it is important in the regulation of metabolism and it has been suggested that it contributes to energy resource distribution, linking nutrients to growth and development of the organs. Ghrelin levels vary during pregnancy, reaching the highest peak at mid-gestation, and then declining up to term [143]. Ghrelin is present in the cord blood and inversely correlates with fetal growth. Moreover, intrauterine ghrelin levels have been linked to programming body weight in the postnatal period [144]. FGR fetuses present high ghrelin levels in response to intrauterine malnutrition, which might contribute to increase neonate appetite, which suggests a role of ghrelin in catch-up growth [145,146]. Nevertheless, more recently, others have shown that ghrelin levels are reduced in "small for gestational age" fetuses [146], and this is in accordance with increased levels of cortisol in FGR fetuses due to the stress in the intrauterine environment. It has been shown that there is a negative correlation between cortisol and ghrelin levels [147]. Despite there being few studies about ghrelin's involvement in lung function and development, the reported results suggest it has a relevant role. The action mechanisms underlying the effects of ghrelin in the lungs will need some more studies to be revealed.

GLP-1 is the least studied metabolic hormone, here presented in relation with pregnancy. GLP-1 could compensate pregnancy-related alterations in metabolism, such as an increase in glycaemia and the development of insulin resistance, based on the increase of fasted active GLP-1 levels in the third trimester of gestation [148]. This increase in GLP-1 secretion is a product of gastrointestinal tissue expansion, rather than satiety [149]. GLP-1 circulating levels are reduced in pregnant mothers with gestational diabetes [150,151]. However, we have no data about changes in GLP-1 levels during normal pregnancy. It is important to emphasize that GLP-1 half-life is very short, lower than 2 min. Therefore, GLP-1 levels may change very fast after meals, and so to study GLP-1 variations will demand to do repeated short-interval blood sampling in every individual. In a recent study, it has been reported that

GLP-1 and GIP circulating levels in mothers and cord blood negatively correlate with 25OHD, and, surprisingly, GLP-1, GIP, and ghrelin positively correlate with glycated albumin maternal/cord ratio, highlighting the relevance of these hormones and their interplay in the complex control of metabolism, especially in pregnancy.

Ghrelin and GLP-1 are secreted in relation to meals and, since they may serve as a link between maternal food intake and metabolism, may possibly modulate the exchange of nutrients through the placenta. However, and as described above, both hormones have direct and important effects in lung development. It must be highlighted that GLP-1 modulates many different functions of the lung, including key processes such as the production of surfactant components, or the modulation of vascular tone of pulmonary vessels by controlling the renin–angiotensin system local activation. In addition, it should of the greatest interest to study whether the placenta, as the maternal/fetal interchange organ, is a target for GLP-1 modulatory actions, as we have no data in this respect.

Finally, clinicians dedicated to pregnancy must be conscious of the delay in lung maturity in all of the five clinical situations mentioned above, which include: Persistent severe vomiting beyond first trimester; "Maternal Depletion Syndrome", especially in susceptible populations; teenager pregnancy; use of tobacco and abuse of alcohol and drugs [119]; but also in obese and diabetic mothers. In all of these cases, a complete, well balanced, and eventually supplemented diet of mothers will guarantee normal lung development of fetuses and newborns, contributing to prevent lung pathology in infancy and adult life. This diet should provide enough, but not an excessive amount of, calories and calcitriol and retinoid sources, in addition to other known nutrients needed for organogenesis, such as good quality protein, iodine, and iron. Although, correct attention to the diet of pregnant women is included in current gestational protocols in occidental medicine, it appears that this is not so general in many countries, and thus should be regarded as a priority objective of preventive health policies.

In conclusion, the reduction of food intake during pregnancy may not just directly affect tissue development because insufficient resources, but also undernutrition modifies the hormonal milieu, which is critical for many organs, including lung. Retinol and cholecalciferol are hormones synthetized from precursors obtained from diet; therefore, reductions in food intake limit the availability of these hormones. In fact, the deficit in cholecalciferol is one of the most frequent in pregnancy, especially in susceptible populations. Gestational undernutrition also reduces fat storage, as well as leptin circulating levels in the medium-term; and daily-reduced caloric intake may affect the levels of hormones regulated in the short-term, linked to meals such as ghrelin and GLP-1. The mentioned hormones have key roles in lung development and maturity, including morphogenesis and structure development, cell proliferation and apoptosis, and many functional processes such as production of surfactant components, activity of the local renin–angiotensin system, and vascular tone of pulmonary vessels (see Table 1). Moreover, undernutrition in pregnancy affects all of these hormonal systems at once, in addition to others also relevant such as insulin and IGFs, thyroid hormones, and glucocorticoids. Therefore, the correction of known specific deficits with diet supplementation during gestation is mandatory and should be included in clinical protocols. The disruption of the hormonal environment during pregnancy becomes especially important when the mothers present metabolic diseases such as diabetes and obesity, despite that caloric intake may be preserved. The dysregulation in hormonal control in altered metabolism in mothers may affect lung development and maturity of the fetus to different degrees, also conditioning higher risk to lung pathology in adult life. In this case, the correction during pregnancy of diet and food intake, in proper amounts and composition, is so important to lung development, like it might be in caloric restriction and undernutrition.

Table 1. Summary of the effects of the different hormones over lung development.

Hormone	Action in Lung Development	References
Ghrelin	Fetal lung branching	[15,16]
	Upregulating RA receptors/ sensitizing RA action	[17]
Leptin	Enhance lung maturity	[28,31–34]
	In vitro phosphatidylcholine secretion	[28]
	In vitro SFTPs expression	[28,32–34]
GLP-1	In vitro phosphatidylcholine secretion	[43,44]
	In vivo SFTPs expression	[42,46,47]
	Increase ACE2/Ang (1-7)/MasR branch of the renin-angiotensin system	[46,47]
Retinoic acid	Formation of bronchial tubules during pseudoglandular phase	[57]
	Lung maturation	[62,69,70,72,77–79]
	In vitro Proliferation of ATII cells and differentiation to ATI cells	[62,81]
	In vitro and in vivo SFTPs expression	[62,63]
Cholecalciferol	Branching morphogenesis	[91]
	In vitro proliferation of ATII cells	[96]
	In vitro surfactant phospholipids secretion	[96]
	In vitro SFTPs expression	[96]
	Lung maturation	[95,96]

Abbreviations: RA, retinoic acid; SFTPs, surfactant-associated proteins; ACE2, angiotensin-converting enzyme 2; Ang (1-7), angiotensin 1-7; MAS1, Mas proto-oncogene, G protein-coupled receptor; ATII cells, alveolar type II cells; ATI cells, alveolar type I cells.

Author Contributions: Conceptualization, L.C.G.-M. and F.M.; writing, J.F., L.T., Y.D.-C., and F.M.; figure designing, J.F. and L.T.; review and editing, J.F., Y.D.-C., L.C.G.-M., and F.M.

References

1. Kelly, R.W. Nutrition and placental development. *Proc. Nutr. Soc. Aust.* **1992**, *17*, 203–211.
2. McCance, R.A.; Widdowson, E.M. The determinants of growth and form. *Proc. R. Soc. Lond. B Biol. Sci.* **1974**, *185*, 1–17. [CrossRef] [PubMed]
3. Barker, D.J.; Clark, P.M. Fetal undernutrition and disease in later life. *Rev. Reprod.* **1997**, *2*, 105–112. [CrossRef] [PubMed]
4. Sharma, D.; Shastri, S.; Sharma, P. Intrauterine Growth Restriction: Antenatal and Postnatal Aspects. *Clin. Med. Insights Pediatr.* **2016**, *10*, 67–83. [CrossRef] [PubMed]
5. DiFiore, J.W.; Wilson, J.W. Lung development. *Semin. Pediatr. Surg.* **1994**, *3*, 221–232. [PubMed]
6. Burri, P.H. Structural aspects of postnatal lung development – alveolar formation and growth. *Biol. Neonate* **2006**, *89*, 313–322. [CrossRef] [PubMed]
7. Chen, L.; Zosky, G.R. Lung development. *Photochem. Photobiol. Sci.* **2017**, *16*, 339–346. [CrossRef] [PubMed]
8. Stocks, J.; Hislop, A.; Sonnappa, S. Early lung development: Lifelong effect on respiratory health and disease. *Lancet Respir. Med.* **2013**, *9*, 728–742. [CrossRef]
9. Kojima, M.; Hosoda, H.; Date, Y.; Nakazato, M.; Matsuo, H.; Kangawa, K. Ghrelin is a growth-hormone-releasing acylated peptide from stomach. *Nature* **1999**, *402*, 656–660. [CrossRef]

10. Wang, G.; Lee, H.M.; Englander, E.; Greeley, G.H., Jr. Ghrelin—not just another stomach hormone. *Regul. Pept.* **2002**, *105*, 75–81. [CrossRef]
11. Wren, A.M.; Small, C.J.; Ward, H.L.; Murphy, K.G.; Dakin, C.L.; Taheri, S.; Kennedy, A.R.; Roberts, G.H.; Morgan, D.G.; Ghatei, M.A.; et al. The novel hypothalamic peptide ghrelin stimulates food intake and growth hormone secretion. *Endocrinology* **2000**, *141*, 4325–4328. [CrossRef] [PubMed]
12. Cortelazzi, D.; Cappiello, V.; Morpurgo, P.S.; Ronzoni, S.; Nobile De Santis, M.S.; Cetin, I.; Beck-Peccoz, P.; Spada, A. Circulating levels of ghrelin in human fetuses. *Eur. J. Endocrinol.* **2003**, *149*, 111–116. [CrossRef]
13. Volante, M.; Fulcheri, E.; Allìa, E.; Cerrato, M.; Pucci, A.; Papotti, M. Ghrelin expression in fetal, infant and adult human lung. *J. Histochem. Cytochem.* **2002**, *50*, 1013–1021. [CrossRef] [PubMed]
14. Nakahara, K.; Nakagawa, M.; Baba, Y.; Sato, M.; Toshinai, K.; Date, Y.; Nakazato, M.; Kojima, M.; Miyazato, M.; Kaiya, H.; et al. Maternal ghrelin plays an important role in rat fetal development during pregnancy. *Endocrinology* **2006**, *147*, 1333–1342. [CrossRef]
15. Nunes, S.; Nogueira-Silva, C.; Dias, E.; Moura, R.S.; Correia-Pinto, J. Ghrelin and obestatin: Different role in fetal lung development? *Peptides* **2008**, *29*, 2150–2158. [CrossRef]
16. Santos, M.; Bastos, P.; Gonzaga, S.; Roriz, J.M.; Baptista, M.J.; Nogueira-Silva, C.; Melo-Rocha, G.; Henriques-Coelho, T.; Roncon-Albuquerque, R., Jr.; Leite-Moreira, A.F.; et al. Ghrelin expression in human and rat fetal lungs and the effect of ghrelin administration in nitrofen-induced congenital diaphragmatic hernia. *Pediatr. Res.* **2006**, *59*, 531–537. [CrossRef]
17. Pereira-Terra, P.; Moura, R.S.; Nogueira-Silva, C.; Correia-Pinto, J. Neuroendocrine factors regulate retinoic acid receptors in normal and hypoplastic lung development. *J. Physiol.* **2015**, *593*, 3301–3311. [CrossRef]
18. Xu, Y.P.; Zhu, J.J.; Cheng, F.; Jiang, K.W.; Gu, W.Z.; Shen, Z.; Wu, Y.D.; Liang, L.; Du, L.Z. Ghrelin ameliorates hypoxia-induced pulmonary hypertension via phosphor-GSK3 β/β-catenin signalling in neonatal rats. *J. Mol. Endocrinol.* **2011**, *47*, 33–43. [CrossRef]
19. Zhang, Y.; Proenca, R.; Maffei, M.; Barone, M.; Leopold, L.; Friedman, J.M. Positional cloning of the mouse obese gene and its human homologue. *Nature* **1994**, *372*, 425–432. [CrossRef]
20. Friedman, J.M.; Halaas, J.L. Leptin and the regulation of body weight in mammals. *Nature* **1998**, *395*, 763–770. [CrossRef]
21. Malli, F.; Papaiopannou, A.L.; Gourgoulianis, K.L.; Daniil, Z. The role of leptin in the respiratory system: An overview. *Respir. Res.* **2010**, *11*, 152. [CrossRef] [PubMed]
22. Tartaglia, L.A.; Dembski, M.; Weng, X.; Deng, N.; Culpepper, J.; Devos, R.; Richards, G.J.; Campfield, L.A.; Clarck, F.T.; Deeds, J.; et al. Identification and expression cloning of a leptin receptor, OB-R. *Cell* **1995**, *83*, 1263–1271. [CrossRef]
23. Gorska, E.; Popko, K.; Stelmaszczyk-Emmel, A.; Ciepiela, O.; Kucharska, A.; Wasik, M. Leptin receptors. *Eur. J. Med. Res.* **2010**, *15*, 50–54. [CrossRef] [PubMed]
24. Hoggard, N.; Mercer, J.G.; Rayner, D.V.; Moar, K.; Trayhurn, P.; Williams, L.M. Localization of leptin receptor mRNA splice variants in murine peripheral tissues by RT-PCR and in situ hybridization. *Biochem. Biophys. Res. Commun.* **1997**, *232*, 383–387. [CrossRef]
25. Masuzaki, H.; Ogawa, Y.; Sagawa, N.; Hosoda, K.; Matsumoto, T.; Mise, H.; Nishimura, H.; Yoshimasa, Y.; Tanaka, I.; Mori, T.; et al. Nonadipose tissue production of leptin: Leptin as a novel placenta-derived hormone in humans. *Nat. Med.* **1997**, *3*, 1023–1033. [CrossRef]
26. Vernooy, J.H.; Drummen, N.E.; van Suylen, R.J.; Cloots, R.H.; Möller, G.M.; Bracke, K.R.; Zuyderduyn, S.; Dentener, M.A.; Brusselle, G.G.; Hiemstra, P.S.; et al. Enhanced pulmonary leptin expression in patients with severe COPD and asymptomatic smokers. *Thorax* **2009**, *64*, 26–32. [CrossRef]
27. Belmeyer, A.; Martino, J.M.; Chandel, N.S.; Scott Budinger, G.R.; Dean, D.A.; Mutlu, G.M. Leptin resistance protects mice from hyperoxia-induced acute lung injury. *Am. J. Respir. Crit. Care Med.* **2007**, *175*, 587–594. [CrossRef]
28. Torday, J.S.; Sun, H.; Wang, L.; Torres, E.; Sunday, M.E.; Rubin, L.P. Leptin mediates the parathyroid hormone-related protein paracrine stimulation of fetal lung maturation. *Am. J. Physiol. Lung Cell Mol. Physiol.* **2002**, *282*, L405–L410. [CrossRef]
29. Hoggard, N.; Hunter, L.; Duncan, J.S.; Williams, L.M.; Trayhurn, P.; Mercer, J.G. Leptin and leptin receptor mRNA and protein expression in the murine fetus and placenta. *Proc. Natl. Acad. Sci. USA* **1997**, *94*, 11073–11078. [CrossRef]

30. Bergen, H.T.; Cherlet, T.C.; Manuel, P.; Scott, J.E. Identification of leptin receptors in lung and isolated fetal type II cells. *Am. J. Respir. Cell Mol. Biol.* **2002**, *27*, 71–77. [CrossRef]
31. Henson, M.C.; Swan, K.F.; Edwards, D.E.; Hoyle, G.W.; Purcell, J.; Castracane, V.D. Leptin receptor expression in fetal lung increases in late gestation in the baboon: A model for human pregnancy. *Reproduction* **2004**, *127*, 87–94. [CrossRef] [PubMed]
32. Chen, H.; Zhang, J.P.; Huang, H.; Wang, Z.H.; Cheng, R.; Cai, W.B. Leptin promotes fetal lung maturity and upregulats SP-A expression in pulmonary alveoli type-II epithelial cells involving TTF-1 activation. *PLoS ONE* **2013**, *8*, e69297. [CrossRef]
33. Kirwin, S.M.; Bhandari, V.; Dimatteo, D.; Barone, C.; Johnson, L.; Paul, S.; Spitzer, A.R.; Chander, A.; Hassink, S.G.; Funanage, V.L. Leptin enhances lung maturity in the fetal rat. *Pediatr. Res.* **2006**, *60*, 200–204. [CrossRef] [PubMed]
34. Sato, A.; Schehr, A.; Ikegami, M. Leptin does not influence surfactant synthesis in fetal sheep and mice lungs. *Am. J. Physiol. Lung Cell Mol. Physiol.* **2011**, *300*, L498–L505. [CrossRef] [PubMed]
35. De Blasio, M.J.; Boije, M.; Kempster, S.L.; Smith, G.C.; Charnock-Jones, D.S.; Denyer, A.; Hughes, A.; Wooding, F.B.; Blache, D.; Fowden, A.L.; et al. Leptin Matures Aspects of Lung Structure and Function in the Ovine Fetus. *Endocrinology* **2016**, *157*, 395–404. [CrossRef]
36. Ingalls, A.M.; Dickie, M.M.; Snell, G.D. Obese, a new mutation in the house mouse. *J. Hered.* **1950**, *41*, 317–318. [CrossRef]
37. Huang, K.; Rabold, R.; Abston, E.; Schofield, B.; Misra, V.; Galdzicka, E.; Lee, H.; Biswal, S.; Mitzner, W.; Tankersley, C.G. Effects of leptin deficiency on postnatal lung development in mice. *J. Appl. Physiol.* **2008**, *105*, 249–259. [CrossRef]
38. Song, Y.; Yu, Y.; Wang, D.; Chai, S.; Liu, D.; Xiao, X.; Huang, Y. Maternal high-fat diet feeding during pregnancy and lactation augments lung inflammation and remodelling in offspring. *Respir. Physiol. Neurobiol.* **2015**, *207*, 1–6. [CrossRef]
39. Khrisanapant, W.; Sengmeuang, P.; Kukongviriyapan, U.; Pasurivong, O.; Pakdeechotel, P. Plasma leptin levels and a restrictive lung in obese thai children and adolescents. *Southeast Asian J. Trop. Med. Public Health* **2015**, *46*, 116–124.
40. Holst, J.J. From the Incretin Concept and the Discovery of GLP-1 to Today's Diabetes Therapy. *Front. Endocrinol.* **2019**, *10*, 260. [CrossRef]
41. Bullock, B.P.; Heller, R.S.; Habener, J.F. Tissue distribution of messenger ribonucleic acid encoding the rat glucagon-like peptide-1 receptor. *Endocrinology* **1996**, *137*, 2968–2978. [CrossRef] [PubMed]
42. Romaní-Pérez, M.; Outeiriño-Iglesias, V.; Gil-Lozano, M.; González-Matías, L.C.; Mallo, F.; Vigo, E. Pulmonary GLP-1 receptor increases at birth and exogenous GLP-1 Receptor agonists augmented surfactant-protein levels in litters from normal and nitrofen-treated pregnant rats. *Endocrinology* **2013**, *154*, 1144–1155. [CrossRef] [PubMed]
43. Benito, E.; Blazquez, E.; Bosch, M.A. Glucagon-like peptide-1-(7–36) amide increases pulmonary surfactant secretion through a cyclic adenosine 3′, 5′-monophosphate-dependent protein kinase mechanism in rat type II pneumocytes. *Endocrinology* **1998**, *139*, 2363–2368. [CrossRef] [PubMed]
44. Vara, E.; Arias-Díaz, J.; Garcia, C.; Balibrea, J.L.; Blázquez, E. Glucagon-like peptide-1 (7–36) amide stimulates surfactant secretion in human type II pneumocytes. *Am. J. Respir. Crit. Care Med.* **2001**, *163*, 840–846. [CrossRef] [PubMed]
45. Eastwood, M.P.; Kampmeijer, A.; Jimenez, J.; Zia, S.; Vanbree, R.; Verbist, G.; Toelen, J.; Deprest, J.A. The Effect of Transplacental Administration of Glucagon-Like Peptide-1 on Fetal Lung Development in the Rabbit Model of Congenital Diaphragmatic Hernia. *Fetal Diagn. Ther.* **2016**, *39*, 125–133. [CrossRef]
46. Fandiño, J.; Vaz, A.A.; Toba, L.; Romaní-Pérez, M.; González-Matías, L.C.; Mallo, F.; Diz-Chaves, Y. Liraglutide Enhances the Activity of the ACE/Ang(1–7)/Mas Receptor Pathway in Lungs of Male Pups from Food-Restricted Mothers and Prevents the Reduction of SP-A. *Int. J. Endocrinol.* **2018**, *2018*, 6920620. [CrossRef]
47. Romaní-Pérez, M.; Outeiriño-Iglesias, V.; Moya, C.M.; Santisteban, P.; González-Matías, L.C.; Vigo, E.; Mallo, F. Activation of the GLP-1 Receptor by Liraglutide Increases ACE2 Expression, Reversing Right Ventricle Hypertrophy, and Improving the Production of SP-A and SP-B in the Lungs of Type 1 Diabetes Rats. *Endocrinology* **2015**, *156*, 3559–3569. [CrossRef]

48. Ross, A.C.; Ternus, M.E. Vitamin A as a hormone: Recent advances in understanding the actions of retinol, retinoic acid, and beta carotene. *J. Am. Diet. Assoc.* **1993**, *93*, 1285–1290. [CrossRef]
49. Conaway, H.H.; Henning, P.; Lerner, U.H. Vitamin a metabolism, action, and role in skeletal homeostasis. *Endocr. Rev.* **2013**, *34*, 766–797. [CrossRef]
50. Marill, J.; Idres, N.; Capron, C.C.; Nguyen, E.; Chabot, G.G. Retinoica cid metabolism and mechanism of action: A review. *Curr. Drug Metab.* **2003**, *4*, 1–10. [CrossRef]
51. Bastien, J.; Rochette-Egly, C. Nuclear retinoid receptors and the reanscription of retinoid-target genes. *Gene* **2004**, *328*, 1–17. [CrossRef] [PubMed]
52. Ross, S.A.; McCaffery, P.J.; Drager, U.C.; De Luca, L.M. Retinoids in embryonal development. *Physiol. Rev.* **2000**, *80*, 1021–1054. [CrossRef] [PubMed]
53. Wilson, J.G.; Roth, C.B.; Warkany, J. An analysis of the syndrome of malformations induced by maternal vitamin a deficiency. Effects of restoration of vitamin A at various times during gestation. *Am. J. Anat.* **1953**, *92*, 189–217. [CrossRef]
54. Lammer, E.J.; Chen, D.T.; Hoar, R.M.; Agnish, N.D.; Benke, P.J.; Braun, J.T.; Curry, C.T.; Fernhoff, P.M.; Grix, A.W., Jr.; Lott, I.T.; et al. Retinoid acid embryopathy. *N. Engl. J. Med.* **1985**, *313*, 837–841. [CrossRef] [PubMed]
55. Mollard, R.; Viville, S.; Ward, S.J.; Décimo, D.; Chambon, P.; Dollé, P. Tissue-specific expression of retinoic acid receptor isoform transcripts in the mouse embryo. *Mech. Dev.* **2000**, *94*, 223–232. [CrossRef]
56. Malpel, S.; Mendelsohn, C.; Cardoso, W.V. Regulation of retinoic acid signalling during lung morphogenesis. *Development* **2000**, *127*, 3057–3067.
57. Chazaud, C.; Dollé, P.; Rossant, J.; Mollard, R. Retinoic acid signalling regulates murine bronchial tubule. *Mech. Dev.* **2003**, *120*, 691–700. [CrossRef]
58. Timoneda, J.; Rodríguez-Fernández, L.; Zaragozá, R.; Marín, M.P.; Cabezuelo, M.T.; Torres, L.; Viña, J.R.; Barber, T. Vitamin A Deficiency and the Lung. *Nutrients* **2018**, *10*, 1132. [CrossRef]
59. Mendelsohn, C.; Lohnes, D.; Décimo, D.; Lufkin, T.; LeMeur, M.; Chambon, P.; Mark, M. Function of the retinoic acid receptors (RARs) during development (II). Multiple abnormalities at various stages of organogenesis in RAR double mutants. *Development* **1994**, *120*, 2749–2771.
60. Geevarghese, S.K.; Chytil, F. Depletion of retinyl esters in the lungs coincides with lung prenatal morphological maturation. *Biochem. Biophys. Res. Commun.* **1994**, *200*, 529–535. [CrossRef]
61. Hind, M.; Corcoran, J.; Maden, M. Temporal/spatial expression of retinoid binding proteins and RAR isoforms in the postnatal lung. *Am. J. Physiol. Lung Cell. Mol. Physiol.* **2002**, *282*, L468–L476. [CrossRef] [PubMed]
62. Gao, R.W.; Kong, X.Y.; Zhu, X.X.; Zhu, G.Q.; Ma, J.S.; Liu, X.X. Retinoic acid promotes primary fetal alveolar epithelial type II cell proliferation and differentiation to alveolar epithelial type I cells. *In Vitro Cell. Dev. Biol. Anim.* **2015**, *51*, 479–487. [CrossRef] [PubMed]
63. Grubor, B.; Meyerholtz, D.K.; Lazic, T.; DeMacedo, M.M.; Derscheid, R.J.; Hostetter, J.M.; Gallup, J.M.; DeMartini, J.C.; Ackermann, M.R. Regulation of surfactant protein and defensin mRNA expression in cultured ovine type II pneumocytes by all-trans retinoic acid and VEGF. *Int. J. Exp. Pathol.* **2006**, *87*, 393–403. [CrossRef] [PubMed]
64. Bohn, D.; Tamura, M.; Perrin, D.; Barker, G.; Rabinovitch, M. Ventilatory predictors of pulmonary hypoplasia in congenital diaphragmatic hernia, confirmed by morphologic assessment. *J. Pediatr.* **1987**, *11*, 423–431. [CrossRef]
65. Greer, J.J.; Babiuk, R.P.; Thebaud, B. Etiology of congenital diaphragmatic hernia: The retinoid hypothesis. *Pediatr. Res.* **2003**, *53*, 726–730. [CrossRef] [PubMed]
66. Andersen, D.H. Incidence of congenital diaphragmatic hernia in the young of rats bred on a diet deficient in Vitamin A. *Am. J. Dis. Child.* **1941**, *62*, 888–889.
67. Major, D.; Cadenas, M.; Fournier, L.; Leclerc, S.; Lefebvre, M.; Cloutier, R. Retinol status of newborn infants with congenital diaphragmatic hernia. *Pediatr. Surg. Int.* **1998**, *13*, 547–549. [CrossRef]
68. Nardiello, C.; Miziková, I.; Silva, D.M.; Ruiz-Camp, J.; Mayer, K.; Vadász, I.; Herold, S.; Seeger, W.; Morty, R.E. Standardisation of oxygen exposure in the development of mouse models for brochopulmonary dysplasia. *Dis. Model. Mech.* **2017**, *10*, 185–196. [CrossRef]
69. Veness-Meehan, K.A.; Botone, F.G., Jr.; Stiles, A.D. Effects of retinoic acid on airspace development and lung collagen in hyperoxia-exposed newborn rats. *Pediatr. Res.* **2000**, *48*, 434–444. [CrossRef]

70. Veness-Meehan, K.A.; Pierce, R.A.; Moats-Staats, B.M.; Stiles, A.D. Retinoic acid attenuates O2-induced inhibition of lung septation. *Am. J. Physiol. Lung Cell. Mol. Physiol.* **2002**, *283*, L971–L980. [CrossRef]
71. Ozer, E.A.; Kumral, A.; Ozer, E.; Duman, N.; Yilmaz, O.; Ozkal, S.; Ozkan, H. Effect of retinoic acid on oxygen-induced lung injury in the newborn rat. *Pediatr. Pulmonol.* **2005**, *39*, 35–40. [CrossRef] [PubMed]
72. Londhe, V.A.; Maisonet, T.M.; Lopez, B.; Shin, B.C.; Huynh, J.; Devaskar, S.U. Retinoic acid rescues alveolar hypoplasia in the calorie-restricted developing rat lung. *Am. J. Respir. Cell. Mol. Biol.* **2013**, *48*, 179–187. [CrossRef] [PubMed]
73. Van Loenhout, R.B.; Tibboel, D.; Post, M.; Keijzer, R. Congenital diaphragmatic hernia: Comparisons of animal models and relevance to the human situation. *Neonatology* **2009**, *96*, 137–149. [CrossRef] [PubMed]
74. Mey, J.; Babiuk, R.P.; Clugston, R.; Zhang, W.; Greer, J.J. Retinal dehydrogenase-2 is inhibited by compounds that induce congenital diaphragmatic hernias in rodents. *Am. J. Pathol.* **2003**, *162*, 673–679. [CrossRef]
75. Chen, M.H.; MacGowan, A.; Ward, S.; Bavik, C.; Greer, J.J. The activation of the retinoic acid response element is inhibited in an animal model of congenital diaphragmatic hernia. *Biol. Neonate* **2003**, *83*, 157–161. [CrossRef] [PubMed]
76. Nakazawa, N.; Montedonico, S.; Takayasu, H.; Paradisi, F.; Puri, P. Disturbance of retinol transportation causes nitrofen-induced hypoplastic lung. *J. Pediatr. Surg.* **2007**, *42*, 345–349. [CrossRef] [PubMed]
77. Montedonico, S.; Nakazawa, N.; Puri, P. Retinoic acid rescues lung hypoplasia in nitrofen-induced hypoplastic foetal rat lung explants. *Pediatr. Surg. Int.* **2006**, *22*, 2–8. [CrossRef]
78. Thébaud, B.; Tibboel, D.; Rambaud, C.; Mercier, J.C.; Bourbon, J.R.; Dinh-Xuan, A.T.; Archer, S.L. Vitamin A decreases the incidence and severity of nitrofen-induced congenital diaphragmatic hernia in rats. *Am. J. Physiol.* **1999**, *277*, L423–L429. [CrossRef]
79. Thébaud, B.; Barlier-Mur, A.M.; Chailley-Heu, B.; Henrion-Caude, A.; Tibboel, D.; Dinh-Xuan, A.T.; Bourbon, J.R. Restoring effects of vitamin A on surfactant synthesis in nitrofen-induced congenital diaphragmatic hernia in rats. *Am. J. Respir. Crit. Care Med.* **2001**, *164*, 1083–1089. [CrossRef]
80. Montedonico, S.; Sugimoto, K.; Felle, P.; Bannigan, J.; Puri, P. Prenatal treatment with retinoic acid promotes pulmonary alveologenesis in the nitrofen model of congenital diaphragmatic hernia. *J. Pediatr. Surg.* **2008**, *43*, 500–507. [CrossRef]
81. Sugimoto, K.; Takayasu, H.; Nakazawa, N.; Montedonico, S.; Puri, P. Prenatal treatment with retinoic acid accelerates type 1 alveolar cell proliferation of the hypoplastic lung in the nitrofen model of congenital diaphragmatic hernia. *J. Pediatr. Surg.* **2008**, *43*, 367–372. [CrossRef]
82. Bikle, D.D. Vitamin D metabolism, mechanism of action, and clinical applications. *Chem. Biol.* **2014**, *21*, 319–329. [CrossRef] [PubMed]
83. Haussler, M.R.; Whitfield, G.K.; Haussler, C.A.; Hsieh, J.C.; Thompson, P.D ; Selznick, S.H.; Dominguez, C.E.; Jurutka, P.W. The nuclear vitamin D receptor: Biological and molecular regulatory properties revealed. *J. Bone Miner. Res.* **1998**, *13*, 325–349. [CrossRef] [PubMed]
84. Bouillon, R.; Carmeliet, G.; Verlinden, L.; van Etten, E.; Verstuyf, A.; Luderer, H.F.; Lieben, L.; Mathieu, C.; Demay, M. Vitamin D and human health: Lessons from vitamin D receptor null mice. *Endocr. Rev.* **2008**, *29*, 726–776. [CrossRef] [PubMed]
85. Nguyen, M.; Guillozo, H.; Garabédian, M.; Balsan, S. Lung as a possible additional target organ for vitamin D during fetal life in the rat. *Biol. Neonate* **1987**, *52*, 232–240. [CrossRef]
86. Marin, L.; Dufour, M.E.; Tordet, C.; Nguyen, M. 1, 25(OH) 2D3 stimulates phospholipid biosynthesis and surfactant release in fetal rat lung explants. *Biol. Neonate* **1990**, *57*, 257–260. [CrossRef]
87. Edelson, J.D.; Chan, S.; Jassal, D.; Post, M.; Tanswell, A.K. Vitamin D stimulates DNA synthesis in alveolar type-II cells. *Biochim. Biophys. Acta* **1994**, *1221*, 159–166. [CrossRef]
88. Nguyen, T.M.; Guillozo, H.; Marin, L.; Tordet, C.; Koite, S.; Garabedian, M. Evidence for a vitamin D paracrine system regulating maturation of developing rat lung epithelium. *Am. J. Physiol.* **1996**, *271*, L392–L399. [CrossRef]
89. Nguyen, M.; Trubert, C.L.; Rizk-Rabin, M.; Rehan, V.K.; Besançon, F.; Cayre, Y.E.; Garabédian, M. 1, 25-Dihydroxyvitamin D3 and fetal lung maturation: Immunogold detection of VDR expression in pneumocytes type II cells and effect on fructose 1, 6 bisphosphatase. *J. Steroid. Biochem. Mol. Biol.* **2004**, *89–90*, 93–97. [CrossRef]

90. Phokela, S.S.; Peleg, S.; Moya, F.R.; Alcorn, J.L. Regulation of human pulmonart surfactant protein gene expression by 1alpha, 25-dihydroxyvitamin D3. *Am. J. Physiol. Lung Cell Mol. Physiol.* **2005**, *289*, L617–L626. [CrossRef]
91. Foong, R.E.; Bosco, A.; Jones, A.C.; Gout, A.; Gorman, S.; Hart, P.H.; Zosky, G.R. The effects of in utero vitamin D deficiency on airway smooth muscle mass and lung function. *Am. J. Respir. Cell Mol. Biol.* **2015**, *53*, 664–675. [CrossRef] [PubMed]
92. Zosky, G.R.; Berry, L.J.; Elliot, J.G.; James, A.L.; Gorman, S.; Hart, P.H. Vitamin D deficiency causes deficits in lung function and alters lung structure. *Am. J. Respir. Crit. Care Med.* **2011**, *183*, 1336–1343. [CrossRef] [PubMed]
93. Lykkedegn, S.; Sorensen, G.L.; Beck-Nielsen, S.S.; Pilecki, B.; Duelund, L.; Marcussen, N.; Christesen, H.T. Vitamin D Depletion in Pregnancy Decreases Survival Time, Oxygen Saturation, Lung Weight and Body Weight in Preterm Rat Offspring. *PLoS ONE* **2016**, *11*, e0155203. [CrossRef] [PubMed]
94. Wagner, C.L.; Hollis, B.W. The Implications of Vitamin D Status during Pregnancy on Mother and her Developing Child. *Front. Endocrinol.* **2018**, *9*, 500. [CrossRef] [PubMed]
95. Saadoon, A.; Ambalavanan, N.; Zink, K.; Ashraf, A.P.; MacEwen, M.; Nicola, T.; Fanucchi, M.V.; Harris, W.T. Effect of Prenatal versus Postnatal Vitamin D Deficiency on Pulmonary Structure and Function in Mice. *Am. J. Respir. Cell Mol. Biol.* **2017**, *56*, 383–392. [CrossRef]
96. Taylor, S.K.; Sakurai, R.; Sakurai, T.; Rehan, V.K. Inhaled Vitamin D: A Novel Strategy to Enhance Neonatal Lung Maturation. *Lung* **2016**, *194*, 931–943. [CrossRef]
97. Zosky, G.R.; Hart, P.H.; Whitehouse, A.J.; Kusel, M.M.; Ang, W.; Foong, R.E.; Chen, L.; Holt, P.G.; Sly, P.D.; Hall, G.L. Vitamin D deficiency at 16 to 20 weeks' gestation is associated with impaired lung function and asthma at 6 years of age. *Ann. Am. Thorac. Soc.* **2014**, *11*, 571–577. [CrossRef]
98. Ataseven, F.; Aygün, C.; Okuyucu, A.; Bedir, A.; Kücük, Y.; Kücüködük, S. Is vitamin d deficiency a risk factor for respiratory distress syndrome? *Int. J. Vitam. Nutr. Res.* **2013**, *83*, 232–237. [CrossRef]
99. Backström, M.C.; Mäki, R.; Kuusela, A.L.; Sievänen, H.; Koivisto, A.M.; Ikonen, R.S.; Kouri, T.; Mäki, M. Randomised controlled trial of vitamin D supplementation on bone density and biochemical indices in preterm infants. *Arch. Dis. Child. Fetal Neonatal Ed.* **1999**, *80*, F161–F166. [CrossRef]
100. Yurt, M.; Liu, J.; Sakurai, R.; Gong, M.; Husain, S.M.; Siddiqui, M.A.; Husain, M.; Villareal, P.; Akcay, F.; Torday, J.S.; et al. Vitamin D supplementation blocks pulmonary structural and functional changes in a rat model of perinatal vitamin D deficiency. *Am. J. Physiol. Lung Cell. Mol. Physiol.* **2014**, *307*, L859–L867. [CrossRef]
101. Swanson, A.M.; David, A.L. Animal models of fetal growth restriction: Considerations for translational medicine. *Placenta* **2015**, *36*, 623–630. [CrossRef] [PubMed]
102. Rees, S.; Ng, J.; Dickson, K.; Nicholas, T.; Harding, R. Growth retardation and the development of the respiratory system in fetal sheep. *Early Hum. Dev.* **1991**, *26*, 13–27. [CrossRef]
103. Cock, M.L.; Albuquerque, C.A.; Joyce, B.J.; Hooper, S.B.; Harding, R. Effects of intrauterine growth restriction on lung liquid dynamics and lung development in fetal sheep. *Am. J. Obstet. Gynecol.* **2001**, *184*, 209–216. [CrossRef] [PubMed]
104. Maritz, G.S.; Cock, M.L.; Louey, S.; Joyce, B.J.; Albuquerque, C.A.; Harding, R. Effects of fetal growth restriction on lung development before and after birth: A morphometric analysis. *Pediatr. Pulmonol.* **2001**, *32*, 201–210. [CrossRef]
105. Rozance, P.J.; Seedorf, G.J.; Brown, A.; Roe, G.; O'Meara, M.C.; Gien, J.; Tang, J.R.; Abman, S.H. Intrauterine growth restriction decreases pulmonary alveolar and vessel growth and causes pulmonary artery endothelial cell dysfunction in vitro in fetal sheep. *Am. J. Physiol. Lung Cell Mol. Physiol.* **2011**, *301*, L860–L871. [CrossRef]
106. Maritz, G.S.; Cock, M.L.; Louey, S.; Suzuki, K.; Harding, R. Fetal growth restriction has long-term effects on postnatal lung structure in sheep. *Pediatr. Res.* **2004**, *55*, 287–295. [CrossRef]
107. Cock, M.L.; Joyce, B.J.; Hooper, S.B.; Wallace, M.J.; Gagnon, R.; Brace, R.A.; Louey, S.; Harding, R. Pulmonary elastin synthesis and deposition in developing and mature sheep: Effects of intrauterine growth restriction. *Exp. Lung Res.* **2004**, *30*, 405–418. [CrossRef]
108. Orgeig, S.; Crittenden, T.A.; Marchant, C.; McMillen, I.C.; Morrison, J.L. Intrauterine growth restriction delays surfactant protein maturation in the sheep fetus. *Am. J. Physiol. Lung Cell. Mol. Physiol.* **2010**, *298*, L575–L583. [CrossRef]

109. Soo, J.Y.; Orgeig, S.; McGillick, E.V.; Zhang, S.; McMillen, I.C.; Morrison, J.L. Normalisation of surfactant protein –A and –B expression in the lungs of low birth weight lambs by 21 days old. *PLoS ONE* **2017**, *12*, e0181185. [CrossRef]
110. Deng, F.T.; Ouyang, W.X.; Ge, L.F.; Zhang, L.; Chai, X.Q. Expression of lung surfactant proteins SP-B and SP-C and their modulating factors in fetal lung of FGT rats. *J. Huazhong Univ. Sci. Technol. Med. Sci.* **2015**, *35*, 122–128. [CrossRef]
111. Gortner, L.; Hilhendorff, A.; Bähner, T.; Ensen, M.; Reiss, I.; Rudloff, S. Hypoxia-induced intrauterine growth retardation: Effects on pulmonary development and surfactant protein transcription. *Biol. Neonate* **2005**, *88*, 129–135. [CrossRef] [PubMed]
112. Chen, C.M.; Wang, L.F.; Su, B. Effects of maternal undernutrition during late gestation on the lung surfactant system and morphometry in rats. *Pediatr. Res.* **2004**, *56*, 329–335. [CrossRef] [PubMed]
113. Karadag, A.; Sakurai, R.; Wang, Y.; Guo, P.; Desai, M.; Ross, M.G.; Torday, J.S.; Rehan, V.K. Effect of maternal food restriction on fetal rat lung lipid differentiation program. *Pediatr. Pulmonol.* **2009**, *44*, 635–644. [CrossRef] [PubMed]
114. Joss-Moore, L.A.; Wang, Y.; Yu, X.; Campbell, M.S.; Callaway, C.W.; McKnight, R.A.; Wint, A.; Dahl, M.J.; Dull, R.O.; Albertine, K.H.; et al. IUGR decreases elastin mRNA expression in the developing rat lung and alters elastin content and lung compliance in the mature rat lung. *Physiol. Genomics* **2011**, *43*, 499–505. [CrossRef]
115. Snell, L.H.; Haughey, B.P.; Buck, G.; Marecki, M.A. Metabolic crisis: Hyperemesis gravidarum. *J. Perinat. Neonatal Nurs.* **1998**, *12*, 26–37. [CrossRef]
116. Wendt, A.; Gibbs, C.M.; Peters, S.; Hogue, C.J. Impact of increasing inter-pregnancy interval on maternal and infant health. *Paediatr. Perinat. Epidemiol.* **2012**, *26*, 239–258. [CrossRef]
117. Scholl, T.O.; Hediger, M.L. A review of the epidemiology of nutrition and adolescent pregnancy: Maternal growth during pregnancy and its effect on the fetus. *J. Am. Coll. Nutr.* **1993**, *12*, 101–107. [CrossRef]
118. McEwoy, C.T.; Spindel, E.R. Pulmonary Effects of Maternal Smoking on the Fetus and Child: Effects on Lund Development, Respiratory Morbidities, and Life Long Lung Health. *Paediatr. Respir. Rev.* **2017**, *21*, 27–33. [CrossRef]
119. Sebastiani, G.; Borrás-Novell, C.; Casanova, M.A.; Pascual Tutusaus, M.; Ferrero Martínez, S.; Gómez Roig, M.D.; García-Algar, O. The Effects of Alcohol and Drugs of Abuse on Maternal Nutritional Profile during Pregnancy. *Nutrients* **2018**, *10*, 1008. [CrossRef]
120. Sharma, P.; McKay, K.; Rosenkrantz, T.S.; Hussain, N. Comparisons of mortality and pre-discharge respiratory outcomes in small-for-gestational-age and appropriate-for-gestational-age premature infants. *BMC Pediatr.* **2004**, *8*, 4–9. [CrossRef]
121. Torrance, H.L.; Voorbij, H.A.; Wijnberger, L.D.; van Bel, F.; Visser, G.H. Lung maturation in small for gestational age foetuses from pregnancies complicated by placental insufficiency or maternal hypertension. *Early Hum. Dev.* **2008**, *84*, 465–469. [CrossRef] [PubMed]
122. Tyson, J.E.; Kennedy, K.; Broyles, S.; Rosenfeld, C.R. The small for gestational age infant: Accelerated or delayed pulmonary maturation? Increased or decreased survival? *Pediatrics* **1995**, *95*, 534–538. [PubMed]
123. Giapros, V.; Drougia, A.; Krallis, V.; Theocharis, P.; Andronikou, S. Morbidity and mortality patterns in small-for-gestational age infants born preterm. *J. Maternal. Fetal Neonatal Med.* **2012**, *25*, 153–157. [CrossRef] [PubMed]
124. Eriksson, L.; Haglund, B.; Odlind, V.; Altman, M.; Ewald, U.; Kieler, H. Perinatal conditions related to growth restriction and inflammation are associated with an increased risk of bronchopulmonary dysplasia. *Acta Paediatr.* **2015**, *104*, 259–263. [CrossRef]
125. Wjst, M.; Popescu, M.; Trepka, M.J.; Heinrich, J.; Wichmann, H.E. Pulmonary function in children with initial low birth weight. *Pediatr. Allergy Immunol.* **1998**, *9*, 80–90. [CrossRef]
126. Matharu, K.; Ozanne, S.E. The Fetal Origins of Disease and Associations with Low Birthweight. *NeoReviews* **2004**, *5*, e522–e526. [CrossRef]
127. Briana, D.D.; Malamitsi-Puchner, A. Small for gestational age birth weight: Impact on lung structure and function. *Paediatr. Respir. Rev.* **2013**, *14*, 256–262. [CrossRef]
128. Saad, N.J.; Patel, J.; Burney, P.; Minelli, C. Birth Weight and Lung Function in Adulthood: A Systematic Review and Meta-analysis. *Ann. Am. Thorac. Soc.* **2017**, *14*, 994–1004. [CrossRef]

129. Lelijveld, N.; Kerac, M.; Seal, A.; Chimwezi, E.; Wells, J.C.; Heyderman, R.S.; Nyirenda, M.J.; Stocks, J.; Kirkby, J. Long-term effect of severe acute malnutrition on lung function in Malawian children: A cohort study. *Eur. Respir. J.* **2017**, *49*, 1601301. [CrossRef]
130. Lopuhaä, C.E.; Roseboom, T.J.; Osmond, C.; Barker, D.J.; Ravelli, A.C.; Bleker, O.P.; van der Zee, J.S.; van der Meulen, J.H. Atopy, lung function, and obstructive airways disease after prenatal exposure to famine. *Thorax* **2000**, *55*, 555–561. [CrossRef]
131. Wang, Z.; Zou, Z.; Yang, Z.; Dong, Y.; Ma, J. Association between exposure to the Chinese famine during infancy and the risk of self-reported chronic lung diseases in adulthood: A cross-sectional study. *BMJ Open* **2017**, *7*, e015476. [CrossRef] [PubMed]
132. Shaheen, S.O.; Sterne, J.A.; Montgomery, S.M.; Azima, H. Birth weight, body mass index and asthma in young adults. *Thorax* **1999**, *54*, 396–402. [CrossRef] [PubMed]
133. Hagström, B.; Nyberg, P.; Nilsson, P.M. Asthma in adult life—is there an association with birth weight? *Scand. J. Prim. Health Care* **1998**, *16*, 117–120. [CrossRef] [PubMed]
134. Black, R.E.; Allen, L.H.; Bhutta, Z.A.; Caulfield, L.E.; de Onis, M.; Ezzati, M.; Mathers, C.; Rivera, J. Maternal and child undernutrition: Global and regional exposures and health consequences. *Lancet* **2008**, *371*, 243–260. [CrossRef]
135. Bastos Maia, S.; Rolland Souza, A.S.; Costa Caminha, M.F.; Lins da Silva, S.; Callou Cruz, R.S.B.L.; Carvalho Dos Santos, C.; Batista Filho, M. Vitamin A and Pregnancy: A Narrative Review. *Nutrients* **2019**, *11*, 681. [CrossRef]
136. Ahima, R.S.; Prabakaran, D.; Mantzoros, C.; Qu, D.; Lowell, B.; Maratos-Flier, E.; Flier, J.S. Role of leptin in the neuroendocrine response to fasting. *Nature* **1996**, *382*, 250–252. [CrossRef]
137. Pérez-Pérez, A.; Toro, A.; Vilariño-García, T.; Maymó, J.; Guadix, P.; Dueñas, J.L.; Fernández-Sánchez, M.; Varone, C.; Sánchez-Margalet, V. Leptin action in normal and pathological pregnancies. *J. Cell. Mol. Med.* **2018**, *22*, 716–727. [CrossRef]
138. Catov, J.M.; Patrick, T.E.; Powers, R.W.; Ness, R.B.; Harger, G.; Roberts, J.M. Maternal leptin across pregnancy in women with small-for-gestational-age-infants. *Am. J. Obstet. Gynecol.* **2007**, *196*, 558-e1. [CrossRef]
139. Laivuori, H.; Gallaher, M.J.; Collura, L.; Crombleholme, W.R.; Markovic, N.; Rajakumar, A.; Hubel, C.A.; Roberts, J.M.; Powers, R.W. Relationships between maternal plasma leptin, placental leptin mRNA and protein in normal pregnancy, pre-eclampsia and intrauterine growth restriction without pre-eclampsia. *Mol. Hum. Reprod.* **2006**, *12*, 551–556. [CrossRef]
140. Jaquet, D.; Leger, J.; Tabone, M.D.; Czernichow, P.; Levy-Marchal, C. High serum leptin concentrations during catch-up growth of children born with intrauterine growth retardation. *J. Clin. Endocrinol. Metab.* **1999**, *84*, 1949–1953. [CrossRef]
141. Guler, N.; Kirerleri, E.; Ones, U.; Tamay, Z.; Salmayenli, N.; Darendeliler, F. Leptin: Does it have any role in childhood asthma? *J. Allergy Clin. Immunol.* **2004**, *114*, 254–259. [CrossRef] [PubMed]
142. Muccioli, G.; Tschöp, M.; Papotti, M.; Deghenghi, R.; Heiman, M.; Ghigo, E. Neuroendocrine and peripheral activities of ghrelin: Implications in metabolism and obesity. *Eur. J. Pharmacol.* **2002**, *440*, 235–254. [CrossRef]
143. Fuglsang, J. Ghrelin in pregnancy and lactation. *Vitam. Horm.* **2008**, *77*, 259–284. [CrossRef] [PubMed]
144. Torres, P.J.; Luque, E.M.; Ponzio, M.F.; Cantarelli, V.; Diez, M.; Figueroa, S.; Vicenti, L.M.; Carlini, V.P.; Martini, A.C. The role of intragestational ghrelin on postnatal development and reproductive programming in mice. *Reproduction* **2018**, *156*, 331–341. [CrossRef] [PubMed]
145. Onal, E.E.; Cinaz, P.; Atalay, Y.; Türkyilmaz, C.; Bideci, A.; Aktürk, A.; Okumus, N.; Unal, S.; Koç, E.; Ergenekon, E. Umbilical cord ghrelin concentrations in small- and appropriate-for-gestational age newborns infants: Relationship to anthropometric markers. *J. Endocrinol.* **2004**, *180*, 267–271. [CrossRef] [PubMed]
146. Yalinbas, E.E.; Binay, C.; Simsek, E.; Aksit, M.A. The Role of Umbilical Cord Blood Concentration of IGF-I, IGF-II, Leptin, Adiponectin, Ghrelin, Resistin, and Visfatin in Fetal Growth. *Am. J. Perinatol.* **2019**, *36*, 600–608. [CrossRef]
147. Otto, B.; Tschöp, M.; Heldwein, W.; Pfeiffer, A.F.; Diederich, S. Endogenous and exogenous glucocorticoids decrease plasma ghrelin in humans. *Eur. J. Endocrinol.* **2004**, *151*, 113–117. [CrossRef]
148. Valsamakis, G.; Margeli, A.; Vitoratos, N.; Boutsiadis, A.; Sakkas, E.G.; Papadimitriou, G.; Al-Daghri, N.M.; Botsis, D.; Kumar, S.; Papassotiriou, I.; et al. The role of maternal gut hormones in normal pregnancy: Fasting plasma active glucagon-like peptide 1 level is a negative predictor of fetal abdomen circumference and maternal weight change. *Eur. J. Endocrinol.* **2010**, *162*, 897–903. [CrossRef]

149. Johnson, M.L.; Saffrey, M.J.; Taylor, V.J. Gastrointestinal capacity, gut hormones and appetite change during rat pregnancy and lactation. *Reproduction* **2019**, *157*, 431–443. [CrossRef]
150. Bonde, L.; Vilsboll, T.; Nielsen, T.; Bagger, J.I.; Svare, J.A.; Holst, J.J.; Larsen, S.; Knop, F.K. Reduced postprandial GLP-1 responses in women with gestational diabetes mellitus. *Diabetes Obes. Metab.* **2013**, *15*, 713–720. [CrossRef]
151. Sukumar, N.; Bagias, C.; Goljan, I.; Weldeselassie, Y.; Gharanei, S.; Tan, B.K.; Holst, J.J.; Saravanan, P. Reduced GLP-1 Secretion at 30 Minutes After a 75-g Oral Glucose Load Is Observed in Gestational Diabetes Mellitus: A Prospective Cohort Study. *Diabetes* **2018**, *67*, 2650–2656. [CrossRef] [PubMed]

11

Role of Diet in Chronic Obstructive Pulmonary Disease Prevention and Treatment

Egeria Scoditti [1,*], Marika Massaro [1], Sergio Garbarino [2] and Domenico Maurizio Toraldo [3]

1 National Research Council (CNR), Institute of Clinical Physiology (IFC), 73100 Lecce, Italy; marika.massaro@ifc.cnr.it

2 Department of Neuroscience, Rehabilitation, Ophthalmology, Genetics and Maternal/Child Sciences, University of Genoa, 16132 Genoa, Italy; sgarbarino.neuro@gmail.com

3 Rehabilitation Department, Cardio-Respiratory Care Unit, "V Fazzi" Hospital, ASL Lecce, 73100 Lecce, Italy; d.torald@tin.it

* Correspondence: egeria.scoditti@ifc.cnr.it

Abstract: Chronic obstructive pulmonary disease is one of the leading causes of morbidity and mortality worldwide and a growing healthcare problem. Identification of modifiable risk factors for prevention and treatment of COPD is urgent, and the scientific community has begun to pay close attention to diet as an integral part of COPD management, from prevention to treatment. This review summarizes the evidence from observational and clinical studies regarding the impact of nutrients and dietary patterns on lung function and COPD development, progression, and outcomes, with highlights on potential mechanisms of action. Several dietary options can be considered in terms of COPD prevention and/or progression. Although definitive data are lacking, the available scientific evidence indicates that some foods and nutrients, especially those nutraceuticals endowed with antioxidant and anti-inflammatory properties and when consumed in combinations in the form of balanced dietary patterns, are associated with better pulmonary function, less lung function decline, and reduced risk of COPD. Knowledge of dietary influences on COPD may provide health professionals with an evidence-based lifestyle approach to better counsel patients toward improved pulmonary health.

Keywords: antioxidant; chronic obstructive pulmonary disease; dietary pattern; inflammation; lung function; Mediterranean diet; nutrition; oxidative stress; polyphenol; polyunsaturated fatty acid

---

1. Introduction

Chronic obstructive pulmonary disease (COPD) is a major cause of morbidity and mortality and healthcare burden worldwide, affecting around 10% of the adult populations aged 40 years and older [1]. According to WHO estimates mainly from high-income countries, 65 million people have moderate to severe COPD, but a great proportion of COPD worldwide may be underdiagnosed, mostly in low- and middle-income countries. COPD burden is projected to dramatically increase due to chronic exposure to risk factors and the changing age structure of the world population and is expected to be the third leading cause of death worldwide by 2030 (WHO 2019. Burden of COPD https://www.who.int/respiratory/copd/burden/en). Therefore, prevention and management of COPD is currently considered a major health problem, with important social and economic issues.

COPD encompasses a group of disorders, including small airway obstruction, emphysema, and chronic bronchitis, and is characterized by chronic inflammation of the airways and lung parenchyma with progressive and irreversible airflow limitation [2]. Symptoms of COPD include dyspnea (distress with breathing), cough, and sputum production. The natural history of COPD is punctuated by recurrent episodes of acute exacerbations, which often require hospitalization and negatively affect patients' quality of life, accelerate the rate of decline in lung function, and are associated with mortality.

Diagnosis, assessment, and management of COPD are mostly guided by the degree of airflow limitation as assessed by the forced expiratory volume in one second (FEV1), forced vital capacity (FVC), and FEV1/FVC ratio, although other physiological measurements such as the inspiratory capacity to total lung capacity (TLC) ratio, arterial blood gases, and exercise capacity provide complementary information on the severity of the disease [3]. To account for the complexity of the disease and aiding in disease severity assessment, multidimensional indices mainly based on clinical and functional parameters have been developed. However, significant heterogeneity in terms of clinical presentation, physiology, imaging, response to therapy, lung function decline, and survival exists in COPD, challenging the oversimplification regarding definition and assessment of COPD and leading to effort in identifying subgroups of patients called phenotypes, resulting from different endotypes (biologic mechanisms) and displaying distinct prognostic and therapeutic value. Accordingly, several COPD phenotypes have been recently described, which exhibit significant differences in age, symptoms, co-morbidities, and predicted mortality [4–7]. Most studies described COPD heterogeneity using a limited range of variables, and in some cases the clinical relevance of identified phenotypes needs to be determined [8]. Despite these current limitations, the phenotypic characterization of COPD patients with insight into the underlying biological processes and related biomarkers may ultimately allow for a better risk stratification and personalization of therapies [9].

The predominant risk factor for COPD development is former or current tobacco smoking. However, not all smokers develop COPD, suggesting that other environmental factors are also involved, including outdoor and indoor air pollution (e.g., biomass fuel exposure), occupational hazards, infections, and second-hand smoke during pregnancy or early childhood. Furthermore, genetic susceptibility (e.g., deficiency in α1-antitrypsin) and epigenetic influences have also been implicated in the pathogenesis of COPD [10]. Recent new insights suggest that these different factors may impinge on lung function and reciprocally interact starting early in life (i.e., in utero and during early childhood), thus determining many potential trajectories of the natural course of the disease, which ultimately predispose to the development of COPD and its different clinical appearances as well as of other coexisting chronic diseases in later life [10,11].

With regard to COPD management, the most important public health message remains smoking cessation, but the multifactorial nature of COPD requires attention to other modifiable risk factors. Compared with other chronic diseases with similar burdens on quality of life and healthcare costs, such as cancer and cardiovascular disease (CVD), less is known about how lifestyle factors other than—and independent of—smoking influence pulmonary function and the development of COPD. Diet has been recognized as a modifiable risk factor for chronic diseases development and progression [12], and recent evidence has also increasingly pointed to a role in obstructive lung diseases, including COPD [13–15]. Importantly, changes in diet over the past few decades, with decreased consumption of fruits, vegetables, wholegrains, and fish, and increased consumption of processed and refined foods, have been invocated to contribute to the increased prevalence of chronic diseases, including COPD, mainly in developing countries.

Dietary factors may modulate the impact of adverse environmental exposures or genetic predisposition on the lung [16] but can also have direct (protective or harmful) effects on the biological processes involved in lung function, disease development, and outcomes [17,18]. The impact exerted by early-life and cumulative dietary choices on later-life health has been increasingly recognized for respiratory diseases, thus offering a greater window of opportunity for disease prevention [19]. Furthermore, the abnormal nutritional status observed in advanced COPD patients, with unintended weight loss, muscle loss, low fat, and fat-free mass associated with the presence of emphysema is a recognized independent determinant of COPD outcomes and provides targets for nutritional interventions [20]. On the other hand, although the phenomenon of the obesity paradox, i.e., the prognostic advantage of increased body mass index (BMI) in COPD (due to the reduction in static volume), has been reported, the role of abdominal visceral adiposity compared with subcutaneous fat in exacerbating the pro-inflammatory state and the CV risk in patients with COPD deserves clinical attention and treatment [21], mostly because a fat redistribution toward more visceral fat and an associated increased systemic inflammatory status have been shown in mild-to-moderate nonobese patients with COPD compared to control subjects [21].

Therefore, improved understanding of dietary impact on prevention and/or outcomes of COPD may increase scientific and clinical awareness about the importance of nutritional approaches as well as provide directions for future research and strategies to promote lung health and prevent disease onset and progression.

There is an expanding literature on the topic regarding diet–COPD relation. A literature search performed with the PubMed database to identify papers with the following terms "diet" and "chronic obstructive pulmonary disease risk" retrieved 233 manuscripts (from 1989 to 2019). The resulted manuscripts were analyzed using the bio-informatic data analysis tool VOSviewer [22], which extracts and analyzes the words in the titles and abstracts of the publications, relates them to citation counts, and visualizes the results as a bubble or term map, based on the strength of the co-occurrence links within the terms. The terms with greatest total link strength were selected and highlighted as bubbles. The analysis returned 750 words, of which 127 met the threshold levels (minimum number of occurrence of a term = 5). As shown in Figure 1, diet has been the focus of relevant scientific attention, and several of the words retrieved from the analysis were connected to diet, feeding behaviors, and specific foods and nutrients (fruits and vegetables, antioxidants, unsaturated fatty acids, meat products), suggesting some of the main key research categories that have been the attention focus in the topic diet and COPD risk.

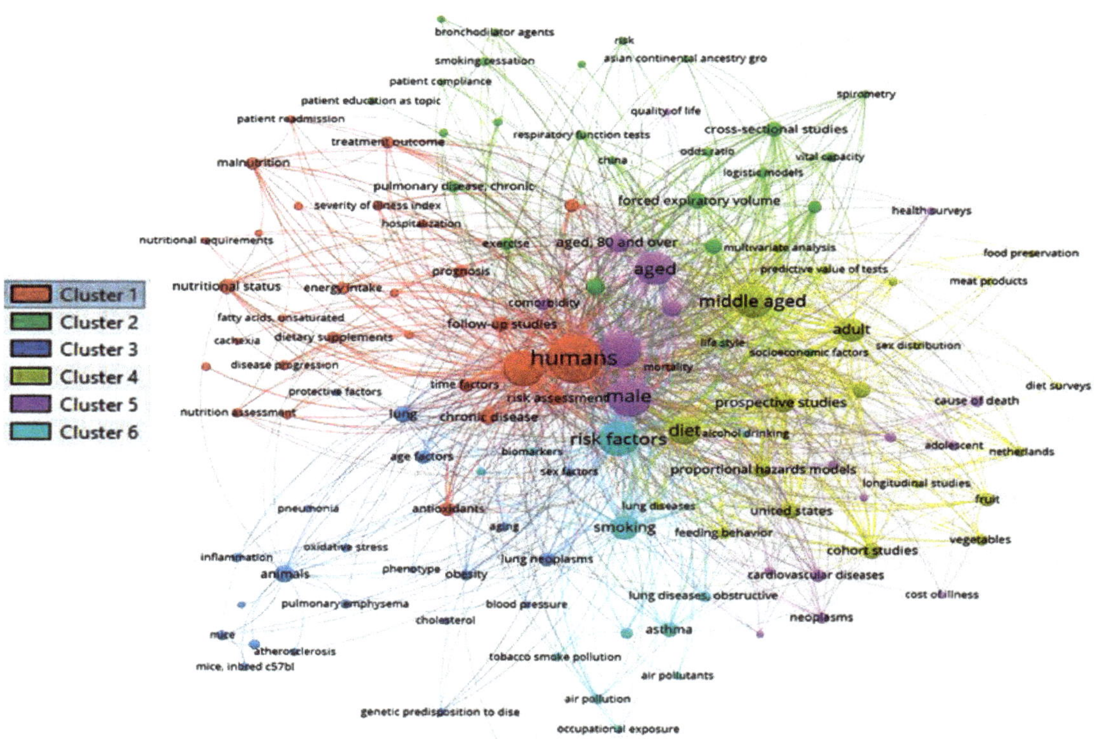

Figure 1. The bubble map visualizes 127 keywords extracted from published papers retrieved in PubMed under the search terms "diet" and "chronic obstructive pulmonary disease risk" between 1989 and 2019. Bubble size indicates the frequency of occurrence of the words, while bubble color represents the cluster of belonging. Words are clustered based on direct citation relations; thus, each cluster corresponds to a set of closely related words. Two bubbles are in closer proximity if the two words had more frequent co-occurrence.

The present narrative review aimed at assessing the available evidence from observational and intervention studies to summarize current understanding of the associations between dietary pattern, individual foods, nutrients and lung function, and prevention and improvements of COPD. The benefit of nutritional supplementation (e.g., high protein/high energy) in undernourished COPD subjects is beyond the scope of the present review, and the readers are directed to other papers on the topic (see [20,23] and references therein).

2. Pathophysiological Aspects in COPD

Several pathogenic processes are thought to be involved in COPD development and progression, including local and systemic oxidative stress (i.e., oxidants in excess compared with antioxidant capacity) and inflammation (neutrophils, macrophages, eosinophils, cytokines, chemokines, eicosanoids, Toll-like receptors, acute phase proteins), procatabolic status, protease/antiprotease imbalance, alteration of immune responses and cell proliferation, apoptosis, and cellular senescence, and remodeling of the small-airway compartment and loss of elastic recoil by emphysematous destruction of parenchyma [2]. Oxidative stress may directly cause lung damage through modification of DNA, lipids or proteins, as well as initiate cellular responses that can drive the inflammatory response within the lung, leading to lung tissue degradation (emphysema). Molecular switches triggering inflammatory responses in COPD involve the activation of redox-sensitive transcription factors (e.g., nuclear factor (NF)-κB), induction of autophagy, and unfolded protein response [24]. In particular, NF-κB plays a crucial role in the chronic inflammatory responses found in COPD, regulating the expression of genes for pro-inflammatory mediators (e.g., IL-1, IL-6, IL-8, MCP-1, TNF-α) and chemotactic factors (e.g., IL-17A and MIP-1a) involved in triggering lung infiltration by inflammatory cells, thus amplifying oxidative stress and inflammation, as well as causing emphysema, fibrosis of small airways and remodeling of airway walls, ultimately impairing lung function. Indeed, the number of NF-κB-positive epithelial cells and macrophages increased in smokers and COPD patients and correlated with the degree of airflow limitation [25].

Although primarily affecting the lungs, COPD is associated with extra-pulmonary (systemic) manifestations such as weight loss, malnutrition, and skeletal muscle dysfunction, which contribute to the morbidity, reduced quality of life, and, possibly, mortality of this disease. Furthermore, other chronic diseases (also called co-morbidities), including CVD and especially coronary artery disease (CAD), osteoporosis, metabolic syndrome, depression, and lung cancer, among others, are highly prevalent in patients with COPD, can be considered part of the nonpulmonary sequelae of the disease, with the low-grade systemic inflammation playing a decisive role in their pathogenesis, and importantly contribute to worsening health status and vital prognosis of COPD patients. In particular, CV-related co-morbidities are the leading cause of morbidity and mortality in patients with COPD, sharing various risk factors and pathophysiological aspects (inflammation-associated oxidative stress) [26]. Reduced lung function is a marker for all-cause, respiratory- and CV-related mortality [27], thus representing a clinically relevant therapeutic target for preventing the development of COPD and its life-threatening complications.

3. Literature Search Strategy

An electronic literature search of MEDLINE/Pubmed, ISI Web of Knowledge, Scopus, EMBASE, and Google Scholar was conducted by two separate investigators to retrieve relevant studies written in English and published between January 1990 and January 2019, using the following keywords: diet, dietary factor, food, nutrition, nutrient, antioxidant, fatty acid, dietary pattern, food pattern, eating habit, lung function, FEV1, chronic obstructive pulmonary disease, COPD. In addition, the references of selected original studies and reviews were scrutinized for further relevant evidence.

4. Epidemiological Studies on Diet and Pulmonary Function: Some Methodological Issues

The methodological approaches used and the specific challenges of nutrition research should be taken into consideration when evaluating single study findings and, most importantly, their potential contribution to evidence-based recommendations. Apart from a few randomized intervention trials, most of the available evidence on the impact of diet on outcomes, such as lung function (FEV1, FVC, FEV1/FVC), symptoms, incidence, prevalence or severity of COPD, and its progression over time, largely comes from observational studies, either cross-sectional or, to a lesser extent, longitudinally in both the general population and at-risk or diseased subjects. The strength of some studies is the use of objective measures of lung function that limit the bias arising from self-reported or physician-diagnosed disease: Post-bronchodilator spirometry is the gold standard for the diagnosis of COPD, minimizing misclassification.

Assessment of dietary intake usually included a 24 h recall and food-frequency questionnaire, both with inherent limitations, including the poor measurement of usual intake due to daily variation in food intake (mostly for 24 h recall), the semiquantitative nature of the assessment, the measurement error, the variation in diet definitions, and the lack of generalizability of study findings among different populations [12]. To estimate the independent association of diet with lung function and COPD, in most studies, the confounding bias is tackled by performing the adjustment for multiple confounding factors known to influence pulmonary function or dietary behavior, including age, gender, BMI, physical activity, intake of other foods or nutrients, energy intake, educational level, and most importantly, tobacco exposure. Sex differences in susceptibility to COPD have been increasingly recognized, with evidence that women are at a greater risk of smoking-induced lung function impairment [28] and poorer health status for the same level of tobacco exposure compared to men [29], and that gender differences may also extend to different food choices [30]. Furthermore, the increased tobacco use recently registered in women likely contributes to the epidemic of COPD in women and influences interpretation of study results. Notably, smokers tend to follow an unhealthy diet compared to ex-smokers [31] and have a higher level of oxidative stress, which is targetable by diet. Moreover, a healthy diet may be associated with other beneficial lifestyles (e.g., higher level of physical activity, higher education, lower BMI, less smoking). Even after adjustment, residual confounding of dietary associations still remains possible and contributes to some inconsistencies across studies.

Many studies have focused on the effects of individual foods or nutrients in relation to respiratory outcomes. However, this information may not completely capture the overall effect of diet on respiratory health nor reflect real life conditions where foods or nutrients are eaten in multiple combinations [32]. Moreover, nutrient and food intakes are closely correlated in the diet, so it can be difficult to disentangle their independent effects. As an example, the lack of benefit of vitamin supplementation on lung function and hospitalization for COPD [33] may be explained, at least in part, by the fact that antioxidant regimens could be effective when adopted in the form of dietary patterns rather than individual nutrients. Dietary pattern analysis captures the quantities, proportions, variety, or combination of different foods and beverages in the diets and provides a framework to evaluate the health effects of the whole diet. This may increase the ability to highlight a stronger impact due to the cumulative effects of many features of the diet and to assess the interaction among synergistic components. This comprehensive approach is emphasized by prevailing dietary guidelines and has been used in several clinical settings, including CVD, cancer, and type 2 diabetes [12].

It should be acknowledged, however, that the evaluation of overall dietary patterns could mask the effects of individual foods or nutrients and disregard potential effects of foods or nutrients not included as components of the pattern. Therefore, the best option could be to complement and integrate data on eating patterns with those of individual components as much as possible in the same study population.

Numerous different combinations of foods and nutrients may be potentially investigated as patterns of food intake, and approaches to rank and quantify adherence of study participants to these patterns have been developed to evaluate their association with disease risk. These approaches [12] include: (1) a priori-defined (hypothesis-driven) indices or scores designed to capture specific dietary patterns defined a priori on the basis of scientific evidence on the relation between food and nutrient intakes and health outcomes; these scores also allow measuring conformity to nutritional requirements and dietary guidelines, with the drawback of considerable variation in the composition of patterns across studies; and (2) data-driven (exploratory) statistical methods (cluster analysis, principal component and factor analysis, and reduced rank regression) to derive existing major patterns of food intake, with the limitation of being specific to the population investigated.

5. Oxidant–Antioxidant Imbalance and Diet Quality in COPD

Oxidative stress and associated inflammation in the lung and in the circulation in response to exposure to air pollution, tobacco smoke, infection, or potentially obesity are leading pathogenic processes in COPD. Compared to healthy controls, patients with COPD tend to have increased systemic and airway oxidative damage markers (relative to DNA, lipid, and proteins) [34], coupled to altered antioxidant defense, as evidenced by marked reduction in both plasma antioxidant capacity and soluble and enzymatic antioxidants levels [34–36]. Moreover, oxidative stress persists long after smoking cessation as a result of continuous production of pro-oxidants [37]. Low serum antioxidant vitamin levels appeared to increase the risk of obstructive airways diseases associated to smoking exposure [38]. In accordance, higher levels of oxidative markers in COPD were correlated with decreased lung function [39–41], while higher serum levels of antioxidant enzymes (catalase, superoxide dismutase, glutathione peroxidase) [40,41], as well as of soluble antioxidants (vitamins, carotenoids, etc.) [35,42,43], were positively associated with lung function. Therefore, it can be hypothesized that targeting oxidative stress with antioxidants or boosting endogenous levels of antioxidants might be beneficial in COPD.

Diet may contribute to antioxidant/oxidant and inflammatory status in COPD. Compared to healthy controls, COPD subjects have diets with lower fruit and vegetable intake [44] and with poorer antioxidant content, which was correlated with impaired lung function and risk of having COPD [35,36]. Moreover, lower energy intake (accompanied by elevated resting energy expenditure), unbalanced intake of macronutrients (e.g., low proteins), and defective intake of several micronutrients (minerals and vitamins, e.g., iron, calcium, potassium, zinc, folate, vitamin B6, retinol, niacin) have been documented in COPD patients compared to healthy controls [45], mostly in the presence of obesity [46], suggesting an increased risk of malnutrition and related adverse consequences in COPD.

The poor diet quality and the nutrient deficiencies in COPD, which are related to disease-specific factors such as symptoms (e.g., dyspnea, fatigue, anxiety, depression, anorexia, periodontal disease, loss of taste, poor dentition, dysphagia, poor chewing and swallowing ability) or social problems (e.g., living or eating alone, or poverty) [47], require improvement through dietary intervention to satisfy nutritional requirements and even to supplement further protective factors able to counteract disease pathogenesis. The inflammatory/oxidative status in COPD and the associated procatabolic state contributing to weight loss and muscle wasting in severe COPD represent further possible targets for nutritional intervention.

6. Individual Foods and Nutrients, Lung Function, and COPD

6.1. *Role of Antioxidant and Anti-Inflammatory Foods: Fruits and Vegetables*

The dietary quality and the nutritional status of COPD patients as well as the oxidative–inflammatory pathogenic basis of COPD provided the rationale to verify the respiratory effects of antioxidant and anti-inflammatory dietary components. Consistent epidemiologic evidence from cross-sectional [36,38,48–51] and longitudinal studies [42,52–55] reported potential beneficial effects of a high intake of antioxidant nutrients (vitamins and nonvitamins) and of foods rich in antioxidants, mostly fresh, hard fruits and, to a lesser extent, vegetables, on lung function and COPD symptoms [35,36,49–51], decline in lung function [42,49,56], incidence of COPD [52,54,55], and mortality [53].

Two recent large population-based prospective studies in Swedish men [54] and women [55] confirmed the inverse and independent association between high long-term consumption of fruits (in both men and women) and vegetables (only in men) and incidence of COPD (35% lower risk in men, p for trend <0.0001 [54]; 37% lower risk in women, p for trend <0.0001 [55]). These beneficial dietary associations were particularly evident among smokers. Specifically, in the cohort of men (with higher smoking intensity than women), the protective effect was restricted to current and ex-smokers (40% lower risk, p for trend <0.0001, and 34% lower risk, p for trend = 0.001, respectively), mostly benefiting from dietary antioxidants, probably as a result of increased oxidative stress level due to smoking compared with never smoking, and the continued oxidative burden even after smoking cessation [54]. Regarding individual food items, intakes of apples, pears, peppers, and green leafy vegetables were negatively associated with the risk of COPD [54].

Few randomized dietary intervention trials have been conducted. In a small 12-week randomized trial including moderate-to-severe COPD patients complying with an intervention to increase fruit intake, no improvement in airways or systemic inflammation and oxidative stress markers was observed, although the follow-up might have been too short to observe any significant effect [57]. In COPD patients, 1-week supplementation with beetroot juice, a dietary source of nitrates that improves mitochondrial respiration and energy production via nitric oxide formation, increased plasma nitrate levels and decreased diastolic blood pressure (mean difference 4.6 mmHg, 95% CI: 0.1, 9.1, $p < 0.05$) without any effect on walking capacity, physical activity level, or oxygen consumption of submaximal exercise [58]. However, another randomized trial reported that COPD patients following a diet rich in fruits and vegetables (>1 portion/day) showed an annual increase in FEV1 compared with the control group following a free diet over 3 years ($p = 0.03$), after adjustment for physical activity, alcohol intake, co-morbidities, and exacerbation frequency [59].

Collectively, these observations suggest fruit and vegetable consumption as an important determinant of pulmonary function and COPD risk. It should be noted that fresh fruit intake may be one component of an overall healthier lifestyle, including less smoking, more physical activity, low consumption of Western foods (e.g., meat), and increased consumption of vegetables [54,55,59], and other not checked nutrients may mediate the observed beneficial effects. Furthermore, assessment of blood, urine or exhaled breath condensate biomarkers of endogenous oxidative stress is generally lacking in most longitudinal studies, thus limiting the possibility to more accurately select subjects more susceptible to antioxidant dietary regimens and to appraise the antioxidant efficacy of tested foods over time.

6.2. *Vitamin and Nonvitamin Antioxidants*

Plausible mechanisms underlying fruit and vegetable protective effects include their antioxidant and anti-inflammatory activities, as suggested by the epidemiologic association observed between fruit and vegetable consumption and lower markers of oxidative stress and inflammation, and higher levels of antioxidant markers [60,61]. Fruits' and vegetables' beneficial effects on respiratory function may be partially contributed by their high content in vitamin and nonvitamin antioxidants. Accordingly, higher dietary intakes of vitamin C, a hydrophilic antioxidant, were associated with higher levels of FEV1 [35,62] and with a lower rate of decline in FEV1 after a 9-year follow-up period [62]. Other studies did not confirm a significant effect of vitamin C dietary intake on lung function (FEV1), its longitudinal decline [49], COPD incidence [52] or mortality [53]. Although not consistently [62], a protective role has also been credited to other vitamins such as vitamin E or tocopherol, a lipid soluble antioxidant acting in synergy with vitamin C and able of breaking lipid peroxidation chain reaction and protecting the lung against oxidative damage [36,53]. Lower serum vitamin E levels have been observed in COPD during exacerbation compared to stable condition [63]. Randomized trials of vitamin E supplementation in clinical populations have, however, reported mixed results, including both protective [64] and no effects [33] on the risk of developing COPD.

Butland et al. [49] found a positive cross-sectional association between higher consumption of hard fruits, such as apples (5 or more apples per week) and lung function (FEV1) (138 mL higher FEV1 for those eating 5 or more apples per week compared with nonconsumers, 95% CI: 58.1, 218.1, p for trend <0.001), more strongly than soft or citrus fruits and independent of vitamin E and vitamin C intakes. Similarly, Miedema et al. [52] found a stronger inverse association with 25-year incidence of COPD for solid fruits (apples, pears) than for other types of fruits. Other nonvitamin dietary components may therefore exert protective effects. These include the fat-soluble antioxidant carotenoids (lycopene, lutein, zeaxanthin, and the provitamin A carotenoids α-carotene, β-carotene, and β-cryptoxanthin), whose serum and dietary levels have been positively correlated to lung function indicators (FEV1, FVC) [35,42,65]. However, long-term supplementation with β-carotene or α-tocopherol failed to reduce COPD symptoms in a large cohort of male smokers randomized into the α-tocopherol and β-carotene Cancer Prevention (ATBC) Study [66]. Notably, strong evidence from randomized controlled trials conducted in heavy smokers and asbestos-exposed workers, i.e., the β-carotene and retinol efficacy trial (CARET) [67] and the abovementioned ATBC study [68], showed that high-dose β-carotene supplements may increase the risk of lung cancer and of death from lung cancer, CVD, and any cause. Contrarily, this harmful effect was not observed among healthy male physicians in the Physicians' Health Study in the USA [69]. An interaction of carotenoids with cigarette smoking has been proposed to explain the shifting of carotenoid antioxidant potential into a pro-oxidant detrimental effect on the lung: β-carotene can easily form oxidation products with pro-oxidant effects, especially at high concentrations in the oxidative environment of the smoker's lung characterized by increased cell oxidative stress and decreased antioxidant defense [70]. Against this background, according to the 2018 report of the World Cancer Research Fund/American Institute for Cancer Research (https://www.wcrf.org/dietandcancer), β-carotene supplements (and dietary supplements in general) are not recommended for cancer prevention (especially in smokers), while intake of natural micronutrients through diet is advisable. Therefore, caution should be taken, especially in smokers, when considering dietary supplementation with β-carotene.

Other potentially protective dietary factors include polyphenols, the most abundant antioxidants in human diets naturally present in plant foods, and exhibiting potent anti-inflammatory properties. Polyphenols, including phenolic acids, flavonoids (flavonols, flavones, isoflavones, flavanones, flavanols, and anthocyanidins), stilbenes (resveratrol, etc.), lignans, and secoiridoids, have been reportedly associated with prevention of chronic diseases, including CV and neurodegenerative diseases and cancer, and with the promotion of healthy aging [71]. Beneficial effects on respiratory function have been reported for the flavonoid class of polyphenols: In an earlier Dutch study, the intake of catechins was positively associated with FEV1 (mean difference in FEV1 comparing high vs. low intake of catechins = 130 mL, 95% CI: 101–159, $p < 0.05$) and negatively associated with all three COPD symptoms (odds ratio (OR) of phlegm, breathlessness and cough, comparing high vs. low intake of catechins = 0.60–0.72, $p < 0.001$) [50]; concordantly, slower longitudinal decline in lung function was observed with higher intake of anthocyanidins in US elderly men [72], and a beneficial association of dietary intakes of isoflavones as well as of soy, which is a rich food source of isoflavones, with lung function and COPD prevalence was also observed in Japanese adults [73,74]. In a recent randomized trial in COPD patients, supplementation with flavonoids in the form of oligomeric pro-anthocyanidins extracted from grape seeds was effective in improving oxidative stress and lipid profile, but not lung function parameters after 8 weeks [75]. More recent observational findings in a Mediterranean population confirmed protective effects of the intake of various polyphenol classes on pulmonary function parameters [76]. In a cross-sectional study in 267 Spanish COPD patients, dietary intakes of vitamin E as well as vegetables and olive oil, rich in vitamin E and polyphenols, have been shown to be inversely correlated with serum markers of oxidative stress, especially in current smokers [77]. In an Asian population-based cross sectional study, a diet rich in the potent antioxidant and anti-inflammatory turmeric-derived polyphenol curcumin was significantly and independently associated with improved lung function measures, and smokers with the highest curcumins intake had levels of lung function greater than smokers not consuming curcumins and similar to those of nonsmokers, supporting the antioxidant and anti-inflammatory dietary hypothesis [78].

6.3. Minerals

Among micronutrients, cross-sectional studies have found deficient intake of some minerals in COPD patients. Indeed, dietary intakes and serum levels of calcium, magnesium, and selenium were found to be below the recommended values in older, underweight patients with severe COPD [79]. Lower intakes of calcium and zinc were observed in elderly COPD patients compared with non-COPD subjects [45]. Some minerals have been studied in relation to lung function and COPD risk and symptoms. A case-control study in Japanese adults found a positive association between intake of calcium, phosphorus, iron, potassium, and selenium and lung function measures (e.g., FEV1), and an inverse association between dietary calcium intake and COPD risk (35% reduction) [80]. FEV1 was independently and positively associated with serum levels of selenium, normalized calcium, chloride, and iron, and was inversely related to potassium and sodium in the general population [43]. Other cross-sectional studies confirmed the association between serum levels of selenium as well as copper and higher lung function [81]. A randomized placebo-controlled trial reported that selenium supplementation (200 μg/d L-selenomethionine), either alone or in combination with vitamin E (400 IU/d all rac-α-tocopheryl acetate), did not affect decline in FEV1 or FEF25–75, a marker of airflow, but attenuated decline in FEF25–75 (by 59 mL/second/year) in current smokers, who may benefit most from selenium supplementation due to its potent antioxidant properties linked to the glutathione peroxidase activity [82].

Early population-based studies reported a strong association between magnesium intake and lung function, airway hyper-responsiveness, and wheeze [83], although this result was not consistently found [49]. More recently, in a general UK population cohort intake of magnesium was cross-sectionally related to higher FEV1 (a 100 mg/day higher magnesium intake was associated with a 52.9 ml higher FEV1 (95% CI, 9.6–96.2)), but no relationship between intake of magnesium and longitudinal decline in FEV1 was seen [62]. Similar results were recently obtained by Leng et al. [84] in New Mexico white smokers. Magnesium may play a beneficial role in respiratory function and COPD, through its protective effects against inflammation and bronchoconstriction [85]. Although the limited evidence suggests protective effects of some minerals on lung function and COPD, mostly for those endowed with antioxidant and anti-inflammatory properties, further prospective studies are warranted.

6.4. Wholegrains and Fibers

Among dietary factors largely investigated, mostly in relation to CVD and cancer, research has also focused on wholegrains. Observational studies reported an independent beneficial effect of a high wholegrain intake on lung function [51,86], and against mortality from chronic respiratory disease [87]. Wholegrains are rich in phenolic acids, flavonoids, phytic acid, vitamin E, selenium, and essential fatty acids, which may additively or synergistically contribute to wholegrain documented beneficial effect on respiratory as well as nonrespiratory diseases.

Part of the protective action of wholegrains as well as of fruits and vegetables is attributable to the antioxidant and anti-inflammatory properties of their fiber content [88]. Indeed, epidemiological data indicated that fiber intake is associated with lower serum levels of C-reactive protein and cytokines (IL-6, TNF-α) and higher level of adiponectin, an insulin-sensitizing adipocytokine with anti-inflammatory properties [89]. In line with these beneficial properties, cross-sectional and longitudinal studies found a negative and independent association between total fiber intake and lung function decline, and COPD incidence and prevalence [90–92]. Indeed, higher dietary intake of total fiber reduced by about 40% the risk of COPD in large prospective studies [91,92]. Considering fiber types (cereal, fruit, vegetable), the beneficial association was observed mostly for cereal fiber intake mainly in current smokers and ex-smokers, but evidence exists also for fruit and vegetable fiber intake [91,92].

6.5. Alcohol and Wine

Other significant associations with respiratory health have been documented in the general population for intake of alcohol and wine. Previous epidemiologic studies found that subjects with low alcohol consumption (1–30 g/day) had higher levels of FEV1, lower prevalence of COPD symptoms [51], and a decreased risk of COPD compared to nonconsumers [52]. By contrast, heavy alcohol intake, as assessed by both dietary and serum biomarker measurements, was shown to have negative effects on lung function, additive to that of smoking [93]. Among the different alcohol sources, only wine intake (>7.4 g/day) was found to be positively associated with FEV1 in the general population [94], as well as with a lower risk of airway obstruction, defined as an abnormally low FEV1/FVC ratio, predominantly in smokers [95]. Beyond direct protective effects of alcohol as previously reported [96], putative candidates accounting for the observed beneficial effect of wine are flavonoids [50], as well as the stilbene resveratrol [95], both associated with improved measures of lung function. Congruently, resveratrol has been reported to exert anti-inflammatory properties in airway epithelial cells [97], alveolar macrophages derived from COPD patients [98], and airways smooth muscle cells [99], and the flavonol quercetin has been shown to attenuate rhinovirus-induced lung inflammation and emphysema progression in a mice model of COPD [100].

Interestingly, the independent beneficial effects of a favorable intake of fruits (>180 g/day), wholegrains (>45 g/day), and alcohol (1–30 g/day) on FEV1 and COPD symptoms were additive (favorable vs. unfavorable intake, 139 mL higher FEV1 and COPD symptoms prevalence OR = 0.44, $p < 0.001$) [51], suggesting important interaction among nutrients and food groups. Moreover, findings from the ECLIPSE study in COPD subjects demonstrated that recent consumption of "healthy" foods, such as fruits (grapefruit and bananas), fish, tea, dairy products, and alcohol, was associated with higher lung function and less decline over time, less emphysema and emphysema progression, greater 6-minute walk and St. George's Respiratory Questionnaire (SGRQ) scores, and lower levels of inflammatory markers (C-reactive protein, white blood cells, surfactant protein D, total neutrophils) [101]. These data extend the role for dietary intakes to phenotypic features of COPD patients.

6.6. Vitamin D

Limited evidence also supports a direct correlation between vitamin D levels, which mainly depend on sun exposure in addition to diet, and lung function, COPD incidence, symptoms, severity and progression [102–104]. Genetic variants in the vitamin D-binding protein associated with lower plasma vitamin D levels have also been linked to COPD risk [105]. Mechanistic studies support a role for vitamin D other than calcemic effects and in particular in normal growth and development of the lung as well as in immune responses and COPD progression. Vitamin D supplementation trials to prevent COPD exacerbation reported conflicting results but, collectively, pointed to a benefit only in patients with low baseline vitamin D levels (i.e., levels of active metabolite 25-hydroxyvitamin D <25 nmol/L) [106]. Although further studies are needed, taking into account the highly prevalent osteoporosis and risk of falls in COPD patients and also the supposed beneficial effects of vitamin D beyond bone health, screening for vitamin D deficiency (25-hydroxyvitamin D <50 nmol/L) may be important in COPD patients.

6.7. Coffee and Its Components

Given its widespread consumption, interest has been growing around the potential role of coffee in respiratory health. Findings from literature reviews point to an association between regular (not decaffeinated) coffee intake and improved lung function and reduced mortality from respiratory disease, but not COPD [107], with contributory roles for its constituents, caffeine (bronchodilator, anti-inflammatory) and polyphenols (antioxidant, anti-inflammatory). Smoking is a major confounder in these studies because it may accelerate the hepatic metabolism and clearance of caffeine or may dilute or dampen the beneficial effects of coffee through its potent pro-oxidant and pro-inflammatory action [107].

6.8. Role of Fish and n-3 Polyunsaturated Fatty Acids

α-Linolenic acid (ALA, C18:3) and its long-chain derivatives eicosapentaenoic acid (EPA, C20:5) and docosahexaenoic acid (DHA, C22:6) are polyunsaturated fatty acids (PUFA) of the *n-3* (omega-3) family. Due to the low efficiency of endogenous synthesis from precursors, they are considered nutritionally essential and depend on exogenous source, mainly seafood (fatty fish). *n*-3 PUFAs and fish display potent anti-inflammatory properties with beneficial effects and, in most cases, clinical applications in several chronic inflammatory diseases, including CVD, cancer, rheumatoid arthritis, and diabetes [108]. Opposite effects have been described for *n*-6 PUFAs, including linoleic acid (LA, C18:2) and its long-chain derivative arachidonic acid (AA, C20:4), mainly found in vegetable oils (soybean, corn, and sunflower oils), grain-fed animals, dairy, and eggs. Indeed, metabolism of long-chain *n-6* PUFA produces eicosanoids (such as thromboxane(TX) A2, prostaglandin(PG) E2 and leukotriene(LT) B4) which are more potent mediators of inflammation, thrombosis, and vaso- and bronco-constriction than similar products derived from *n*-3 PUFAs (PGs of the 3-series and LTs of the 5-series) [109]. Some EPA and DHA metabolites via cytochrome P450 enzymes, which are highly expressed in the lungs, are potent vasodilators and bronchodilators and show anti-inflammatory properties. Other metabolites of long-chain *n*-3 PUFAs include the inflammation-resolving eicosanoids resolvins and protectins, which act to remove inflammatory mediators and promote healing.

Increasing the content of *n*-3 PUFA in the diet causes a partial substitution of the *n*-6 PUFA in the cell membranes and competition for the metabolizing enzymes, thus favoring the synthesis of generally less biologically active eicosanoids. In addition to lipid metabolites, *n*-3 PUFA anti-inflammatory mechanisms also include the direct modulation of inflammatory gene expression (adhesion molecules, cytokines, matrix degrading enzymes, cyclooxygenase-2) via the regulation of nuclear transcription factors, mainly the oxidative stress-sensitive pro-inflammatory NF-κB [109], which has also been involved in the pathogenesis of lung inflammation [24].

The secular trend of dietary shift to a more Westernized pattern and the following increased consumption of *n*-6 PUFAs and decreased consumption of *n*-3 PUFAs is thought to have contributed to the rise in chronic inflammatory disease [108]. Given the role of inflammation in COPD and the reported benefits of long-chain *n*-3 PUFAs in many inflammatory diseases, studies have been conducted to verify the ability of dietary PUFAs to also modulate COPD (prevalence, severity, and health outcomes). However, as underlined in a recent systematic review [110], data are conflicting. Some earlier observational studies suggest benefits from increased consumption of *n*-3 PUFA-rich foods, in particular fatty fish, on respiratory function and COPD symptoms, mainly among smokers, but none of the studies adjusted for other dietary intakes [111–113]. Contrarily, in a 25-year prospective study conducted in the Netherlands, the intake of *n*-6 PUFA was positively related to the incidence of chronic lung diseases (defined as chronic productive cough, chronic bronchitis, emphysema, and asthma), but no relation between *n*-3 PUFA intake and the incidence of chronic nonspecific lung disease was observed [52]. Concordantly, other studies did not find any independent beneficial association between fish intake and FEV1, COPD symptoms [51] or mortality [53]. A large population-based cross-sectional study found that higher intake of individual *n-6* PUFAs was associated with lower FEV1 (reduction in FEV1 between the highest vs. lowest quintile of intake = 54.5 mL, 95% CI: –81.6, –27.4, $p < 0.0001$), particularly in smokers, and with increased risk of COPD, while no association between individual *n*-3 PUFAs intake and FEV1 or COPD symptoms was seen [114].

More recently, in two large US cohorts, while an initial analysis showed that higher intake of fish (≥4 servings/week), but not PUFAs, was associated with lower risk of newly diagnosed COPD, after adjustment for overall dietary pattern, this association lost significance, suggesting that potential benefits of fish might be evident within the whole diet [115]. Interestingly, fish intake could reduce the risk of COPD when intake of plant sources of *n*–3 PUFAs is high [115], suggesting that a healthy diet including fish as well as vegetable sources of n-3 PUFAs may be more beneficial for COPD than isolated food or nutrient.

Evidence exists that anti-inflammatory actions of n-3 PUFA may extend and be relevant to COPD pathogenesis. In an in vitro study, shifting the PUFA supply from AA to DHA significantly reduced the release of pro-inflammatory cytokines (TNF-α, IL-6, and IL-8) and increased the release of anti-inflammatory cytokine (IL-10) from human alveolar cells after endotoxin challenge [116]. Resolvin D1 (derived from DHA) has been reported to inhibit cigarette smoke-induced pro-inflammatory response in human lung cells in vitro and in a mouse model of acute cigarette smoke-induced lung inflammation by selectively activating specific anti-inflammatory pathways, including the inhibition of neutrophilic inflammation and the activation of a subset of anti-inflammatory, pro-resolving macrophages [117]. In stable COPD patients, higher circulating inflammatory markers (IL-6, C-reactive protein) were associated with higher dietary intake of n-6 PUFAs (for IL-6, OR = 1.96, $p = 0.034$; for CRP, OR = 1.95, $p = 0.039$), while lower plasma levels of the cytokine TNF-α were related to n-3 PUFAs intake (OR = 0.46, $p = 0.049$) [118]. Results from feeding trials assessed health outcomes in COPD patients. An 8-week supplementation with n-3 PUFA (1200 mg ALA, 700 mg EPA, and 340 mg DHA) in patients with moderate-to-severe COPD reversed muscle wasting and improved the functional capacity compared with placebo, without any effect on FEV1 or systemic inflammatory markers (CRP, IL-6, and TNF-α) [119]. Further studies, especially randomized controlled trials, are therefore needed to appraise the relationships between intake of long-chain n-3 PUFA and/or fish and COPD.

6.9. Foods with Potential Deleterious Effects on Lung Function and COPD

Among potential deleterious foods, a statistically significant inverse association between frequent consumption of cured (bacon, hot dogs, and processed meats) and red meats and pulmonary function has been reported, in agreement with evidence of detrimental effects in other nonrespiratory diseases, including CAD, diabetes, and cancer [120,121], and all-cause mortality [122]. Increased intake of cured meats was independently associated with an obstructive pattern of spirometry in a cross-sectional analysis in the third National Health and Nutrition Examination Survey [123] and with an increased risk of newly diagnosed COPD in both men and women in US prospective cohorts, independent of Western dietary pattern (highly loaded with red meat) or other associated dietary intakes (refined grains, desserts, etc.) [124,125]. Importantly, more recent large Swedish population-based prospective studies confirmed this detrimental effect for both baseline and long-term consumption of processed (not unprocessed) red meat [126,127]. Another study found that cured meat intake increased the risk of COPD readmission [128]. Collectively, as summarized in a recent meta-analysis, available evidence indicated a 40% increased risk of COPD with higher consumption of processed red meat (>75–785.5 g/week) [129].

These data suggest that health-promoting activities should include specific advice on lowering red/processed meat consumption. It would be important to confirm these results in those populations experiencing nutrition transition with an increased consumption of Westernized foods, including processed meats.

In addition to the high content in cholesterol and saturated fatty acids, drawbacks of processed red meat include the presence of nitrites, which are added to processed meat during the manufacturing process as a preservative, antimicrobial, and color fixative. Nitrites generate reactive nitrogen species, such as peroxynitrite, with the subsequent nitrosative stress that can contribute to, and amplify, inflammatory processes in the airways and lung parenchyma, causing DNA damage, inhibition of mitochondrial respiration, and cell dysfunction. Moreover, tyrosine nitration in connective tissue proteins, including collagen and elastin, can alter their function. Higher levels of nitrotyrosine have been observed in subjects with COPD and were correlated to disease severity [130]. Accordingly, in animal models, chronic exposure to nitrite caused emphysema-like pathological changes in the lungs [131]. Nitrites are also byproducts of tobacco smoke; thus, nitrite generation may be one of the mechanisms by which tobacco smoke causes COPD. Congruently, the combination of smoking and higher cured meat consumption is indeed associated with the highest risk of newly diagnosed COPD [125]. Cured meats also contain a high amount of sodium that may increase bronchial hyper-reactivity and may elicit inflammation [132]. Sodium dietary intake has been reported to be higher in COPD patients compared to healthy controls and to be associated with lower lung function [80].

Meat is also an important source of saturated fatty acids (SFAs), which can trigger inflammation, also in the airways [133], and have been associated with both impaired lung function [134] and an elevated risk of coronary heart disease and metabolic diseases [135]. This risk seems to be mainly attributable to medium and long chain SFAs (C14:0–C18:0) highly present in meat compared to other animal sources such as dairy products. By contrast, increased intake of low-fat dairy products [136] as well as of short and medium chain SFAs, as assessed by 24 h recall [137], may exert protective effects on lung function, possibly through their anti-inflammatory action.

An important feature of the Western lifestyle and diet is the consumption of foods with high glycemic index, such as refined grains, desserts, sweets, and sweetened beverages. In addition to increasing the risk of obesity, hyperglycemia may trigger oxidative stress-related inflammatory responses [138], is associated with impaired lung function [139] and poor COPD outcomes [140], and may promote pulmonary infection, at least in part, by an effect on airway glucose concentrations [141]. Part of the detrimental effects of hyperglycemia is mediated by the formation of advanced glycation end-products (AGEs), which are elevated in lung tissues of COPD patients and are known to be associated with lung inflammation and pathophysiology [142]. Compared to no consumption, high levels of soft drink consumption (>0.5 L/day, sweetened or not), an important component of the Western lifestyle and diet, were associated with a higher prevalence of COPD (OR = 1.79, 95% CI: 1.32, 2.43, $p < 0.001$) and asthma (OR = 1.26, 95% CI: 1.01, 1.58, $p = 0.014$), in an additive manner with smoking [143]. Moreover, consumption of excess fructose-sweetened soft drink (>5 times/week) was significantly correlated to chronic bronchitis in US adults (OR = 1.80, 95% CI: 1.01, 3.20, $p = 0.047$) [144], as well as to pediatric asthma [145], possibly due to the formation of AGEs from the interaction between unabsorbed free fructose and dietary proteins in the gastrointestinal tract. These results clearly emphasize the public health implication of interventions targeting modern unhealthy lifestyle habits.

7. Dietary Patterns, Lung Function, and COPD

Dietary patterns have been widely investigated in relation to cancer, CVD or diabetes [12], but limited data are available on their association with respiratory outcomes with relevance to COPD. As shown in a recent meta-analysis [14], most studies were performed in Europe and North America, limiting the generalizability of study findings, and were observational in design. Overall, the evidence concordantly indicated that the pattern of dietary intake is an important factor in the pathogenesis and prevention of COPD and provided support for specific dietary modifications as a clinically relevant tool to promote lung health. Moreover, examination of dietary patterns complements the evaluation of the effects of individual food and nutrient intake on COPD. Table 1 summarizes findings from main epidemiological studies addressing the relation between diet and lung function, COPD risk, symptoms, and progression.

Table 1. Main findings from epidemiological studies linking dietary patterns to adult lung function and chronic obstructive pulmonary disease (COPD) (incidence, prevalence, and severity).

Dietary Patterns	Country (Cohort)	Design (Follow-Up)	Population	Sex (Age)	Diet Assessment Method	Outcome	Outcome Assessment	Main Results	Ref
					Data-driven dietary patterns				
Meat–dim sum pattern and vegetable–fruit–soy pattern	China (SCHS)	P (5.3 year)	General population $n = 52{,}325$	F, M (45–74 year)	FFQ and PCA	New onset of cough with phlegm	Self-reported	The meat-dim sum pattern was associated with increased incidence of cough with phlegm (fourth vs. first quartile, OR = 1.43, 95% CI: 1.08, 1.89, p for trend = 0.02))	[146]
Prudent pattern and Western pattern	USA (HPFS)	P (12 year)	Health professionals $n = 42{,}917$	M (40–75 year)	FFQ and PCA	COPD incidence	Self-reported	The prudent pattern was negatively (highest vs. lowest quintile, RR = 0.50, 95% CI: 0.25, 0.98), while the Western pattern was positively (highest vs. lowest quintile, RR = 4.56, 95% CI: 1.95, 10.69) associated with COPD risk	[147]
Prudent pattern and Western pattern	USA (NHS)	P (6 year)	Nurses $n = 72{,}043$	F (30–55 year)	FFQ and PCA	COPD incidence	Self-reported	The prudent pattern was negatively (highest vs. lowest quintile, RR = 0.75, 95% CI: 0.58, 0.98), while the Western pattern was positively (highest vs. lowest quintile, RR = 1.31, 95% CI: 0.94, 1.82) associated with COPD risk	[148]
Prudent pattern and traditional pattern	United Kingdom (HCS)	C	General population $n = 1391$ (F), $n = 1551$ (M)	F, M (mean 66 year)	FFQ and PCA	Primary outcome: FEV1; Secondary outcomes: FVC, FEV1/FVC, COPD prevalence	Spirometry	The prudent pattern was positively associated with FEV1 in M and F (changes in FEV1 between highest vs. lowest quintiles, 180 mL in M, 95% CI: 0.00, 0.16, p for trend<0.001, and 80 mL in F, 95% CI: 0.26, 0.81, p for trend = 0.008), and negatively with COPD in M (top versus bottom quintile, OR = 0.46, 95% CI: 0.26, 0.81, $p = 0.012$)	[149]
Prudent pattern, high-CHO diet, Western pattern	Swiss (SAPALDIA)	C	General population $n = 2178$	F, M (mean 58.6 year)	FFQ and PCA	FEV1, FEV1/FVC, FEF25-75, COPD prevalence	Spirometry	The prudent pattern was positively associated with lung function and negatively with COPD prevalence (NS)	[150]

Table 1. *Cont.*

Dietary Patterns	Country (Cohort)	Design (Follow-Up)	Population	Sex (Age)	Diet Assessment Method	Outcome	Outcome Assessment	Main Results	Ref
					Data-driven dietary patterns				
Western pattern and prudent pattern	USA (ARIC)	C	General population n = 15,256	F, M (mean 54.2 year)	FFQ and PCA	Respiratory symptoms (cough, phlegm, wheeze), FEV1, FEV1/FVC, COPD prevalence	Spirometry	The Western pattern was associated with higher prevalence of COPD (fifth vs. first quintile: OR = 1.62, 95% CI: 1.33, 1.97, $p < 0.001$), respiratory symptoms (wheeze OR = 1.37, 95% CI: 1.11, 1.69, $p = 0.002$; cough OR = 1.32, 95% CI: 1.10, 1.59, $p = 0.001$, phlegm OR = 1.27, 95% CI: 1.05, 1.54, $p = 0.031$), and worse lung function (e.g., percent predicted FEV1: fifth quintile 91.8 vs. first quintile 95.1, $p < 0.001$). The prudent pattern was associated with lower prevalence of COPD (OR = 0.82, 95% CI: 0.70, 0.95, $p = 0.007$), cough (OR = 0.77, 95% CI: 0.67, 0.89, $p < 0.001$), and higher lung function (e.g., percent predicted FEV1: fifth quintile 94.3 vs. first quintile 92.7, $p < 0.001$)	[151]
Cosmopolitan pattern, traditional pattern, and refined food dietary pattern	Netherlands (MORGEN-EPIC)	C	General population n = 12,648	F, M (mean 41 year)	FFQ and PCA	FEV1, wheeze, asthma, COPD prevalence	Spirometry and self-reported symptoms	The traditional pattern was associated with lower FEV1 (fifth vs. first quintile, −94.4 mL, 95% CI:−123.4, −65.5, $p < 0.001$) and increased prevalence of COPD (fifth vs. first quintile, OR = 1.60, 95% CI: 1.1, 2.3, p for trend = 0.001); the cosmopolitan pattern was associated with increased prevalence of asthma (fifth vs. first quintile, OR = 1.4; 95% CI: 1.0, 2.0; p for trend = 0.047) and wheeze (fifth vs. first quintile, OR = 1.3, 95% CI: 1.0, 1.5; p for trend = 0.001)	[152]
		P (5 y)	General population n = 2911	F, M (mean 45 year)	FFQ and PCA	FEV1	Spirometry	The refined food pattern was associated with a nonsignificant greater decline in lung function (−48.5 mL, 95% CI: -80.7, −16.3; p for trend = 0.11)	[152]
Alcohol-consumption pattern, Westernized pattern, and MED-like pattern	Spain	C	Smokers with no respiratory diseases n = 207	F, M (35–70 year)	FFQ and PCA	Impaired lung function	Spirometry	Alcohol-consumption pattern (OR = 4.56, 95% CI: 1.58, 13.18, $p = 0.005$) and Westernized pattern (in F) (OR = 5.62, 95% CI: 1.17, 27.02, $p = 0.031$) were associated with impaired lung function; a nonsignificant trend for preserved lung function was found for MED-like pattern (OR = 0.71, 95% CI: 0.28, 1.79, $p > 0.05$)	[153]

Table 1. *Cont.*

Dietary Patterns	Country (Cohort)	Design (Follow-Up)	Population	Sex (Age)	Diet Assessment Method	Outcome	Outcome Assessment	Main Results	Ref
					Diet quality scores				
Alternate Health Eating Index (AHEI)	USA (NHS and HPFS)	P (16 y NHS; 12 y HPFS)	Nurses n = 73,228 (NHS) Health professionals n = 47,026 (HPFS)	F (30–55 year), M (40–75)	FFQ and diet quality index (AHEI-2010)	COPD incidence	Self-reported	A higher AHEI-2010 diet score was associated with lower COPD risk (for the fourth fifth of the score, HR = 0.67, 95% CI: 0.53, 0.85, p for trend <0.001)	[154]
Health Eating Index (HEI) and MED diet score	Iran	C	Stable COPD n = 121	F, M (mean 66.1 year)	FFQ and diet quality index (HEI, and MED score)	COPD severity	Spirometry	Higher MED score was associated with lower FEV1 and FCV. MED score and AHEI decreased as COPD severity increased (NS)	[155]
MED diet score	Spain (ILERVAS)	C	General population n = 3020	F (50–70 year), M (45–65 year)	FFQ and MED score	FEV1, FVC, FEV1/FVC	Spirometry	A lower MED diet score was associated with impaired lung function in F (low vs. high adherence, OR = 2.07, 95% CI: 1.06, 4.06, p = 0.033) and the presence of obstructive ventilator defects in M (low vs. high adherence, OR = 4.14, 95% CI: 1.42, 12.1, p = 0.009)	[156]

Abbreviations: AHEI = Alternate Healthy Eating Index; ARIC = atherosclerosis risk in communities; C = cross-sectional; CHO = carbohydrate; CI = confidence interval; BMI = body mass index; F = female; FEF25-75 = forced expiratory flow at 25-75%; FEV1 = forced expiratory volume in one second; FFQ = food frequency questionnaire; FVC = forced vital capacity; HCS = Hertfordshire cohort study; HEI = Healthy Eating Index; HPFS = Health Professionals Follow-up Study; HR = hazard ratio; ILERVAS = Ilerda vascular project; M = male; MED = Mediterranean; MORGEN-EPIC = Monitoring Project on Risk Factors and Chronic Diseases in the Netherlands—European Prospective Investigation into Cancer and Nutrition; NHS = Nurses' Health Study; NS = not significant; OR = odds ratio; P = prospective; PCA = principal component analysis; RR = relative risk; SAPALDIA = Swiss Cohort Study on Air Pollution and Lung and Heart Diseases in Adults; SCHS = Singapore Chinese Health Study.

7.1. Data-Driven Dietary Patterns and COPD

A cohort study in Chinese Singaporeans found that the meat–dim sum dietary pattern (red meat, preserved foods, rice, noodles, deep-fried foods) was associated with an increased incident cough with phlegm (odds ratio (OR) = 1.43 comparing fourth to first quartile, p for trend = 0.02) [146], indicating a deleterious effect of a diet rich in meat, starchy foods, and high-fat dairy products on respiratory symptoms. Two prospective studies in US health professionals identified two distinct major dietary patterns, the "prudent pattern", loaded by a high intake of fruits and vegetables, oily fish, poultry, wholegrain products, and low-fat dairy products, and the "Western pattern", characterized by a high consumption of refined grains, cured and red meats, desserts, French fries, and high-fat dairy products [147,148]. Both studies consistently found that the "prudent" pattern was negatively and the Western pattern positively associated with the risk of self-reported newly diagnosed COPD in women [148] and men [147] after adjustment for several potential confounders, including measures of tobacco exposures. In contrast with findings for COPD, the dietary patterns were not associated with the risk of adult-onset asthma. Notably, the effect of each dietary pattern was stronger in men than in women [147,148]. For the prudent pattern, the relative risk (RR) for highest vs. lowest quintile was 0.50 (p for trend = 0.02) in the men cohort [147], and 0.75 (p for trend = 0.02) in the women cohort [148]. For the Western pattern, the RR for highest vs. lowest quintile was 4.56 (p for trend <0.001) in the men cohort [147], and 1.31 (p for trend = 0.02) in the women cohort [148]. As several individual foods of the "prudent" or the "Western" diet might be related to COPD, as discussed in previous paragraphs, the "prudent" and the "Western" diet patterns reflect the possible combinatory effects of these diverse but highly correlated foods.

Cross-sectional studies confirmed the associations between dietary patterns and respiratory symptoms, lung function, and COPD. A study in the UK population observed that a similar "prudent" dietary pattern was positively associated with lung function (FEV1) in males and females (difference in mean FEV1 between highest vs. lowest quintiles of pattern score = 180 mL in men, p for trend <0.001, and 80 mL in females, p for trend = 0.008), and negatively associated with COPD prevalence in males (54% reduction, p for trend = 0.012) [149]. Associations in males were stronger among smokers than nonsmokers [149]. In this study, the second dietary pattern identified in the study subjects, i.e., the "traditional" pattern, was similar to the unhealthy Western dietary pattern of other studies [147,148], but here, it was not associated with any negative outcome, probably because of its relatively high fish and vegetables content. A "prudent" diet was confirmed to be associated positively with FEV1 and negatively with COPD prevalence, not significantly in a large sample (n = 2,178) of Swiss adults (changes in FEV1 per unit increment in the dietary pattern score = 23 mL, p = 0.08; COPD prevalence OR = 0.90, p = 0.21) [150], as well as in a significant manner in a US population-based study (COPD prevalence OR = 0.82, p for trend = 0.007) where protective effects by the prudent pattern were also observed on respiratory symptoms (cough), whereas a Western diet was associated with higher prevalence of COPD (OR = 1.62, p for trend <0.001), worse respiratory symptoms, and lower lung function [151].

In a population of around 12,000 adults from the Netherlands, McKeever et al. [152] identified three major dietary patterns, the "cosmopolitan pattern" (higher intakes of vegetables, fish, chicken, wine, and lower intakes of high-fat dairy products, added fat, added sugar, and potato), the "traditional pattern" (higher intakes of red meat, processed meat, potato, boiled vegetables, added fat, coffee, and beer and lower intakes of soy products, low-fat dairy products, tea, breakfast cereal, brown rice, pizza, juice, and fruit), and the "refined food dietary pattern" (higher intakes of mayonnaise, salty snacks, candy, high-sugar beverages, French fries, white bread, and pizza and lower intake of boiled vegetables, wholegrains, fruit, and cheese). These dietary patterns were analyzed for their relation to lung function (FEV1) and symptoms of COPD as well as to longitudinal change in FEV1. When nutrient intake associated with the diets was analyzed, the "cosmopolitan" diet was positively correlated with intake of alcohol, vitamin C, and beta-carotene, the "traditional" diet was positively associated with alcohol and total fat intake, and negatively with carbohydrate intake, and the "refined food" diet was negatively associated with magnesium, fiber, and vitamin C intake [152]. In the cross-sectional analysis, the "traditional" diet was associated with a lower lung function (−94.4 mL, p for trend <0.001) and an higher prevalence of COPD (OR = 1.6, p for trend = 0.001), while the "cosmopolitan" diet was associated with a small increased prevalence of asthma and wheeze. None of the dietary patterns were associated with a decline in lung function over 5 years, although a higher intake of refined foods was associated with a greater decline in lung function (−48.5 mL, p for trend = 0.11) [152].

Accordingly, in a Spanish population of adult smokers without respiratory diseases, three major dietary patterns were derived: alcohol-consumption pattern (loaded by intake of wine, beer, and/or distilled drinks), Westernized pattern (loaded by high consumption of cured and red meats, dairy products, and sugary drinks, desserts and sweets, and low in fruits, vegetables, legumes, and fish), and Mediterranean-like pattern (loaded by high intake of poultry, eggs, fish, vegetables, legumes, potatoes, dairy desserts, fruits, nuts, and dried fruit) [153]. When the prevalence of impaired lung function (as determined by spirometry) across tertiles of dietary patterns was analyzed, impaired lung function was observed in all participants with an alcohol consumption pattern (OR = 4.56, p for trend = 0.005) especially in women (OR = 11.47, p for trend = 0.003), and in women with the Westernized pattern (OR = 5.62, p for trend = 0.031). By contrast, the Mediterranean-like dietary pattern was not significantly associated with impaired lung function, but with a trend for preserved lung function (OR = 0.71, p for trend >0.05), suggesting that it may protect lung function against the deleterious effects of smoking [153].

The study by Sorli-Aguilar et al. [153] provides some new information: (1) it restricted the observation to smokers, thus stressing the importance of eating pattern, in addition to smoking cessation, as a possible preventive measure for improving lung health; (2) it provides a first report on the association between a Mediterranean-like diet and lung function. An impressive and unprecedented accrual of high-quality evidence from observational and interventional studies converges to the recognition of the traditional Mediterranean diet as one of the healthiest dietary patterns, being protective against incidence and mortality of major chronic diseases, mainly CVD and cancer [157,158]. However, limited evidence exists for a role in obstructive respiratory diseases and mostly regards asthma [159]. As discussed above, many individual foods and nutrients characteristic of the Mediterranean diet and endowed with anti-inflammatory, antioxidant, and beneficial metabolic properties (fruits, vegetables, seafood, nuts, legumes, vitamins, polyphenols, etc.) have been associated to improved lung function and COPD prevention in several studies. The Mediterranean-like diet pattern described by Sorli-Aguilar et al., the healthiest one compared to the other dietary patterns identified, included key foods of the traditional Mediterranean diet (fruits, vegetables, legumes, wholegrains, nuts, olive oil, fish) [160] and was similar to the "prudent" patterns that have been previously found to protect against impaired lung function and COPD risk [147–149]. However, it cannot be strictly defined as a traditional Mediterranean diet because it also included non-Mediterranean diet/unhealthy components, such as red and processed meats, desserts, sweets, and refined grains [153]. This may have diluted or masked the possible positive effect on lung function by other beneficial components. Of course, more investigations (mostly interventional in design) in different populations and countries are needed to confirm Mediterranean diet health benefits in COPD.

7.2. Diet Quality Scores and COPD

In addition to data-driven approaches to derive dietary pattern, a priori-defined diet quality scores have also been used to assess and/or confirm the relationship of diet with lung function and risk and outcomes of COPD (Table 1). In order to measure compliance to the Dietary Guidelines for Americans (DGAs) and provide dietary guidance for healthy eating, two dietary indices, the Healthy Eating Index (HEI) [161] and the Alternate Healthy Eating Index (AHEI) (2005 and 2010 editions) [162], a modified version of the HEI, have been developed and used in the US population and subpopulations. Apart from some distinctive features, such as more attention to fat quality, inclusion of moderate alcohol intake, cereal fiber, red-to-white meat ratio, and duration of multivitamin use in the AHEI compared to the original HEI, both scores reflect a dietary pattern characterized by high intakes of wholegrains, PUFAs, nuts, and long-chain n-3 fats and low intakes of red/processed meats, refined grains, and sugar sweetened beverages, and have been found to beneficially impact health outcomes. Indeed, the AHEI was inversely associated with incidence and mortality from chronic diseases (CVD, diabetes, and cancer) [163,164]. Using the AHEI-2010 score, a recent several year-long prospective study in participants of the US Nurses' Health Study (NHS, n = 73,000 women) and Health Professionals Follow-up Study (HPFS, n = 47,000 men) [154] found that higher AHEI-2010 diet score was associated with a 33% lower risk of newly diagnosed COPD in both men and women, without any effects by smoking status and after adjustment for several confounding factors (multivariable HR for eating the healthiest diet compared to eating the least healthy diet = 0.67, p for trend <0.001). This negative association also persisted after excluding participants with cancer and CVD at baseline (multivariable HR for eating the healthiest diet compared with eating the least healthy diet = 0.71, p for trend = 0.007), indicating a direct effect of a healthy diet on COPD beyond its association with other chronic diseases. Contrarily, no association was found between AHEI and the risk of adult onset asthma. Although obtained in health professionals with differences in health awareness, socioeconomic status, and smoking behavior compared to the general population, these results extend the relevance of the AHEI-2010 diet score and its main dietary features to COPD. When the association between individual components of the score and the risk of COPD was analyzed, high intake of fruit and wholegrains, and low intake of red and processed meat and sugar sweetened drinks and fruit juice were associated with lower risk of COPD [154], confirming some previous findings about the respiratory benefits of similar dietary patterns, in agreement with the antioxidant and anti-inflammatory diet hypothesis [148,149].

Another more recent study used the HEI (2005 and 2010 editions) diet score and a modified version of the Mediterranean diet score [165] to assess the cross-sectional association of these two diet quality scores with COPD severity (according to GOLD stages) and parameters of lung function (FEV1 and FVC) in 121 patients with stable COPD [155]. Both scores reflected high intakes of fruits, vegetables, wholegrains, PUFAs, MUFA, nuts, legumes, and low intakes of refined grains, red/cured meat (and red meat to white meat ratio), saturated fat, empty calories, and sodium. In particular, the Mediterranean diet score, from its original conception [165] to the latest modifications [166], is intended to capture compliance to the plant-based eating patterns of olive tree-growing areas of the Mediterranean basin. According to both HEI and Mediterranean diet scores, the diet quality of the study subjects appeared to need improvements. Although not reaching significance, reduced HEI and Mediterranean diet scores were observed with increased COPD severity, mostly stage 4, and a one-unit increase of the Mediterranean diet score was significantly associated with 2.9 (p = 0.002) and 2.8 (p = 0.007) increase of FEV1 and FVC, respectively [155]. Although obtained in a small sample of already diseased subjects, these results further suggest protective effects on lung function by the Mediterranean diet pattern. Further high-powered confirmatory studies as well as the evaluation of diet effect on COPD progression over time are highly warranted.

In a very recent cross-sectional study conducted in middle-aged healthy subjects at low-to-moderate CV risk but without pulmonary diseases (Ilerda Vascular Project, ILERVAS) [156], low adherence to the Mediterranean diet as well as low physical activity practice were independently associated with the presence of impaired spirometric values and with ventilatory defects, compared with high adherence to the Mediterranean diet and vigorous physical activity. Therefore, although we are still awaiting interventional studies providing causality, these results agree with those previously obtained with dietary pattern analysis [153] and collectively suggest a beneficial association between the Mediterranean diet and lung function with relevance to both the prevention of respiratory diseases as well as the improvement of COPD.

In a large prospective Asian cohort study, adherence to several recommended dietary patterns as reflected in the AHEI-2010, the alternate Mediterranean diet score, the dietary approaches to stop hypertension (DASH) score, and the healthy diet indicator (HDI), and based on healthy plant-based foods and fish, was associated with a substantially lower risk of 17-year all-cause and disease-specific

(CVD, cancer and respiratory disease) mortality, specifically with a 14–28% lower risk of mortality for respiratory diseases [167]. Interestingly, COPD was one of the predominant respiratory conditions contributing to respiratory disease mortality in the study cohort. These results agree with earlier reports of an inverse association between intake of single dietary components of these dietary patterns, such as fruits, and COPD mortality [53]. Other studies in different populations confirmed the beneficial association between adherence to the DASH diet and COPD risk [168], and adherence to the healthy Dutch dietary guideline and the risk of all-cause mortality and COPD development [169].

Collectively, although needing further confirmations, published studies concordantly suggest a significant role for high-quality whole diet on lung function outcomes and COPD incidence and prevalence, as well as on mortality. Adhering to dietary patterns resembling the general principles of the Mediterranean diet and the prudent diets, which emphasize a variety of healthy plant-based foods (vegetables, fruit, nuts, wholegrains) and fish, avoidance of heavy alcohol intake, and low consumption of foods typical of Westernized patterns (red/processed meat, refined grains, sweets/desserts), exerts beneficial effects in contrast with Western diets (Figure 2). Interestingly, the Western diet has been shown to be positively associated while the prudent/Mediterranean diet inversely associated with serum levels of inflammatory markers [170,171]. Moreover, beneficial effects have also been documented for bioactive nutrients of the healthy diets, such as polyphenols and PUFAs, against visceral adiposity and related inflammation/oxidative stress, mitochondrial dysfunction, as well as insulin resistance [172], thus potentially providing the opportunity to favorably manage the risk associated with metabolic derangements observed in some patients with COPD (obesity and/or abdominal visceral adiposity).

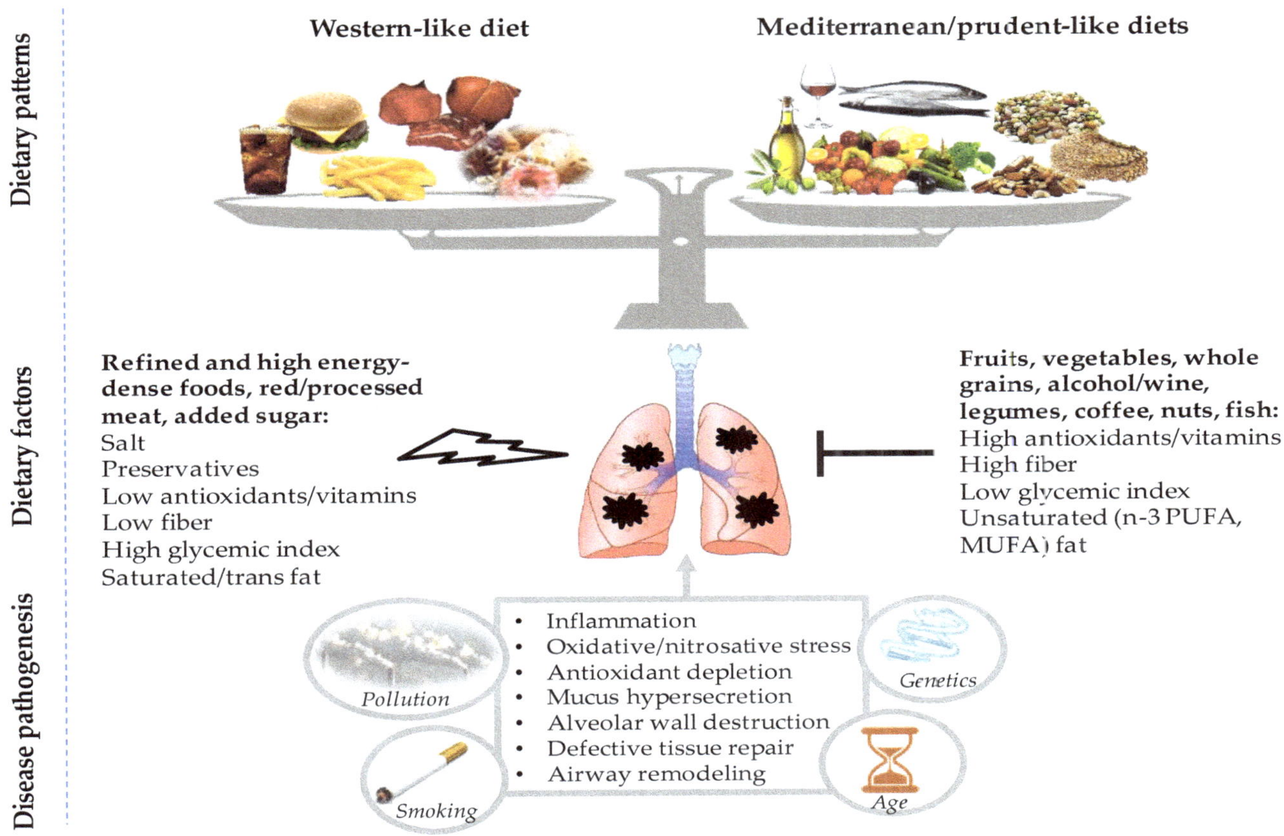

Figure 2. A framework model of the interactions of diets and dietary factors with lung function and COPD development and progression.

In addition to directly improving inflammation, oxidative stress, and immune and metabolic deregulation, dietary factors may act by inducing modification of gut microbiota, which can influence immune system, systemic inflammation, and metabolism through the production of locally- and systemically-active metabolites, such as the fiber fermentation-derived short chain fatty acids (SCFAs) (butyrate, propionate and acetate) or the carnitine/choline-derived trimethylamine-N-oxide (TMAO). Human studies have found that plant-based diets such as the Mediterranean diet (rich in fiber) shaped the composition of gut microbiota so as to increase the circulating levels of anti-inflammatory SCFAs, while animal-based diets such as the Western diet (rich in carnitine and choline from meat, egg yolks, and high-fat dairy products) were associated with increased levels of the pro-inflammatory TMAO, which is linked to risk of atherosclerosis, CV disorders, and mortality [173]. An emerging concept and potential therapeutic opportunity for dietary modulation is the gut–lung axis, where intestinal microbial modulation can influence the respiratory system [174]. Indeed, high dietary fiber intake was shown to protect against inflammatory airways disease via systemic SCFAs [175]. Moreover, increased circulating TMAO levels were associated with long-term all-cause mortality in patients with COPD [176]. Of course, further studies are required to address whether gut–lung axis modulation by nutrition would beneficially impact lung function and the risk or evolution of COPD.

8. Conclusions and Perspectives

Given the alarming increasing burden of COPD worldwide, identification of modifiable risk factors for prevention and treatment of COPD is highly in demand. Based on the available evidence, greater awareness of diet and dietary factors influencing respiratory health may be of interest for public health due to their disease-modifying effects. Many studies in the general population and in subjects with respiratory disease have reported that current dietary habits are qualitatively poor and therefore leave plenty of opportunities for improvements and interventions. Taking into account the increasing smoking habit in developing countries and the worldwide unstoppable phenomenon of Westernization of lifestyle factors, including a more processed and convenience-orientated diet, a two-hit lifestyle burden (smoking and unhealthy diet) is currently rising.

Based on strong evidence of association with improved cardiometabolic health, including lower risk of CV disease, diabetes, and obesity, many scientific organizations recommend the prudent/Mediterranean-like diets as healthy dietary patterns. Published studies also consistently show the adverse effects of the Western diet, rich in refined foods, saturated fat, meat, and sugar, on lung function and the risk of COPD, and, by contrast, the ability of specific dietary factors and diets, mostly the prudent/Mediterranean-like diets loaded by plant-based foods and healthy fats, to preserve lung function and prevent COPD or its evolution over time. Interestingly, the magnitude of effect of diet on lung function is estimated to be comparable to that of chronic smoking [51], underscoring that healthy dietary approaches may have a great impact jointly on COPD development and the associated metabolic and CV risk.

Interestingly, in many studies, specific dietary patterns and/or nutrients exerted benefits on lung function and the risk of COPD, but not asthma, strongly suggesting a true underlying effect rather than a generalized and most probably confounded effect. COPD as well as CV diseases share a systemic inflammatory pathogenesis differently from the immune pathogenesis of asthma. Nutritional targeting of oxidative balance and overwhelming inflammation may therefore represent a unique opportunity to prevent/treat COPD and its related CV co-morbidities.

Of course, there is not a single diet identified as a magic pill for respiratory health. Food groups, including fruits, vegetables, fish, and wholegrain products, contributing to basic nutraceutical ingredients, such as antioxidants, vitamins, fiber, and PUFAs, may vary across the dietary patterns documented to be beneficial for lung function, according to the populations studied. However, some unifying principles of all the healthful diets may be recognized and emphasized in designing preventive nutritional measures. In many studies, dietary factors documented to improve several processes (inflammation, oxidative stress ad immune dysfunction) and co-morbidities (CVD, obesity) of respiratory diseases translate into improved respiratory outcomes. Importantly, considering the early origin of COPD [10] and the profound impact of diet on lung function and later respiratory health, nutrition intervention offers the opportunity for early strategies of primary prevention and/or targeted early therapeutic approaches.

The negative results of supplementation trials with single antioxidant nutrients suggest that the effect of single nutrients may be too small to be observed, reinforcing the notion that combination of nutrients and foods within a dietary pattern may allow cumulative/synergic effects to become apparent. Moreover, since diet tends to track throughout life, this means that exposure to (or lack of) certain nutrients may occur over a long period of time (as captured in observational studies). Therefore, observational studies of dietary benefits may not always translate into positive results from clinical trials (performed in a specific age group with single nutrients and for a limited follow-up).

With regard to disease treatment, several therapeutic strategies, including smoking cessation, pharmacological interventions, and rehabilitation programs, are implemented in COPD patients to improve quality of life, decelerate lung function decline, and prevent major complications. As malnutrition associated with skeletal muscle impairment is an important systemic and disabling consequence of COPD, nutritional support (e.g., energy-enriched diet) has been recently suggested as a valuable adjuvant tool in the management of COPD patients at risk of malnutrition, mainly in combination with physical exercise [177], suggesting that at least some of the adverse functional consequences of severe COPD are reversible by nutritional support [20].

More animal experimentations and human intervention studies are needed to confirm the effectiveness and mechanisms of diet in preventing and treating COPD. A new area of investigation is the microbiota modulation by diet, which offers the prospect of increasing health and mitigating disease risk. However, the field of nutrigenetics (i.e., the relationship between genetic variants and diet) also deserves attention to address the inter-individual variability in response to diet and improve a personalized nutrition intervention to prevent/treat COPD. Moreover, it is possible that diet influences may be different across different clinical phenotypes of COPD, as some evidence suggests [101]. Therefore, more studies are needed to ascertain the effect of diet on different COPD phenotypes and to develop tailored nutritional strategies. Although evidence for the role of diet in COPD is clearly available, smoking cessation and the appropriate pharmacologic therapy remain key measures for the prevention and treatment of COPD.

Although current nutritional guidelines for COPD management do not formally include specific dietary recommendations other than nutritional counseling for malnourished patients, the available scientific evidence provides new directions for future research to substantiate the role of nutrition in lung function maintenance, respiratory disease prevention, and treatment, leading to the ultimate positioning of nutrition on the roadmap to optimal respiratory health.

Based on the evidence presented in this review and pending further evidence from basic science and interventional studies, a pragmatic view for managing respiratory health and COPD, as well as many other aspects of health, would be to recommend (along with physical exercise) a healthy balanced diet characterized by high consumption of fresh fruits, vegetables, wholegrains, plant oils and fish, low intake of alcohol (preferably wine), and avoidance of processed, refined, high-saturated fat foods, sweets, cured/red meats, and sugar-containing beverages.

Most importantly in current times, there may be a wide range of appropriate approaches to diet that should be considered and include social, cultural, and psychological aspects of eating. Moreover, nutrition-based measures for health maintenance and disease management are complicated by issues such as food production and processing technologies that need careful attention and convergent efforts by health policy makers, the food industry, health professionals, and consumers, in order to align nutritional health also with a sustainable food system. All these considerations and achievements have the great potential to improve evidence-based public health recommendations for a healthier eating pattern to adopt early in life as part of a healthy lifestyle in order to preserve lung function and prevent or improve COPD, in addition to encouraging smoking avoidance or cessation, and especially in smokers who are unable to quit smoking.

Author Contributions: Conceptualization, E.S. and D.M.T.; investigation, E.S. and M.M.; writing—original draft preparation, E.S; writing—review and editing, S.G. and D.M.T.; supervision, S.G. and D.M.T.

References

1. Adeloye, D.; Chua, S.; Lee, C.; Basquill, C.; Papana, A.; Theodoratou, E.; Nair, H.; Gasevic, D.; Sridhar, D.; Campbell, H.; et al. Global and regional estimates of COPD prevalence: Systematic review and meta-analysis. *J. Glob. Health* **2015**, *5*, 020415. [CrossRef] [PubMed]
2. Barnes, P.J.; Shapiro, S.D.; Pauwels, R.A. Chronic obstructive pulmonary disease: Molecular and cellular mechanisms. *Eur. Respir. J.* **2003**, *22*, 672–688. [CrossRef] [PubMed]
3. Vestbo, J.; Hurd, S.S.; Agusti, A.G.; Jones, P.W.; Vogelmeier, C.; Anzueto, A.; Barnes, P.J.; Fabbri, L.M.; Martinez, F.J.; Nishimura, M.; et al. Global strategy for the diagnosis, management, and prevention of chronic obstructive pulmonary disease: GOLD executive summary. *Am. J. Respir. Crit. Care Med.* **2013**, *187*, 347–365. [CrossRef] [PubMed]
4. Vestbo, J.; Edwards, L.D.; Scanlon, P.D.; Yates, J.C.; Agusti, A.; Bakke, P.; Calverley, P.M.; Celli, B.; Coxson, H.O.; Crim, C.; et al. Changes in forced expiratory volume in 1 second over time in COPD. *N. Engl. J. Med.* **2011**, *365*, 1184–1192. [CrossRef] [PubMed]
5. Agusti, A.; Edwards, L.D.; Rennard, S.I.; MacNee, W.; Tal-Singer, R.; Miller, B.E.; Vestbo, J.; Lomas, D.A.; Calverley, P.M.; Wouters, E.; et al. Persistent systemic inflammation is associated with poor clinical outcomes in COPD: A novel phenotype. *PLoS ONE* **2012**, *7*, e37483. [CrossRef]
6. Burgel, P.R.; Paillasseur, J.L.; Peene, B.; Dusser, D.; Roche, N.; Coolen, J.; Troosters, T.; Decramer, M.; Janssens, W. Two distinct chronic obstructive pulmonary disease (COPD) phenotypes are associated with high risk of mortality. *PLoS ONE* **2012**, *7*, e51048. [CrossRef] [PubMed]
7. Burgel, P.R.; Paillasseur, J.L.; Roche, N. Identification of clinical phenotypes using cluster analyses in COPD patients with multiple comorbidities. *BioMed Res. Int.* **2014**, *2014*. [CrossRef]
8. Burgel, P.R.; Roche, N.; Paillasseur, J.L.; Tillie-Leblond, I.; Chanez, P.; Escamilla, R.; Court-Fortune, I.; Perez, T.; Carre, P.; Caillaud, D.; et al. Clinical COPD phenotypes identified by cluster analysis: Validation with mortality. *Eur. Respir. J.* **2012**, *40*, 495–496. [CrossRef]
9. Miravitlles, M.; Calle, M.; Soler-Cataluna, J.J. Clinical phenotypes of COPD: Identification, definition and implications for guidelines. *Arch. Bronconeumol.* **2012**, *48*, 86–98. [CrossRef]
10. Postma, D.S.; Bush, A.; van den Berge, M. Risk factors and early origins of chronic obstructive pulmonary disease. *Lancet* **2015**, *385*, 899–909. [CrossRef]
11. Rabe, K.F.; Watz, H. Chronic obstructive pulmonary disease. *Lancet* **2017**, *389*, 1931–1940. [CrossRef]
12. Schulze, M.B.; Martinez-Gonzalez, M.A.; Fung, T.T.; Lichtenstein, A.H.; Forouhi, N.G. Food based dietary patterns and chronic disease prevention. *BMJ* **2018**, *361*, k2396. [CrossRef] [PubMed]
13. Berthon, B.S.; Wood, L.G. Nutrition and respiratory health—Feature review. *Nutrients* **2015**, *7*, 1618–1643. [CrossRef]
14. Zheng, P.F.; Shu, L.; Si, C.J.; Zhang, X.Y.; Yu, X.L.; Gao, W. Dietary Patterns and Chronic Obstructive Pulmonary Disease: A Meta-analysis. *COPD* **2016**, *13*, 515–522. [CrossRef] [PubMed]
15. Vasankari, T.; Harkanen, T.; Kainu, A.; Saaksjarvi, K.; Mattila, T.; Jousilahti, P.; Laitinen, T. Predictors of New Airway Obstruction—An 11 Year's Population-Based Follow-Up Study. *COPD* **2019**, *16*, 45–50. [CrossRef] [PubMed]
16. Whyand, T.; Hurst, J.R.; Beckles, M.; Caplin, M.E. Pollution and respiratory disease: Can diet or supplements help? A review. *Respir. Res.* **2018**, *19*, 79. [CrossRef] [PubMed]
17. Smit, H.A. Chronic obstructive pulmonary disease, asthma and protective effects of food intake: From hypothesis to evidence? *Respir. Res.* **2001**, *2*, 261–264. [CrossRef]
18. Zhai, T.; Li, S.; Hu, W.; Li, D.; Leng, S. Potential Micronutrients and Phytochemicals against the Pathogenesis of Chronic Obstructive Pulmonary Disease and Lung Cancer. *Nutrients* **2018**, *10*. [CrossRef]
19. Carraro, S.; Scheltema, N.; Bont, L.; Baraldi, E. Early-life origins of chronic respiratory diseases: Understanding and promoting healthy ageing. *Eur. Respir. J.* **2014**, *44*, 1682–1696. [CrossRef]

20. Schols, A.M.; Ferreira, I.M.; Franssen, F.M.; Gosker, H.R.; Janssens, W.; Muscaritoli, M.; Pison, C.; Rutten-van Molken, M.; Slinde, F.; Steiner, M.C.; et al. Nutritional assessment and therapy in COPD: A European Respiratory Society statement. *Eur. Respir. J.* **2014**, *44*, 1504–1520. [CrossRef]
21. van den Borst, B.; Gosker, H.R.; Wesseling, G.; de Jager, W.; Hellwig, V.A.; Snepvangers, F.J.; Schols, A.M. Low-grade adipose tissue inflammation in patients with mild-to-moderate chronic obstructive pulmonary disease. *Am. J. Clin. Nutr.* **2011**, *94*, 1504–1512. [CrossRef] [PubMed]
22. van Eck, N.J.; Waltman, L. Software survey: VOSviewer, a computer program for bibliometric mapping. *Scientometrics* **2010**, *84*, 523–538. [CrossRef]
23. Hsieh, M.J.; Yang, T.M.; Tsai, Y.H. Nutritional supplementation in patients with chronic obstructive pulmonary disease. *J. Formos. Med. Assoc.* **2016**, *115*, 595–601. [CrossRef] [PubMed]
24. Yao, H.; Rahman, I. Current concepts on oxidative/carbonyl stress, inflammation and epigenetics in pathogenesis of chronic obstructive pulmonary disease. *Toxicol. Appl. Pharmacol.* **2011**, *254*, 72–85. [CrossRef]
25. Di Stefano, A.; Caramori, G.; Oates, T.; Capelli, A.; Lusuardi, M.; Gnemmi, I.; Ioli, F.; Chung, K.F.; Donner, C.F.; Barnes, P.J.; et al. Increased expression of nuclear factor-kappaB in bronchial biopsies from smokers and patients with COPD. *Eur. Respir. J.* **2002**, *20*, 556–563. [CrossRef] [PubMed]
26. Brassington, K.; Selemidis, S.; Bozinovski, S.; Vlahos, R. New frontiers in the treatment of comorbid cardiovascular disease in chronic obstructive pulmonary disease. *Clin. Sci. (Lond.)* **2019**, *133*, 885–904. [CrossRef] [PubMed]
27. Sin, D.D.; Wu, L.; Man, S.F. The relationship between reduced lung function and cardiovascular mortality: A population-based study and a systematic review of the literature. *Chest* **2005**, *127*, 1952–1959. [CrossRef] [PubMed]
28. Gut-Gobert, C.; Cavailles, A.; Dixmier, A.; Guillot, S.; Jouneau, S.; Leroyer, C.; Marchand-Adam, S.; Marquette, D.; Meurice, J.C.; Desvigne, N.; et al. Women and COPD: Do we need more evidence? *Eur. Respir. Rev.* **2019**, *28*. [CrossRef]
29. Han, M.K.; Postma, D.; Mannino, D.M.; Giardino, N.D.; Buist, S.; Curtis, J.L.; Martinez, F.J. Gender and chronic obstructive pulmonary disease: Why it matters. *Am. J. Respir. Crit. Care Med.* **2007**, *176*, 1179–1184. [CrossRef]
30. O'Doherty Jensen, K.; Holm, L. Preferences, quantities and concerns: Socio-cultural perspectives on the gendered consumption of foods. *Eur. J. Clin. Nutr.* **1999**, *53*, 351–359. [CrossRef]
31. Osler, M.; Tjonneland, A.; Suntum, M.; Thomsen, B.L.; Stripp, C.; Gronbaek, M.; Overvad, K. Does the association between smoking status and selected healthy foods depend on gender? A population-based study of 54 417 middle-aged Danes. *Eur. J. Clin. Nutr.* **2002**, *56*, 57–63. [CrossRef] [PubMed]
32. Hu, F.B. Dietary pattern analysis: A new direction in nutritional epidemiology. *Curr. Opin. Lipidol.* **2002**, *13*, 3–9. [CrossRef] [PubMed]
33. Heart Protection Study Collaborative Group. MRC/BHF Heart Protection Study of antioxidant vitamin supplementation in 20,536 high-risk individuals: A randomised placebo-controlled trial. *Lancet* **2002**, *360*, 7–22. [CrossRef]
34. Tavilani, H.; Nadi, E.; Karimi, J.; Goodarzi, M.T. Oxidative stress in COPD patients, smokers, and non-smokers. *Respir. Care* **2012**, *57*, 2090–2094. [CrossRef] [PubMed]
35. Ochs-Balcom, H.M.; Grant, B.J.; Muti, P.; Sempos, C.T.; Freudenheim, J.L.; Browne, R.W.; McCann, S.E.; Trevisan, M.; Cassano, P.A.; Iacoviello, L.; et al. Antioxidants, oxidative stress, and pulmonary function in individuals diagnosed with asthma or COPD. *Eur. J. Clin. Nutr.* **2006**, *60*, 991–999. [CrossRef] [PubMed]
36. Rodriguez-Rodriguez, E.; Ortega, R.M.; Andres, P.; Aparicio, A.; Gonzalez-Rodriguez, L.G.; Lopez-Sobaler, A.M.; Navia, B.; Perea, J.M.; Rodriguez-Rodriguez, P. Antioxidant status in a group of institutionalised elderly people with chronic obstructive pulmonary disease. *Br. J. Nutr.* **2016**, *115*, 1740–1747. [CrossRef]
37. Louhelainen, N.; Rytila, P.; Haahtela, T.; Kinnula, V.L.; Djukanovic, R. Persistence of oxidant and protease burden in the airways after smoking cessation. *BMC Pulm. Med.* **2009**, *9*, 25. [CrossRef]
38. Sargeant, L.A.; Jaeckel, A.; Wareham, N.J. Interaction of vitamin C with the relation between smoking and obstructive airways disease in EPIC Norfolk. European Prospective Investigation into Cancer and Nutrition. *Eur. Respir. J.* **2000**, *16*, 397–403. [CrossRef]

39. Bartoli, M.L.; Novelli, F.; Costa, F.; Malagrino, L.; Melosini, L.; Bacci, E.; Cianchetti, S.; Dente, F.L.; Di Franco, A.; Vagaggini, B.; et al. Malondialdehyde in exhaled breath condensate as a marker of oxidative stress in different pulmonary diseases. *Mediat. Inflamm.* **2011**, *2011*, 891752. [CrossRef]
40. Arja, C.; Surapaneni, K.M.; Raya, P.; Adimoolam, C.; Balisetty, B.; Kanala, K.R. Oxidative stress and antioxidant enzyme activity in South Indian male smokers with chronic obstructive pulmonary disease. *Respirology* **2013**, *18*, 1069–1075. [CrossRef]
41. Ahmad, A.; Shameem, M.; Husain, Q. Altered oxidant-antioxidant levels in the disease prognosis of chronic obstructive pulmonary disease. *Int. J. Tuberc. Lung Dis.* **2013**, *17*, 1104–1109. [CrossRef] [PubMed]
42. Guenegou, A.; Leynaert, B.; Pin, I.; Le Moel, G.; Zureik, M.; Neukirch, F. Serum carotenoids, vitamins A and E, and 8 year lung function decline in a general population. *Thorax* **2006**, *61*, 320–326. [CrossRef] [PubMed]
43. McKeever, T.M.; Lewis, S.A.; Smit, H.A.; Burney, P.; Cassano, P.A.; Britton, J. A multivariate analysis of serum nutrient levels and lung function. *Respir. Res.* **2008**, *9*, 67. [CrossRef] [PubMed]
44. Lin, Y.C.; Wu, T.C.; Chen, P.Y.; Hsieh, L.Y.; Yeh, S.L. Comparison of plasma and intake levels of antioxidant nutrients in patients with chronic obstructive pulmonary disease and healthy people in Taiwan: A case-control study. *Asia Pac. J. Clin. Nutr.* **2010**, *19*, 393–401. [PubMed]
45. Laudisio, A.; Costanzo, L.; Di Gioia, C.; Delussu, A.S.; Traballesi, M.; Gemma, A.; Antonelli Incalzi, R. Dietary intake of elderly outpatients with chronic obstructive pulmonary disease. *Arch. Gerontol. Geriatr.* **2016**, *64*, 75–81. [CrossRef] [PubMed]
46. van de Bool, C.; Mattijssen-Verdonschot, C.; van Melick, P.P.; Spruit, M.A.; Franssen, F.M.; Wouters, E.F.; Schols, A.M.; Rutten, E.P. Quality of dietary intake in relation to body composition in patients with chronic obstructive pulmonary disease eligible for pulmonary rehabilitation. *Eur. J. Clin. Nutr.* **2014**, *68*, 159–165. [CrossRef] [PubMed]
47. Gronberg, A.M.; Slinde, F.; Engstrom, C.P.; Hulthen, L.; Larsson, S. Dietary problems in patients with severe chronic obstructive pulmonary disease. *J. Hum. Nutr. Diet.* **2005**, *18*, 445–452. [CrossRef] [PubMed]
48. Tabak, C.; Smit, H.A.; Rasanen, L.; Fidanza, F.; Menotti, A.; Nissinen, A.; Feskens, E.J.; Heederik, D.; Kromhout, D. Dietary factors and pulmonary function: A cross sectional study in middle aged men from three European countries. *Thorax* **1999**, *54*, 1021–1026. [CrossRef]
49. Butland, B.K.; Fehily, A.M.; Elwood, P.C. Diet, lung function, and lung function decline in a cohort of 2512 middle aged men. *Thorax* **2000**, *55*, 102–108. [CrossRef]
50. Tabak, C.; Arts, I.C.; Smit, H.A.; Heederik, D.; Kromhout, D. Chronic obstructive pulmonary disease and intake of catechins, flavonols, and flavones: The MORGEN Study. *Am. J. Respir. Crit. Care Med.* **2001**, *164*, 61–64. [CrossRef]
51. Tabak, C.; Smit, H.A.; Heederik, D.; Ocke, M.C.; Kromhout, D. Diet and chronic obstructive pulmonary disease: Independent beneficial effects of fruits, whole grains, and alcohol (the MORGEN study). *Clin. Exp. Allergy* **2001**, *31*, 747–755. [CrossRef] [PubMed]
52. Miedema, I.; Feskens, E.J.; Heederik, D.; Kromhout, D. Dietary determinants of long-term incidence of chronic nonspecific lung diseases. The Zutphen Study. *Am. J. Epidemiol.* **1993**, *138*, 37–45. [CrossRef] [PubMed]
53. Walda, I.C.; Tabak, C.; Smit, H.A.; Rasanen, L.; Fidanza, F.; Menotti, A.; Nissinen, A.; Feskens, E.J.; Kromhout, D. Diet and 20-year chronic obstructive pulmonary disease mortality in middle-aged men from three European countries. *Eur. J. Clin. Nutr.* **2002**, *56*, 638–643. [CrossRef] [PubMed]
54. Kaluza, J.; Larsson, S.C.; Orsini, N.; Linden, A.; Wolk, A. Fruit and vegetable consumption and risk of COPD: A prospective cohort study of men. *Thorax* **2017**, *72*, 500–509. [CrossRef] [PubMed]
55. Kaluza, J.; Harris, H.R.; Linden, A.; Wolk, A. Long-term consumption of fruits and vegetables and risk of chronic obstructive pulmonary disease: A prospective cohort study of women. *Int. J. Epidemiol.* **2018**, *47*, 1897–1909. [CrossRef]
56. Carey, I.M.; Strachan, D.P.; Cook, D.G. Effects of changes in fresh fruit consumption on ventilatory function in healthy British adults. *Am. J. Respir. Crit. Care Med.* **1998**, *158*, 728–733. [CrossRef] [PubMed]
57. Baldrick, F.R.; Elborn, J.S.; Woodside, J.V.; Treacy, K.; Bradley, J.M.; Patterson, C.C.; Schock, B.C.; Ennis, M.; Young, I.S.; McKinley, M.C.; et al. Effect of fruit and vegetable intake on oxidative stress and inflammation in COPD: A randomised controlled trial. *Eur. Respir. J.* **2012**, *39*, 1377–1384. [CrossRef]

58. Friis, A.L.; Steenholt, C.B.; Lokke, A.; Hansen, M. Dietary beetroot juice—Effects on physical performance in COPD patients: A randomized controlled crossover trial. *Int. J. Chron. Obstruct. Pulmon. Dis.* **2017**, *12*, 1765–1773. [CrossRef]
59. Keranis, E.; Makris, D.; Rodopoulou, P.; Martinou, H.; Papamakarios, G.; Daniil, Z.; Zintzaras, E.; Gourgoulianis, K.I. Impact of dietary shift to higher-antioxidant foods in COPD: A randomised trial. *Eur. Respir. J.* **2010**, *36*, 774–780. [CrossRef]
60. Holt, E.M.; Steffen, L.M.; Moran, A.; Basu, S.; Steinberger, J.; Ross, J.A.; Hong, C.P.; Sinaiko, A.R. Fruit and vegetable consumption and its relation to markers of inflammation and oxidative stress in adolescents. *J. Am. Diet. Assoc.* **2009**, *109*, 414–421. [CrossRef]
61. Rink, S.M.; Mendola, P.; Mumford, S.L.; Poudrier, J.K.; Browne, R.W.; Wactawski-Wende, J.; Perkins, N.J.; Schisterman, E.F. Self-report of fruit and vegetable intake that meets the 5 a day recommendation is associated with reduced levels of oxidative stress biomarkers and increased levels of antioxidant defense in premenopausal women. *J. Acad. Nutr. Diet.* **2013**, *113*, 776–785. [CrossRef] [PubMed]
62. McKeever, T.M.; Scrivener, S.; Broadfield, E.; Jones, Z.; Britton, J.; Lewis, S.A. Prospective study of diet and decline in lung function in a general population. *Am. J. Respir. Crit. Care Med.* **2002**, *165*, 1299–1303. [CrossRef] [PubMed]
63. Tug, T.; Karatas, F.; Terzi, S.M. Antioxidant vitamins (A, C and E) and malondialdehyde levels in acute exacerbation and stable periods of patients with chronic obstructive pulmonary disease. *Clin. Investig. Med.* **2004**, *27*, 123–128. [PubMed]
64. Agler, A.H.; Kurth, T.; Gaziano, J.M.; Buring, J.E.; Cassano, P.A. Randomised vitamin E supplementation and risk of chronic lung disease in the Women's Health Study. *Thorax* **2011**, *66*, 320–325. [CrossRef] [PubMed]
65. Grievink, L.; Smit, H.A.; Ocke, M.C.; van't Veer, P.; Kromhout, D. Dietary intake of antioxidant (pro)-vitamins, respiratory symptoms and pulmonary function: The MORGEN study. *Thorax* **1998**, *53*, 166–171. [CrossRef]
66. Rautalahti, M.; Virtamo, J.; Haukka, J.; Heinonen, O.P.; Sundvall, J.; Albanes, D.; Huttunen, J.K. The effect of alpha-tocopherol and beta-carotene supplementation on COPD symptoms. *Am. J. Respir. Crit. Care Med.* **1997**, *156*, 1447–1452. [CrossRef] [PubMed]
67. Omenn, G.S.; Goodman, G.E.; Thornquist, M.D.; Balmes, J.; Cullen, M.R.; Glass, A.; Keogh, J.P.; Meyskens, F.L.; Valanis, B.; Williams, J.H.; et al. Effects of a combination of beta carotene and vitamin A on lung cancer and cardiovascular disease. *N. Engl. J. Med.* **1996**, *334*, 1150–1155. [CrossRef]
68. Alpha-Tocopherol, Beta Carotene Cancer Prevention Study Group. The effect of vitamin E and beta carotene on the incidence of lung cancer and other cancers in male smokers. *N. Engl. J. Med.* **1994**, *330*, 1029–1035. [CrossRef]
69. Hennekens, C.H.; Buring, J.E.; Manson, J.E.; Stampfer, M.; Rosner, B.; Cook, N.R.; Belanger, C.; LaMotte, F.; Gaziano, J.M.; Ridker, P.M.; et al. Lack of effect of long-term supplementation with beta carotene on the incidence of malignant neoplasms and cardiovascular disease. *N. Engl. J. Med.* **1996**, *334*, 1145–1149. [CrossRef]
70. Palozza, P.; Simone, R.; Mele, M.C. Interplay of carotenoids with cigarette smoking: Implications in lung cancer. *Curr. Med. Chem.* **2008**, *15*, 844–854. [CrossRef]
71. Poti, F.; Santi, D.; Spaggiari, G.; Zimetti, F.; Zanotti, I. Polyphenol Health Effects on Cardiovascular and Neurodegenerative Disorders: A Review and Meta-Analysis. *Int. J. Mol. Sci.* **2019**, *20*. [CrossRef] [PubMed]
72. Mehta, A.J.; Cassidy, A.; Litonjua, A.A.; Sparrow, D.; Vokonas, P.; Schwartz, J. Dietary anthocyanin intake and age-related decline in lung function: Longitudinal findings from the VA Normative Aging Study. *Am. J. Clin. Nutr.* **2016**, *103*, 542–550. [CrossRef] [PubMed]
73. Hirayama, F.; Lee, A.H.; Binns, C.W.; Zhao, Y.; Hiramatsu, T.; Tanikawa, Y.; Nishimura, K.; Taniguchi, H. Soy consumption and risk of COPD and respiratory symptoms: A case-control study in Japan. *Respir. Res.* **2009**, *10*, 56. [CrossRef] [PubMed]
74. Hirayama, F.; Lee, A.H.; Binns, C.W.; Hiramatsu, N.; Mori, M.; Nishimura, K. Dietary intake of isoflavones and polyunsaturated fatty acids associated with lung function, breathlessness and the prevalence of chronic obstructive pulmonary disease: Possible protective effect of traditional Japanese diet. *Mol. Nutr. Food Res.* **2010**, *54*, 909–917. [CrossRef] [PubMed]
75. Lu, M.C.; Yang, M.D.; Li, P.C.; Fang, H.Y.; Huang, H.Y.; Chan, Y.C.; Bau, D.T. Effect of Oligomeric Proanthocyanidin on the Antioxidant Status and Lung Function of Patients with Chronic Obstructive Pulmonary Disease. *In Vivo* **2018**, *32*, 753–758. [CrossRef] [PubMed]

76. Pounis, G.; Arcari, A.; Costanzo, S.; Di Castelnuovo, A.; Bonaccio, M.; Persichillo, M.; Donati, M.B.; de Gaetano, G.; Iacoviello, L. Favorable association of polyphenol-rich diets with lung function: Cross-sectional findings from the Moli-sani study. *Respir. Med.* **2018**, *136*, 48–57. [CrossRef]
77. de Batlle, J.; Barreiro, E.; Romieu, I.; Mendez, M.; Gomez, F.P.; Balcells, E.; Ferrer, J.; Orozco-Levi, M.; Gea, J.; Anto, J.M.; et al. Dietary modulation of oxidative stress in chronic obstructive pulmonary disease patients. *Free Radic. Res.* **2010**, *44*, 1296–1303. [CrossRef]
78. Ng, T.P.; Niti, M.; Yap, K.B.; Tan, W.C. Curcumins-rich curry diet and pulmonary function in Asian older adults. *PLoS ONE* **2012**, *7*, e51753. [CrossRef]
79. Andersson, I.; Gronberg, A.; Slinde, F.; Bosaeus, I.; Larsson, S. Vitamin and mineral status in elderly patients with chronic obstructive pulmonary disease. *Clin. Respir. J.* **2007**, *1*, 23–29. [CrossRef]
80. Hirayama, F.; Lee, A.H.; Oura, A.; Mori, M.; Hiramatsu, N.; Taniguchi, H. Dietary intake of six minerals in relation to the risk of chronic obstructive pulmonary disease. *Asia Pac. J. Clin. Nutr.* **2010**, *19*, 572–577.
81. Pearson, P.; Britton, J.; McKeever, T.; Lewis, S.A.; Weiss, S.; Pavord, I.; Fogarty, A. Lung function and blood levels of copper, selenium, vitamin C and vitamin E in the general population. *Eur. J. Clin. Nutr.* **2005**, *59*, 1043–1048. [CrossRef] [PubMed]
82. Cassano, P.A.; Guertin, K.A.; Kristal, A.R.; Ritchie, K.E.; Bertoia, M.L.; Arnold, K.B.; Crowley, J.J.; Hartline, J.; Goodman, P.J.; Tangen, C.M.; et al. A randomized controlled trial of vitamin E and selenium on rate of decline in lung function. *Respir. Res.* **2015**, *16*, 35. [CrossRef] [PubMed]
83. Britton, J.; Pavord, I.; Richards, K.; Wisniewski, A.; Knox, A.; Lewis, S.; Tattersfield, A.; Weiss, S. Dietary magnesium, lung function, wheezing, and airway hyperreactivity in a random adult population sample. *Lancet* **1994**, *344*, 357–362. [CrossRef]
84. Leng, S.; Picchi, M.A.; Tesfaigzi, Y.; Wu, G.; Gauderman, W.J.; Xu, F.; Gilliland, F.D.; Belinsky, S.A. Dietary nutrients associated with preservation of lung function in Hispanic and non-Hispanic white smokers from New Mexico. *Int. J. Chron. Obstruct. Pulmon. Dis.* **2017**, *12*, 3171–3181. [CrossRef] [PubMed]
85. Al Alawi, A.M.; Majoni, S.W.; Falhammar, H. Magnesium and Human Health: Perspectives and Research Directions. *Int. J. Endocrinol.* **2018**, *2018*, 9041694. [CrossRef] [PubMed]
86. Root, M.M.; Houser, S.M.; Anderson, J.J.; Dawson, H.R. Healthy Eating Index 2005 and selected macronutrients are correlated with improved lung function in humans. *Nutr. Res.* **2014**, *34*, 277–284. [CrossRef] [PubMed]
87. Jacobs, D.R., Jr.; Andersen, L.F.; Blomhoff, R. Whole-grain consumption is associated with a reduced risk of noncardiovascular, noncancer death attributed to inflammatory diseases in the Iowa Women's Health Study. *Am. J. Clin. Nutr.* **2007**, *85*, 1606–1614. [CrossRef] [PubMed]
88. Fonseca Wald, E.L.A.; van den Borst, B.; Gosker, H.R.; Schols, A. Dietary fibre and fatty acids in chronic obstructive pulmonary disease risk and progression: A systematic review. *Respirology* **2014**, *19*, 176–184. [CrossRef] [PubMed]
89. Esposito, K.; Giugliano, D. Whole-grain intake cools down inflammation. *Am. J. Clin. Nutr.* **2006**, *83*, 1440–1441. [CrossRef]
90. Kan, H.; Stevens, J.; Heiss, G.; Rose, K.M.; London, S.J. Dietary fiber, lung function, and chronic obstructive pulmonary disease in the atherosclerosis risk in communities study. *Am. J. Epidemiol.* **2008**, *167*, 570–578. [CrossRef]
91. Varraso, R.; Willett, W.C.; Camargo, C.A., Jr. Prospective study of dietary fiber and risk of chronic obstructive pulmonary disease among US women and men. *Am. J. Epidemiol.* **2010**, *171*, 776–784. [CrossRef] [PubMed]
92. Kaluza, J.; Harris, H.; Wallin, A.; Linden, A.; Wolk, A. Dietary Fiber Intake and Risk of Chronic Obstructive Pulmonary Disease: A Prospective Cohort Study of Men. *Epidemiology* **2018**, *29*, 254–260. [CrossRef] [PubMed]
93. Frantz, S.; Wollmer, P.; Dencker, M.; Engstrom, G.; Nihlen, U. Associations between lung function and alcohol consumption–Assessed by both a questionnaire and a blood marker. *Respir. Med.* **2014**, *108*, 114–121. [CrossRef] [PubMed]
94. Schunemann, H.J.; Grant, B.J.; Freudenheim, J.L.; Muti, P.; McCann, S.E.; Kudalkar, D.; Ram, M.; Nochajski, T.; Russell, M.; Trevisan, M. Beverage specific alcohol intake in a population-based study: Evidence for a positive association between pulmonary function and wine intake. *BMC Pulm. Med.* **2002**, *2*, 3. [CrossRef]
95. Siedlinski, M.; Boer, J.M.; Smit, H.A.; Postma, D.S.; Boezen, H.M. Dietary factors and lung function in the general population: Wine and resveratrol intake. *Eur. Respir. J.* **2012**, *39*, 385–391. [CrossRef] [PubMed]

96. Sisson, J.H. Alcohol and airways function in health and disease. *Alcohol* **2007**, *41*, 293–307. [CrossRef] [PubMed]
97. Donnelly, L.E.; Newton, R.; Kennedy, G.E.; Fenwick, P.S.; Leung, R.H.; Ito, K.; Russell, R.E.; Barnes, P.J. Anti-inflammatory effects of resveratrol in lung epithelial cells: Molecular mechanisms. *Am. J. Physiol. Lung Cell. Mol. Physiol.* **2004**, *287*, L774–L783. [CrossRef]
98. Culpitt, S.V.; Rogers, D.F.; Fenwick, P.S.; Shah, P.; De Matos, C.; Russell, R.E.; Barnes, P.J.; Donnelly, L.E. Inhibition by red wine extract, resveratrol, of cytokine release by alveolar macrophages in COPD. *Thorax* **2003**, *58*, 942–946. [CrossRef]
99. Knobloch, J.; Sibbing, B.; Jungck, D.; Lin, Y.; Urban, K.; Stoelben, E.; Strauch, J.; Koch, A. Resveratrol impairs the release of steroid-resistant inflammatory cytokines from human airway smooth muscle cells in chronic obstructive pulmonary disease. *J. Pharmacol. Exp. Ther.* **2010**, *335*, 788–798. [CrossRef]
100. Farazuddin, M.; Mishra, R.; Jing, Y.; Srivastava, V.; Comstock, A.T.; Sajjan, U.S. Quercetin prevents rhinovirus-induced progression of lung disease in mice with COPD phenotype. *PLoS ONE* **2018**, *13*, e0199612. [CrossRef]
101. Hanson, C.; Sayles, H.; Rutten, E.; Wouters, E.F.M.; MacNee, W.; Calverley, P.; Meza, J.L.; Rennard, S. The Association Between Dietary Intake and Phenotypical Characteristics of COPD in the ECLIPSE Cohort. *Chronic Obstr. Pulm. Dis.* **2014**, *1*, 115–124. [CrossRef] [PubMed]
102. Black, P.N.; Scragg, R. Relationship between serum 25-hydroxyvitamin d and pulmonary function in the third national health and nutrition examination survey. *Chest* **2005**, *128*, 3792–3798. [CrossRef] [PubMed]
103. Afzal, S.; Lange, P.; Bojesen, S.E.; Freiberg, J.J.; Nordestgaard, B.G. Plasma 25-hydroxyvitamin D, lung function and risk of chronic obstructive pulmonary disease. *Thorax* **2014**, *69*, 24–31. [CrossRef] [PubMed]
104. Mulrennan, S.; Knuiman, M.; Walsh, J.P.; Hui, J.; Hunter, M.; Divitini, M.; Zhu, K.; Cooke, B.R.; Musk, A.W.B.; James, A.; et al. Vitamin D and respiratory health in the Busselton Healthy Ageing Study. *Respirology* **2018**, *23*, 576–582. [CrossRef] [PubMed]
105. Janssens, W.; Bouillon, R.; Claes, B.; Carremans, C.; Lehouck, A.; Buysschaert, I.; Coolen, J.; Mathieu, C.; Decramer, M.; Lambrechts, D.; et al. Vitamin D deficiency is highly prevalent in COPD and correlates with variants in the vitamin D-binding gene. *Thorax* **2010**, *65*, 215–220. [CrossRef] [PubMed]
106. Jolliffe, D.A.; Greenberg, L.; Hooper, R.L.; Mathyssen, C.; Rafiq, R.; de Jongh, R.T.; Camargo, C.A.; Griffiths, C.J.; Janssens, W.; Martineau, A.R.; et al. Vitamin D to prevent exacerbations of COPD: Systematic review and meta-analysis of individual participant data from randomised controlled trials. *Thorax* **2019**, *74*, 337–345. [CrossRef] [PubMed]
107. Alfaro, T.M.; Monteiro, R.A.; Cunha, R.A.; Cordeiro, C.R. Chronic coffee consumption and respiratory disease: A systematic review. *Clin. Respir. J.* **2018**, *12*, 1283–1294. [CrossRef]
108. Simopoulos, A.P. The importance of the omega-6/omega-3 fatty acid ratio in cardiovascular disease and other chronic diseases. *Exp. Biol. Med. (Maywood)* **2008**, *233*, 674–688. [CrossRef]
109. Massaro, M.; Scoditti, E.; Carluccio, M.A.; De Caterina, R. Basic mechanisms behind the effects of n-3 fatty acids on cardiovascular disease. *Prostaglandins Leukot. Essent. Fatty Acids* **2008**, *79*, 109–115. [CrossRef]
110. Fulton, A.S.; Hill, A.M.; Williams, M.T.; Howe, P.R.; Coates, A.M. Paucity of evidence for a relationship between long-chain omega-3 fatty acid intake and chronic obstructive pulmonary disease: A systematic review. *Nutr. Rev.* **2015**, *73*, 612–623. [CrossRef]
111. Sharp, D.S.; Rodriguez, B.L.; Shahar, E.; Hwang, L.J.; Burchfiel, C.M. Fish consumption may limit the damage of smoking on the lung. *Am. J. Respir. Crit. Care Med.* **1994**, *150*, 983–987. [CrossRef] [PubMed]
112. Shahar, E.; Folsom, A.R.; Melnick, S.L.; Tockman, M.S.; Comstock, G.W.; Gennaro, V.; Higgins, M.W.; Sorlie, P.D.; Ko, W.J.; Szklo, M.; et al. Dietary n-3 polyunsaturated fatty acids and smoking-related chronic obstructive pulmonary disease. Atherosclerosis Risk in Communities Study Investigators. *N. Engl. J. Med.* **1994**, *331*, 228–233. [CrossRef] [PubMed]
113. Schwartz, J.; Weiss, S.T. The relationship of dietary fish intake to level of pulmonary function in the first National Health and Nutrition Survey (NHANES I). *Eur. Respir. J.* **1994**, *7*, 1821–1824. [CrossRef] [PubMed]
114. McKeever, T.M.; Lewis, S.A.; Cassano, P.A.; Ocke, M.; Burney, P.; Britton, J.; Smit, H.A. The relation between dietary intake of individual fatty acids, FEV1 and respiratory disease in Dutch adults. *Thorax* **2008**, *63*, 208–214. [CrossRef]
115. Varraso, R.; Barr, R.G.; Willett, W.C.; Speizer, F.E.; Camargo, C.A., Jr. Fish intake and risk of chronic obstructive pulmonary disease in 2 large US cohorts. *Am. J. Clin. Nutr.* **2015**, *101*, 354–361. [CrossRef] [PubMed]

116. Cotogni, P.; Muzio, G.; Trombetta, A.; Ranieri, V.M.; Canuto, R.A. Impact of the omega-3 to omega-6 polyunsaturated fatty acid ratio on cytokine release in human alveolar cells. *J. Parenter. Enteral Nutr.* **2011**, *35*, 114–121. [CrossRef] [PubMed]
117. Hsiao, H.M.; Sapinoro, R.E.; Thatcher, T.H.; Croasdell, A.; Levy, E.P.; Fulton, R.A.; Olsen, K.C.; Pollock, S.J.; Serhan, C.N.; Phipps, R.P.; et al. A novel anti-inflammatory and pro-resolving role for resolvin D1 in acute cigarette smoke-induced lung inflammation. *PLoS ONE* **2013**, *8*, e58258. [CrossRef]
118. de Batlle, J.; Sauleda, J.; Balcells, E.; Gomez, F.P.; Mendez, M.; Rodriguez, E.; Barreiro, E.; Ferrer, J.J.; Romieu, I.; Gea, J.; et al. Association between Omega3 and Omega6 fatty acid intakes and serum inflammatory markers in COPD. *J. Nutr. Biochem.* **2012**, *23*, 817–821. [CrossRef] [PubMed]
119. Broekhuizen, R.; Wouters, E.F.; Creutzberg, E.C.; Weling-Scheepers, C.A.; Schols, A.M. Polyunsaturated fatty acids improve exercise capacity in chronic obstructive pulmonary disease. *Thorax* **2005**, *60*, 376–382. [CrossRef]
120. Micha, R.; Wallace, S.K.; Mozaffarian, D. Red and processed meat consumption and risk of incident coronary heart disease, stroke, and diabetes mellitus: A systematic review and meta-analysis. *Circulation* **2010**, *121*, 2271–2283. [CrossRef]
121. Johnson, I.T. The cancer risk related to meat and meat products. *Br. Med. Bull.* **2017**, *121*, 73–81. [CrossRef] [PubMed]
122. Larsson, S.C.; Orsini, N. Red meat and processed meat consumption and all-cause mortality: A meta-analysis. *Am. J. Epidemiol.* **2014**, *179*, 282–289. [CrossRef] [PubMed]
123. Jiang, R.; Paik, D.C.; Hankinson, J.L.; Barr, R.G. Cured meat consumption, lung function, and chronic obstructive pulmonary disease among United States adults. *Am. J. Respir. Crit. Care Med.* **2007**, *175*, 798–804. [CrossRef] [PubMed]
124. Varraso, R.; Jiang, R.; Barr, R.G.; Willett, W.C.; Camargo, C.A., Jr. Prospective study of cured meats consumption and risk of chronic obstructive pulmonary disease in men. *Am. J. Epidemiol.* **2007**, *166*, 1438–1445. [CrossRef] [PubMed]
125. Jiang, R.; Camargo, C.A., Jr.; Varraso, R.; Paik, D.C.; Willett, W.C.; Barr, R.G. Consumption of cured meats and prospective risk of chronic obstructive pulmonary disease in women. *Am. J. Clin. Nutr.* **2008**, *87*, 1002–1008. [CrossRef] [PubMed]
126. Kaluza, J.; Larsson, S.C.; Linden, A.; Wolk, A. Consumption of Unprocessed and Processed Red Meat and the Risk of Chronic Obstructive Pulmonary Disease: A Prospective Cohort Study of Men. *Am. J. Epidemiol.* **2016**, *184*, 829–836. [CrossRef]
127. Kaluza, J.; Harris, H.; Linden, A.; Wolk, A. Long-term unprocessed and processed red meat consumption and risk of chronic obstructive pulmonary disease: A prospective cohort study of women. *Eur. J. Nutr.* **2019**, *58*, 665–672. [CrossRef]
128. de Batlle, J.; Mendez, M.; Romieu, I.; Balcells, E.; Benet, M.; Donaire-Gonzalez, D.; Ferrer, J.J.; Orozco-Levi, M.; Anto, J.M.; Garcia-Aymerich, J.; et al. Cured meat consumption increases risk of readmission in COPD patients. *Eur. Respir. J.* **2012**, *40*, 555–560. [CrossRef]
129. Salari-Moghaddam, A.; Milajerdi, A.; Larijani, B.; Esmaillzadeh, A. Processed red meat intake and risk of COPD: A systematic review and dose-response meta-analysis of prospective cohort studies. *Clin. Nutr.* **2018**, *38*, 1109–1116. [CrossRef]
130. Ricciardolo, F.L.; Caramori, G.; Ito, K.; Capelli, A.; Brun, P.; Abatangelo, G.; Papi, A.; Chung, K.F.; Adcock, I.; Barnes, P.J.; et al. Nitrosative stress in the bronchial mucosa of severe chronic obstructive pulmonary disease. *J. Allergy Clin. Immunol.* **2005**, *116*, 1028–1035. [CrossRef]
131. Shuval, H.I.; Gruener, N. Epidemiological and toxicological aspects of nitrates and nitrites in the environment. *Am. J. Public Health* **1972**, *62*, 1045–1052. [CrossRef] [PubMed]
132. Yi, B.; Titze, J.; Rykova, M.; Feuerecker, M.; Vassilieva, G.; Nichiporuk, I.; Schelling, G.; Morukov, B.; Chouker, A. Effects of dietary salt levels on monocytic cells and immune responses in healthy human subjects: A longitudinal study. *Transl. Res.* **2015**, *166*, 103–110. [CrossRef] [PubMed]
133. Tashiro, H.; Takahashi, K.; Sadamatsu, H.; Kato, G.; Kurata, K.; Kimura, S.; Sueoka-Aragane, N. Saturated Fatty Acid Increases Lung Macrophages and Augments House Dust Mite-Induced Airway Inflammation in Mice Fed with High-Fat Diet. *Inflammation* **2017**, *40*, 1072–1086. [CrossRef] [PubMed]

134. Wood, L.G.; Attia, J.; McElduff, P.; McEvoy, M.; Gibson, P.G. Assessment of dietary fat intake and innate immune activation as risk factors for impaired lung function. *Eur. J. Clin. Nutr.* **2010**, *64*, 818–825. [CrossRef] [PubMed]

135. Zong, G.; Li, Y.; Wanders, A.J.; Alssema, M.; Zock, P.L.; Willett, W.C.; Hu, F.B.; Sun, Q. Intake of individual saturated fatty acids and risk of coronary heart disease in US men and women: Two prospective longitudinal cohort studies. *BMJ* **2016**, *355*, i5796. [CrossRef]

136. Jiang, R.; Jacobs, D.R.; He, K.; Hoffman, E.; Hankinson, J.; Nettleton, J.A.; Barr, R.G. Associations of dairy intake with CT lung density and lung function. *J. Am. Coll. Nutr.* **2010**, *29*, 494–502. [CrossRef] [PubMed]

137. Cornell, K.; Alam, M.; Lyden, E.; Wood, L.; LeVan, T.D.; Nordgren, T.M.; Bailey, K.; Hanson, C. Saturated Fat Intake Is Associated with Lung Function in Individuals with Airflow Obstruction: Results from NHANES 2007(-)2012. *Nutrients* **2019**, *11*. [CrossRef]

138. Esposito, K.; Nappo, F.; Marfella, R.; Giugliano, G.; Giugliano, F.; Ciotola, M.; Quagliaro, L.; Ceriello, A.; Giugliano, D. Inflammatory cytokine concentrations are acutely increased by hyperglycemia in humans: Role of oxidative stress. *Circulation* **2002**, *106*, 2067–2072. [CrossRef]

139. Walter, R.E.; Beiser, A.; Givelber, R.J.; O'Connor, G.T.; Gottlieb, D.J. Association between glycemic state and lung function: The Framingham Heart Study. *Am. J. Respir. Crit. Care Med.* **2003**, *167*, 911–916. [CrossRef]

140. Baker, E.H.; Janaway, C.H.; Philips, B.J.; Brennan, A.L.; Baines, D.L.; Wood, D.M.; Jones, P.W. Hyperglycaemia is associated with poor outcomes in patients admitted to hospital with acute exacerbations of chronic obstructive pulmonary disease. *Thorax* **2006**, *61*, 284–289. [CrossRef]

141. Mallia, P.; Webber, J.; Gill, S.K.; Trujillo-Torralbo, M.B.; Calderazzo, M.A.; Finney, L.; Bakhsoliani, E.; Farne, H.; Singanayagam, A.; Footitt, J.; et al. Role of airway glucose in bacterial infections in patients with chronic obstructive pulmonary disease. *J. Allergy Clin. Immunol.* **2018**, *142*, 815–823. [CrossRef] [PubMed]

142. Wu, L.; Ma, L.; Nicholson, L.F.; Black, P.N. Advanced glycation end products and its receptor (RAGE) are increased in patients with COPD. *Respir. Med.* **2011**, *105*, 329–336. [CrossRef] [PubMed]

143. Shi, Z.; Dal Grande, E.; Taylor, A.W.; Gill, T.K.; Adams, R.; Wittert, G.A. Association between soft drink consumption and asthma and chronic obstructive pulmonary disease among adults in Australia. *Respirology* **2012**, *17*, 363–369. [CrossRef] [PubMed]

144. DeChristopher, L.R.; Uribarri, J.; Tucker, K.L. Intake of high fructose corn syrup sweetened soft drinks is associated with prevalent chronic bronchitis in U.S. Adults, ages 20–55 y. *Nutr. J.* **2015**, *14*, 107. [CrossRef] [PubMed]

145. DeChristopher, L.R.; Uribarri, J.; Tucker, K.L. Intakes of apple juice, fruit drinks and soda are associated with prevalent asthma in US children aged 2–9 years. *Public Health Nutr.* **2016**, *19*, 123–130. [CrossRef] [PubMed]

146. Butler, L.M.; Koh, W.P.; Lee, H.P.; Tseng, M.; Yu, M.C.; London, S.J. Singapore Chinese Health Study. Prospective study of dietary patterns and persistent cough with phlegm among Chinese Singaporeans. *Am. J. Respir. Crit. Care Med.* **2006**, *173*, 264–270. [CrossRef] [PubMed]

147. Varraso, R.; Fung, T.T.; Hu, F.B.; Willett, W.; Camargo, C.A. Prospective study of dietary patterns and chronic obstructive pulmonary disease among US men. *Thorax* **2007**, *62*, 786–791. [CrossRef] [PubMed]

148. Varraso, R.; Fung, T.T.; Barr, R.G.; Hu, F.B.; Willett, W.; Camargo, C.A., Jr. Prospective study of dietary patterns and chronic obstructive pulmonary disease among US women. *Am. J. Clin. Nutr.* **2007**, *86*, 488–495. [CrossRef] [PubMed]

149. Shaheen, S.O.; Jameson, K.A.; Syddall, H.E.; Aihie Sayer, A.; Dennison, E.M.; Cooper, C.; Robinson, S.M. Hertfordshire Cohort Study Group. The relationship of dietary patterns with adult lung function and COPD. *Eur. Respir. J.* **2010**, *36*, 277–284. [CrossRef]

150. Steinemann, N.; Grize, L.; Pons, M.; Rothe, T.; Stolz, D.; Turk, A.; Schindler, C.; Brombach, C.; Probst-Hensch, N. Associations between Dietary Patterns and Post-Bronchodilation Lung Function in the SAPALDIA Cohort. *Respiration* **2018**, *95*, 454–463. [CrossRef]

151. Brigham, E.P.; Steffen, L.M.; London, S.J.; Boyce, D.; Diette, G.B.; Hansel, N.N.; Rice, J.; McCormack, M.C. Diet Pattern and Respiratory Morbidity in the Atherosclerosis Risk in Communities Study. *Ann. Am. Thorac. Soc.* **2018**, *15*, 675–682. [CrossRef] [PubMed]

152. McKeever, T.M.; Lewis, S.A.; Cassano, P.A.; Ocke, M.; Burney, P.; Britton, J.; Smit, H.A. Patterns of dietary intake and relation to respiratory disease, forced expiratory volume in 1 s, and decline in 5-y forced expiratory volume. *Am. J. Clin. Nutr.* **2010**, *92*, 408–415. [CrossRef] [PubMed]

153. Sorli-Aguilar, M.; Martin-Lujan, F.; Flores-Mateo, G.; Arija-Val, V.; Basora-Gallisa, J.; Sola-Alberich, R.; RESET Study Group Investigators. Dietary patterns are associated with lung function among Spanish smokers without respiratory disease. *BMC Pulm. Med.* **2016**, *16*, 162. [CrossRef] [PubMed]
154. Varraso, R.; Chiuve, S.E.; Fung, T.T.; Barr, R.G.; Hu, F.B.; Willett, W.C.; Camargo, C.A. Alternate Healthy Eating Index 2010 and risk of chronic obstructive pulmonary disease among US women and men: Prospective study. *BMJ* **2015**, *350*, h286. [CrossRef] [PubMed]
155. Yazdanpanah, L.; Paknahad, Z.; Moosavi, A.J.; Maracy, M.R.; Zaker, M.M. The relationship between different diet quality indices and severity of airflow obstruction among COPD patients. *Med. J. Islam. Repub. Iran* **2016**, *30*, 380. [PubMed]
156. Gutierrez-Carrasquilla, L.; Sanchez, E.; Hernandez, M.; Polanco, D.; Salas-Salvado, J.; Betriu, A.; Gaeta, A.M.; Carmona, P.; Purroy, F.; Pamplona, R.; et al. Effects of Mediterranean Diet and Physical Activity on Pulmonary Function: A Cross-Sectional Analysis in the ILERVAS Project. *Nutrients* **2019**, *11*. [CrossRef]
157. Scoditti, E.; Capurso, C.; Capurso, A.; Massaro, M. Vascular effects of the Mediterranean diet-part II: Role of omega-3 fatty acids and olive oil polyphenols. *Vasc. Pharmacol.* **2014**, *63*, 127–134. [CrossRef]
158. Sofi, F.; Macchi, C.; Abbate, R.; Gensini, G.F.; Casini, A. Mediterranean diet and health status: An updated meta-analysis and a proposal for a literature-based adherence score. *Public Health Nutr.* **2014**, *17*, 2769–2782. [CrossRef]
159. Papamichael, M.M.; Itsiopoulos, C.; Susanto, N.H.; Erbas, B. Does adherence to the Mediterranean dietary pattern reduce asthma symptoms in children? A systematic review of observational studies. *Public Health Nutr.* **2017**, *20*, 2722–2734. [CrossRef]
160. Davis, C.; Bryan, J.; Hodgson, J.; Murphy, K. Definition of the Mediterranean Diet; a Literature Review. *Nutrients* **2015**, *7*, 9139–9153. [CrossRef]
161. Guenther, P.M.; Casavale, K.O.; Reedy, J.; Kirkpatrick, S.I.; Hiza, H.A.; Kuczynski, K.J.; Kahle, L.L.; Krebs-Smith, S.M. Update of the Healthy Eating Index: HEI-2010. *J. Acad. Nutr. Diet.* **2013**, *113*, 569–580. [CrossRef] [PubMed]
162. McCullough, M.L.; Feskanich, D.; Stampfer, M.J.; Giovannucci, E.L.; Rimm, E.B.; Hu, F.B.; Spiegelman, D.; Hunter, D.J.; Colditz, G.A.; Willett, W.C.; et al. Diet quality and major chronic disease risk in men and women: Moving toward improved dietary guidance. *Am. J. Clin. Nutr.* **2002**, *76*, 1261–1271. [CrossRef] [PubMed]
163. Chiuve, S.E.; Fung, T.T.; Rimm, E.B.; Hu, F.B.; McCullough, M.L.; Wang, M.; Stampfer, M.J.; Willett, W.C. Alternative dietary indices both strongly predict risk of chronic disease. *J. Nutr.* **2012**, *142*, 1009–1018. [CrossRef] [PubMed]
164. Schwingshackl, L.; Bogensberger, B.; Hoffmann, G. Diet Quality as Assessed by the Healthy Eating Index, Alternate Healthy Eating Index, Dietary Approaches to Stop Hypertension Score, and Health Outcomes: An Updated Systematic Review and Meta-Analysis of Cohort Studies. *J. Acad. Nutr. Diet.* **2018**, *118*, 74–100. [CrossRef] [PubMed]
165. Trichopoulou, A.; Costacou, T.; Bamia, C.; Trichopoulos, D. Adherence to a Mediterranean diet and survival in a Greek population. *N. Engl. J. Med.* **2003**, *348*, 2599–2608. [CrossRef]
166. Hernandez-Ruiz, A.; Garcia-Villanova, B.; Guerra Hernandez, E.J.; Amiano, P.; Azpiri, M.; Molina-Montes, E. Description of Indexes Based on the Adherence to the Mediterranean Dietary Pattern: A Review. *Nutr. Hosp.* **2015**, *32*, 1872–1884. [CrossRef] [PubMed]
167. Neelakantan, N.; Koh, W.P.; Yuan, J.M.; van Dam, R.M. Diet-Quality Indexes Are Associated with a Lower Risk of Cardiovascular, Respiratory, and All-Cause Mortality among Chinese Adults. *J. Nutr.* **2018**, *148*, 1323–1332. [CrossRef]
168. Ardestani, M.E.; Onvani, S.; Esmailzadeh, A.; Feizi, A.; Azadbakht, L. Adherence to Dietary Approaches to Stop Hypertension (DASH) Dietary Pattern in Relation to Chronic Obstructive Pulmonary Disease (COPD): A Case-Control Study. *J. Am. Coll. Nutr.* **2017**, *36*, 549–555. [CrossRef]
169. Voortman, T.; Kiefte-de Jong, J.C.; Ikram, M.A.; Stricker, B.H.; van Rooij, F.J.A.; Lahousse, L.; Tiemeier, H.; Brusselle, G.G.; Franco, O.H.; Schoufour, J.D.; et al. Adherence to the 2015 Dutch dietary guidelines and risk of non-communicable diseases and mortality in the Rotterdam Study. *Eur. J. Epidemiol.* **2017**, *32*, 993–1005. [CrossRef]
170. Lopez-Garcia, E.; Schulze, M.B.; Fung, T.T.; Meigs, J.B.; Rifai, N.; Manson, J.E.; Hu, F.B. Major dietary patterns are related to plasma concentrations of markers of inflammation and endothelial dysfunction. *Am. J. Clin. Nutr.* **2004**, *80*, 1029–1035. [CrossRef]

171. Bonaccio, M.; Pounis, G.; Cerletti, C.; Donati, M.B.; Iacoviello, L.; de Gaetano, G.; Investigators, M.-S.S. Mediterranean diet, dietary polyphenols and low grade inflammation: Results from the MOLI-SANI study. *Br. J. Clin. Pharmacol.* **2017**, *83*, 107–113. [CrossRef] [PubMed]
172. Schols, A.M. Translating nutritional potential of metabolic remodelling to disease-modifying nutritional management. *Curr. Opin. Clin. Nutr. Metab. Care* **2013**, *16*, 617–618. [CrossRef] [PubMed]
173. De Filippis, F.; Pellegrini, N.; Vannini, L.; Jeffery, I.B.; La Storia, A.; Laghi, L.; Serrazanetti, D.I.; Di Cagno, R.; Ferrocino, I.; Lazzi, C.; et al. High-level adherence to a Mediterranean diet beneficially impacts the gut microbiota and associated metabolome. *Gut* **2015**, *65*, 1812–1821. [CrossRef] [PubMed]
174. Budden, K.F.; Gellatly, S.L.; Wood, D.L.; Cooper, M.A.; Morrison, M.; Hugenholtz, P.; Hansbro, P.M. Emerging pathogenic links between microbiota and the gut-lung axis. *Nat. Rev. Microbiol.* **2017**, *15*, 55–63. [CrossRef] [PubMed]
175. Trompette, A.; Gollwitzer, E.S.; Yadava, K.; Sichelstiel, A.K.; Sprenger, N.; Ngom-Bru, C.; Blanchard, C.; Junt, T.; Nicod, L.P.; Harris, N.L.; et al. Gut microbiota metabolism of dietary fiber influences allergic airway disease and hematopoiesis. *Nat. Med.* **2014**, *20*, 159–166. [CrossRef] [PubMed]
176. Ottiger, M.; Nickler, M.; Steuer, C.; Bernasconi, L.; Huber, A.; Christ-Crain, M.; Henzen, C.; Hoess, C.; Thomann, R.; Zimmerli, W.; et al. Gut, microbiota-dependent trimethylamine-N-oxide is associated with long-term all-cause mortality in patients with exacerbated chronic obstructive pulmonary disease. *Nutrition* **2018**, *45*, 135–141. [CrossRef] [PubMed]
177. Ferreira, I.M.; Brooks, D.; White, J.; Goldstein, R. Nutritional supplementation for stable chronic obstructive pulmonary disease. *Cochrane Database Syst. Rev.* **2012**, *12*. [CrossRef]

12

Endocrine Disruptor Bisphenol A (BPA) Triggers Systemic Para-Inflammation and is Sufficient to Induce Airway Allergic Sensitization in Mice

Lucas Fedele Loffredo, Mackenzie Elyse Coden and Sergejs Berdnikovs *

Division of Allergy and Immunology, Department of Medicine, Northwestern University Feinberg School of Medicine, Chicago, IL 60611, USA; lucasloffredo@gmail.com (L.F.L.); mackenzie.coden@northwestern.edu (M.E.C.)

* Correspondence: s-berdnikovs@northwestern.edu

Abstract: Allergic airway diseases are accompanied by increased permeability and an inflammatory state of epithelial barriers, which are thought to be susceptible to allergen sensitization. Although exogenous drivers (proteases, allergens) of epithelial barrier disruption and sensitization are well studied, endogenous contributors (diet, xenobiotics, hormones, and metabolism) to allergic sensitization are much less understood. Xenoestrogens are synthetic or natural chemical compounds that have the ability to mimic estrogen and are ubiquitous in the food and water supply of developed countries. By interfering with the estrogen produced by the endocrine system, these compounds have the systemic potential to disrupt the homeostasis of multiple tissues. Our study examined the potential of prototypical xenoestrogen bisphenol A (BPA) to disrupt epithelial homeostasis in vitro and promote allergic responses in vivo. We found that BPA exposure in epithelial cultures in vitro significantly inhibited epithelial cell proliferation and wound healing, as well as promoted the expression of the innate alarmin cytokine TSLP in a time-and dose-dependent manner. In vivo, the exposure to BPA through water supply or inhalation induced a systemic para-inflammatory response by promoting the expression of innate inflammatory mediators in the skin, gut, and airway. In a murine tolerogenic antigen challenge model, chronic systemic exposure to BPA was sufficient to induce airway sensitization to innocuous chicken egg ovalbumin in the complete absence of adjuvants. Mechanistic studies are needed to test conclusively whether endocrine disruptors may play an upstream role in allergic sensitization via their ability to promote a para-inflammatory state.

Keywords: bisphenol A; estrogen; xenoestrogens; para-inflammation; endocrine; alarmins; allergy; asthma

1. Introduction

The epithelium is the first barrier encountered by an inhaled or ingested allergen [1]. Allergic inflammatory diseases are accompanied by the increased permeability and inflammatory state of the epithelial barrier, which is thought to be more susceptible to allergen sensitization [2–5]. Multiple lines of evidence point to the causality of epithelial barrier dysfunction in the development of allergic inflammation. A number of mouse and human models using protease epithelial damage triggers or the targeted deletion of structural or junctional barrier genes report enhanced allergic sensitization and Th2 inflammation [6–9]. Although research shows that exogenous proteases in many allergens themselves are sufficient to disrupt epithelium, this does not explain why only a fraction of the population exposed to the same allergens develops sensitization. Endogenous factors linked to systemic epithelial barrier dysfunction, such as changes in nutrients, hormones, vitamins, chemical exposures, and dysbiosis, are suspected in the origins of allergic disease but are much less understood [10].

Among them, xenoestrogens are receiving attention due to their biological action and ubiquitous human chronic exposure through their release into beverages, food, and the environment [11–13]. Xenoestrogens are synthetic or natural chemical compounds that have the ability to mimic estrogen and have estrogenic effects on biological organisms, thus interfering with the estrogen produced by the endocrine system. For this reason, they are also sometimes called "environmental hormones" or "endocrine disrupting compounds". Synthetic xenoestrogens are widely used industrial compounds that are prevalent in the food and water supply of developed countries because of their widespread use as plasticizers in the production of food packaging. Low but persistent non-toxic exposure to xenoestrogens has been recently shown to be a serious environmental hazard linked to a vast array of human conditions, including allergic diseases [14–17]. Estrogen receptors alpha and beta play a central role in epithelial homeostasis in both sexes, which is independent of their role in reproduction and sexual development [18–20]. In particular, estrogen receptors are essential in the integration of extracellular signals, such as growth factor and WNT/Notch pathways, to properly regulate the expression of genes that control cell fates during epithelial turnover [20–25]. In this manuscript, we tested whether the ubiquitous endocrine disruptor bisphenol A (BPA) is disruptive for epithelial homeostasis with possible in vivo consequences for the initiation of allergic responses. We found that BPA exposure (1) significantly inhibited epithelial cell proliferation and wound healing in vitro as well as promoted the expression of innate alarmin cytokine TSLP in a time- and dose-dependent manner; (2) elevated the systemic expression of innate cytokines and chemokines at skin, gut, and airway barriers when given to mice in water or by inhalation; and (3) in tolerogenic airway antigen challenge protocol was sufficient to induce sensitization to chicken egg ovalbumin in the absence of adjuvants.

2. Materials and Methods

2.1. Animal Experiments

For all in vivo asthma model experiments, we used wild-type adult female littermate mice on the BALB/cJ background (Jackson Laboratories, Bar Harbor, ME, USA). The Institutional Animal Care and Use Committee of Northwestern University approved all animal procedures (protocol IS00001710, original approval date 6/8/2015). For the in vivo experiments, bisphenol A (BPA) (Sigma) was administered at 25 mg/L in drinking water bottles *ad libitum* or intranasally (i.n.) daily at 25 ug/mL (volume administered = 53 μL). This BPA concentration is comparable to human environmental exposure of 5 mg/kg of body weight/day, which is the current NOAEL (no observed adverse effect level) concentration set by the U.S. Food and Drug Administration (FDA) and the European Food Safety Authority (EFSA). This is also the dose typically used in murine studies of low-dose BPA exposures. The BPA was not specifically endotoxin free, but it was ≥ 99.0 pure by HPLC (Sigma). Lung, skin (abdominal), and gut (duodenal) tissues were harvested after seven days of BPA exposure. For the allergic model, mice were maintained on regular drinking water or water with 25 mg/L BPA for 70 days to mimic chronic exposures by ingestion. In the last 10 days of the protocol, mice were administered daily saline or 1% chicken egg ovalbumin (OVA) grade VI (Sigma) with or without BPA (25 ug/mL) by intranasal inhalation. We obtained bronchoalveolar lavage fluid (BALF), lung tissue, and serum 24 h after the last inhalation challenge.

2.2. Bronchoalveolar Lavage, Lung Digestion, and Flow Cytometry

Bronchoalveolar lavage was performed by lavaging lungs with ice-cold 1× phosphate-buffered saline (PBS) through the cannulated trachea. Lungs were digested in 1 mg/mL collagenase D and 0.2 mg/mL DNAse I (Roche, Indianapolis, IN, USA) in preparation for flow cytometry. Digested tissue was filtered through sterile mesh and incubated in 1× BD PharmLyse Lysing Buffer (BD Biosciences, San Jose, CA, USA) to lyse red blood cells. Live/dead exclusion was performed using Aqua dye (Molecular Probes) followed by incubation with CD16/CD32 FC Block (BD Pharmingen, San Jose, CA, USA). Antibody cocktail was added directly to blocked samples and incubated for 30 min at 4 °C.

Antibody cocktail composition was as previously used for leukocyte population characterization during allergic inflammation [26]. Samples were acquired on a BD LSRII flow cytometer (BD Biosciences). BAL cells were pelleted by centrifugation at 300× g for 5 min, washed, and prepared as described above, starting with the live/dead step. Bead compensation (OneComp; eBioscience, San Diego, CA, USA, and ArC; Molecular Probes beads), gating, and data analysis were performed using FlowJo v.10 (TreeStar, Inc., Ashland, OR, USA). Only live, single, hematopoietic (CD45+) cells were used in all analyses. Fluorescence Minus One (FMO) controls were used to set up gate boundaries. Leukocyte populations were identified as follows: (i) eosinophils: CD11b(+)Ly6G(low/-)CD11c(−/low)Siglec-F(med/high); (ii) alveolar macrophages: CD11b(−)Ly6G(−)CD11c(high)Siglec-F(high); and (iii) neutrophils: CD11b(+)Ly6G(high)CD11c(−)Siglec-F(−).

2.3. Cell Culture

For epithelial cultures, we used the commercially available (Sigma) BEAS-2B human cell line originally derived from normal bronchial epithelium obtained from the autopsy of non-cancerous individuals. Cells were cultured in Dulbecco's Modified Eagle Medium (DMEM) with the addition of 1% penicillin–streptomycin and 5% heat-inactivated fetal bovine serum. Cells were treated with BPA dissolved in ethanol (ethanol alone used for vehicle controls). Cells were passaged when reaching 70%–80% confluency to avoid spontaneous transformation. For wound-healing assays, epithelial monolayers were scratched using p10 pipet tips, and wound closure was monitored by bright field microscopy using same field view over a 48 h period. Scratch width was quantified using ImageJ software (NIH).

2.4. Quantitative PCR

RNA was isolated from cells using the Qiagen RNeasy mini kit (Qiagen). cDNA was synthesized using a qScript cDNA synthesis kit (Quanta BioSciences) and analyzed by real-time PCR on a 7500 real-time PCR system (Applied Biosystems) using primers/probes from Integrated DNA Technologies and PrimeTime Gene Expression Master Mix (IDT or Applied Biosystems).

2.5. Cytotoxicity Assay

The Vybrant Cytotoxicity Assay Kit (Thermo Fisher), which detects glucose-6-phosphate dehydrogenase released from damaged cells via the reduction of resazurin into red-fluorescent resorufin, was used to assess cytotoxicity. A total of 7000 BEAS-2B cells were plated in 50 uL of normal media in a 96-well plate and incubated for 24 h to adhere; then, they were changed to 50 uL media with indicated BPA concentrations and incubated for another 24 h. Control wells were lysed with cell lysis buffer from the kit; then, 50 uL of resazurin/enzymatic solution was added to each well, and each plate was incubated on a shaker in the dark for 10 min. Then, fluorescence was measured on a fluorescent plate reader (excitation 560 nm, emission 600 nm).

2.6. Measurements of Serum Proteins and Antibodies

Harvested serum was assayed for cytokine IL-33 using a Ready-SET-Go! ELISA kit purchased from eBioscience (Invitrogen). ELISA assays were performed according to the manufacturer's instructions. OVA-specific IgE was determined by custom ELISA, as previously described [27].

2.7. Statistical Analysis

Statistical significance of all data was determined by an unpaired t-test or one-way ANOVA followed by Tukey's post hoc pairwise testing whenever applicable. All data are represented as mean ± S.E.M. Statistical analysis was performed using GraphPad Prism 7 (GraphPad Software, Inc.). An alpha level of 0.05 was used as a significance cut-off in all tests. For principal component analysis (PCA), PAST v.3 software was used, inputting data as log10-normalized values from the qPCR of alarmin, cytokine, and chemokine gene expression (genes used: *Il33, Tslp, Ifng, Tnfa, Il10, Cxcl9, Cxcl10, Cxcl11, Ccl1, Ccl2,* and *Ccl11*) from the following nine sample groups: non-treated lung tissue, lung tissue from BPA water-treated mice, BPA-i.n. treated lung tissue, non-treated gut tissue, BPA-water treated gut tissue, BPA-i.n. treated gut tissue, non-treated skin tissue, BPA-water treated skin tissue, and BPA-i.n. treated skin tissue.

3. Results

3.1. Bisphenol A Has An Inhibitory Effect on BEAS-2B Epithelial Cell Proliferation and Wound Healing

Estrogen receptors intricately interact with developmental pathway signaling to maintain epithelial homeostasis [21]. Using wound scratch assays, we found that BPA had an inhibitory effect on epithelial wound healing (Figure 1A,B). Our data show that this effect of BPA was likely mediated by the significant inhibition of epithelial cell proliferation, which was both time- and concentration-dependent (Figure 1C). The disruption of epithelial growth by BPA occurred without detectable cytotoxicity at concentrations less than 200 μM (Figure 1E). It is likely that BPA could disrupt epithelium in a non-damaging manner via interfering with the estrogen regulation of epithelial junctions and cell cycle. Moreover, we detected a significant upregulation of the *Tslp* message by BPA-treated epithelial cells in vitro, which was especially evident after 48 h of exposure in culture (Figure 1D). Notably, the highest TSLP expression at 200 µM was at least partially associated with BPA cytotoxicity, which thus can serve as a positive control for levels of death-induced alarmin expression. In summary, BPA directly interferes with homeostatic proliferation and promotes TSLP expression by epithelial cells.

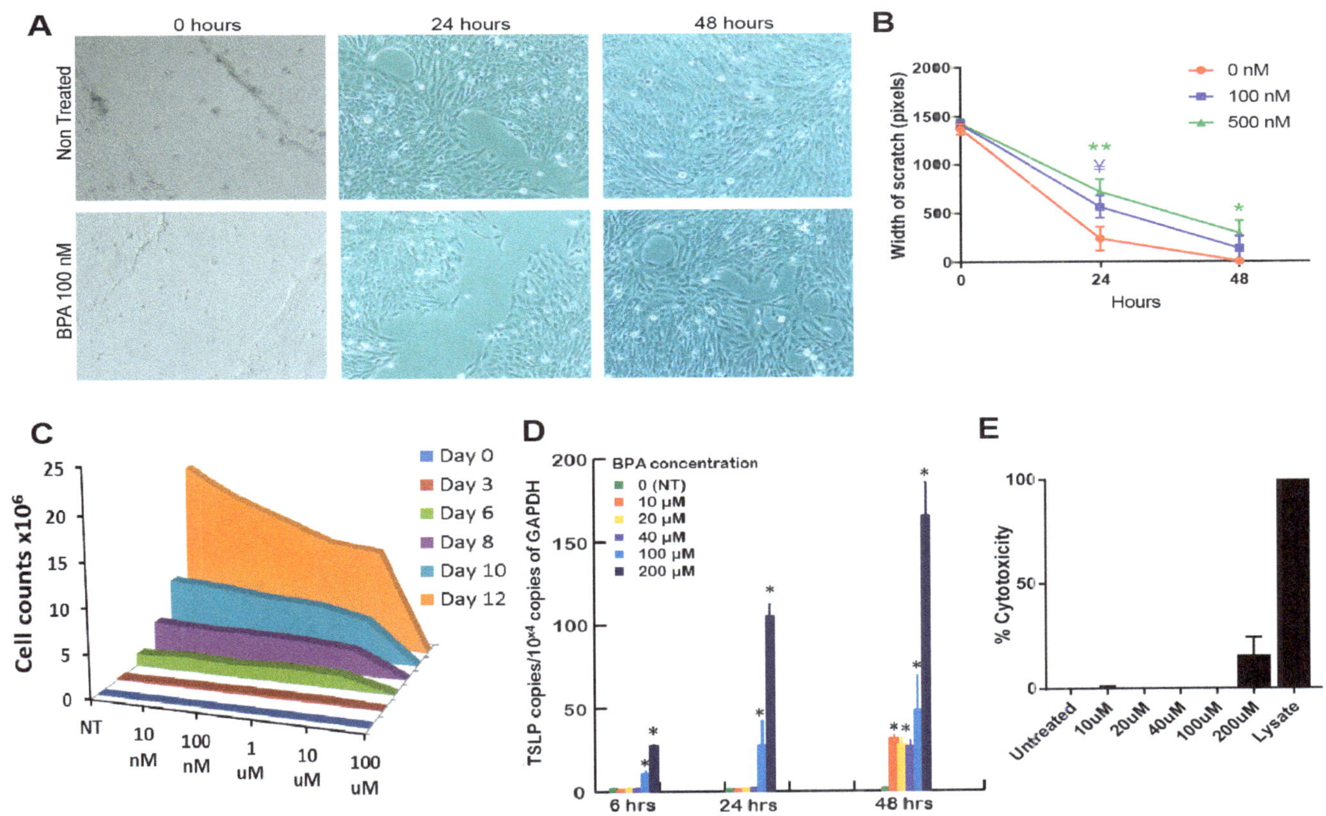

Figure 1. Bisphenol A has an inhibitory effect on BEAS-2B epithelial cell proliferation and wound healing. (**A**) Wound healing assay. Cells were grown to complete confluency, and monolayers were scratched with a p10 pipet tip. Wound closure was monitored over a 48 h period. Representative images from two experiments. (**B**) Quantification of wound closure rates using scratch width measured in ImageJ. Representative quantification from two experiments. (**C**) Inhibitory effect of bisphenol A (BPA)

on long-term BEAS-2B epithelial cells proliferation in culture. Data shown from experiment performed one time. (**D**) BEAS-2B expression of TSLP induced by exposure to BPA. Representative quantification from experiment performed three times. (**E**) Cytotoxicity analysis of BEAS-2B epithelial cell exposure to BPA; cells were cultured for 24 h for adherence, treated with indicated concentrations of BPA for 24 h, and then assessed for cytotoxicity. All values included from experiment performed two times. *, $p < 0.05$ by ANOVA.

3.2. Ingestion of BPA Promotes Systemic Para-Inflammation in Mice

Given the observed effects on epithelial cells in vitro, we proceeded to confirm this in vivo by exposing mice to BPA (5 mg/kg of body weight/day) in water *ad libitum* for seven days (Figure 2A). Another group of mice were exposed to BPA via intranasal inhalation daily at a concentration of 25 ug/mL. The local exposure of epithelial barriers to BPA (airway by inhalation and intestinal barrier by ingestion) promoted the expression of *Ccl1* and *Ifnγ* at several contact sites (Figure 2B). Surprisingly, this was accompanied by significant changes in the expression of these mediators and trends for changes in the expression of multiple other mediators at other barrier sites as well, which were not the result of direct exposure to BPA (Figure 2B,C). In Figure 2C, we used exploratory principal component analysis (PCA) to summarize the variation in expression of all genes measured by qPCR (regardless of significance) at three barrier sites following BPA exposures via water supply or inhalation. It suggests that each barrier site (lung, gut, skin) may promote the expression of innate cytokines and chemokines even if not exposed to BPA directly (Figure 2C), which is consistent with low-grade systemic inflammation.

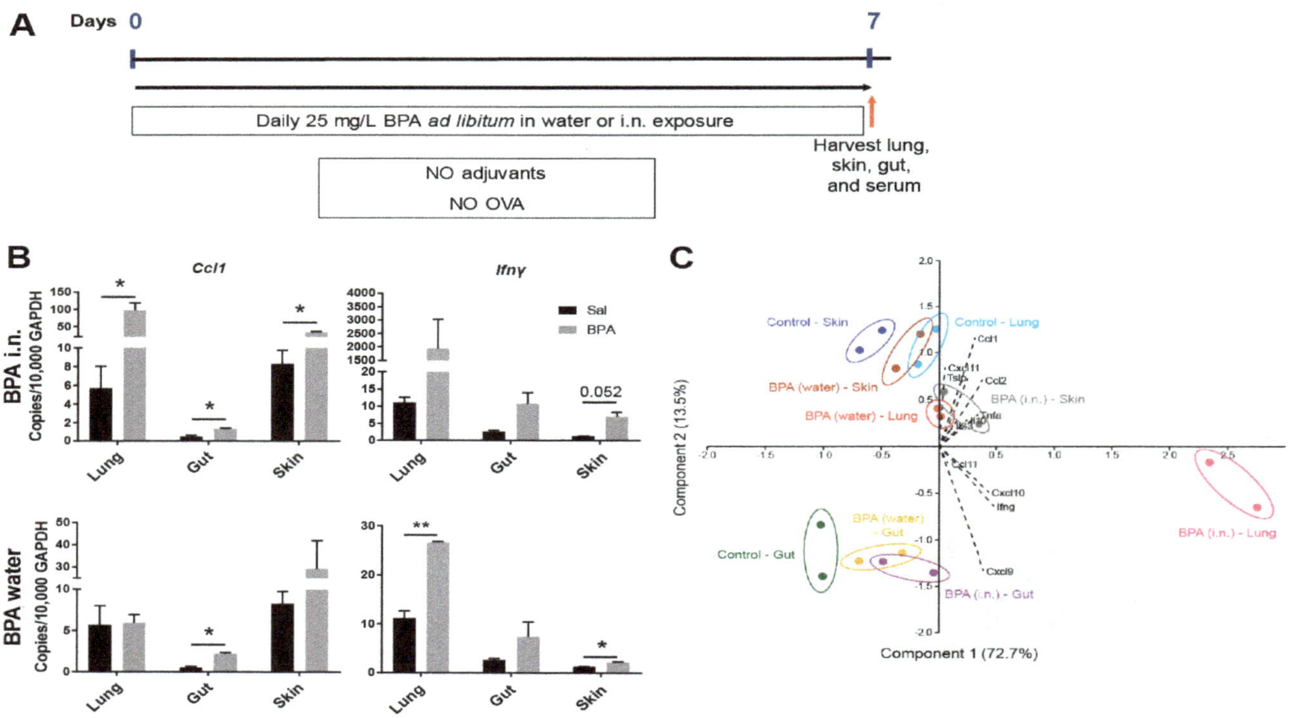

Figure 2. Ingestion of BPA promotes systemic para-inflammation in mice. (**A**) BPA administration protocol. (**B**) Expression of *Ccl1* and *Ifng* in murine lung, gut, and airway after seven days of BPA exposure. Top graphs, exposure by intranasal inhalation; bottom graphs, exposure through *ad libitum* water intake. N = 2 mice/group/9 groups, all data are from one experiment. *, $p < 0.05$, **, $p < 0.01$ by t-test within each tissue compartment. (**C**) Exploratory PCA analysis of log10-normalized values of gene expression measured at all tissue sites (lung, skin, gut) following BPA exposure via water intake or by inhalation (see Methods for list of genes/groups).

3.3. Chronic Systemic BPA Exposure Induces Allergic Sensitization to Innocuous OVA Antigen Exposure and Facilitates the Development of Allergic Inflammation

We further tested whether the para-inflammatory state induced by BPA exposure would facilitate sensitization to chicken egg ovalbumin (OVA) in a tolerogenic antigen exposure protocol. The treatment of mice with 25 ug/mL of BPA in water supply for 10 weeks followed by the daily intranasal treatment of endotoxin-free 1% OVA for 10 days resulted in spontaneous, adjuvant-free sensitization and allergic inflammation development (Figure 3). This OVA treatment protocol is completely tolerogenic and does not result in sensitization or allergic inflammation in the absence of adjuvants. Although there was some non-specific inflammatory response and neutrophil recruitment in control mice (receiving water only, no BPA) challenged with 1% OVA, eosinophils were significantly recruited only in mice treated with BPA plus OVA (Figure 3). Interestingly, the eosinophils in this treatment group showed a CD11c (+) phenotype indicative of their mucosal activation and heightened capacity to migrate to the airway [26] (Figure 3B). The finding that BPA was sufficient to elicit an allergic inflammatory response to innocuous OVA antigen in the complete absence of adjuvant was reinforced by the demonstration that the lung expression of Type 2 cytokines interleukin (IL)-4, IL-5, and IL-13 was significantly upregulated only in mice administered BPA and OVA (Figure 4A). Consistent with the inflammatory response and eosinophil recruitment, we also observed the lung tissue expression of chemokines CCL2 (MCP1) and CCL11/CCL24 (eotaxins 1 and 2) (Figure 4B). There was no difference in the expression of cytokine IL-33 in the lung tissue of mice challenged with BPA and OVA; however, we found significantly elevated serum protein levels of IL-33 in these mice (Figure 4C). Interestingly, BPA administration alone (without OVA) resulted in the marginally significant elevation of IL-33 protein serum, further demonstrating its systemic potential (Figure 4C). To fully demonstrate that BPA promoted allergic sensitization, we measured OVA-specific IgE antibodies in serum. Again, only mice receiving both BPA and OVA showed significant antigen sensitization (Figure 4D).

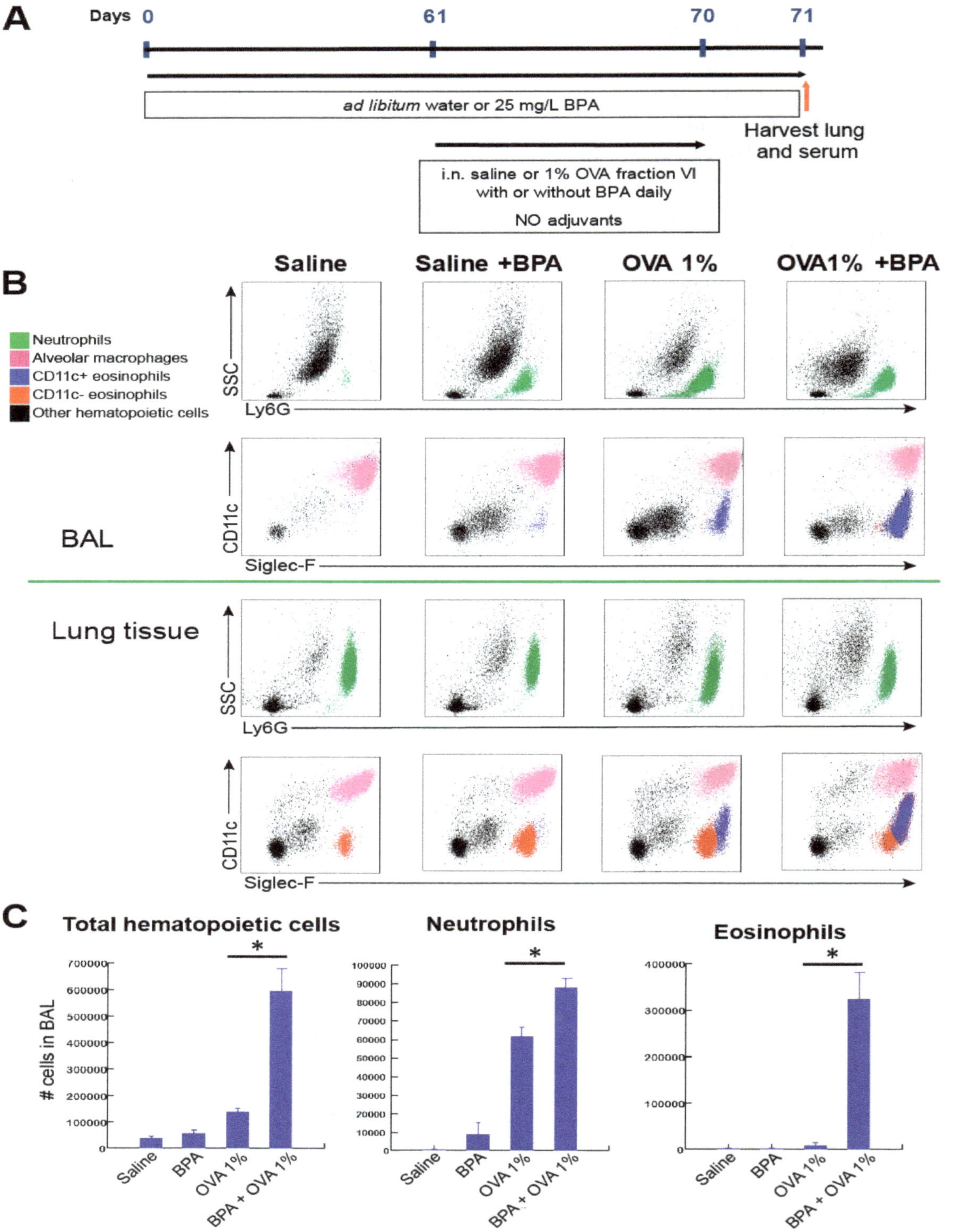

Figure 3. Chronic systemic exposure to BPA facilitates the development of allergic inflammation in a murine tolerogenic ovalbumin (OVA) treatment protocol. (**A**) BPA administration and OVA antigen challenge treatment timeline. (**B**) Flow cytometry analysis of leukocyte inflammatory response. Top charts, leukocyte populations measured in bronchoalveolar lavage; bottom charts, leukocyte responses measured in homogenized lung tissue. (**C**) Quantification of numbers of recruited cells in BALs by flow cytometry. N = 2 in saline group, N = 3-4 mice in treatment groups, all data shown from experiment performed one time. *, $p < 0.05$ by ANOVA.

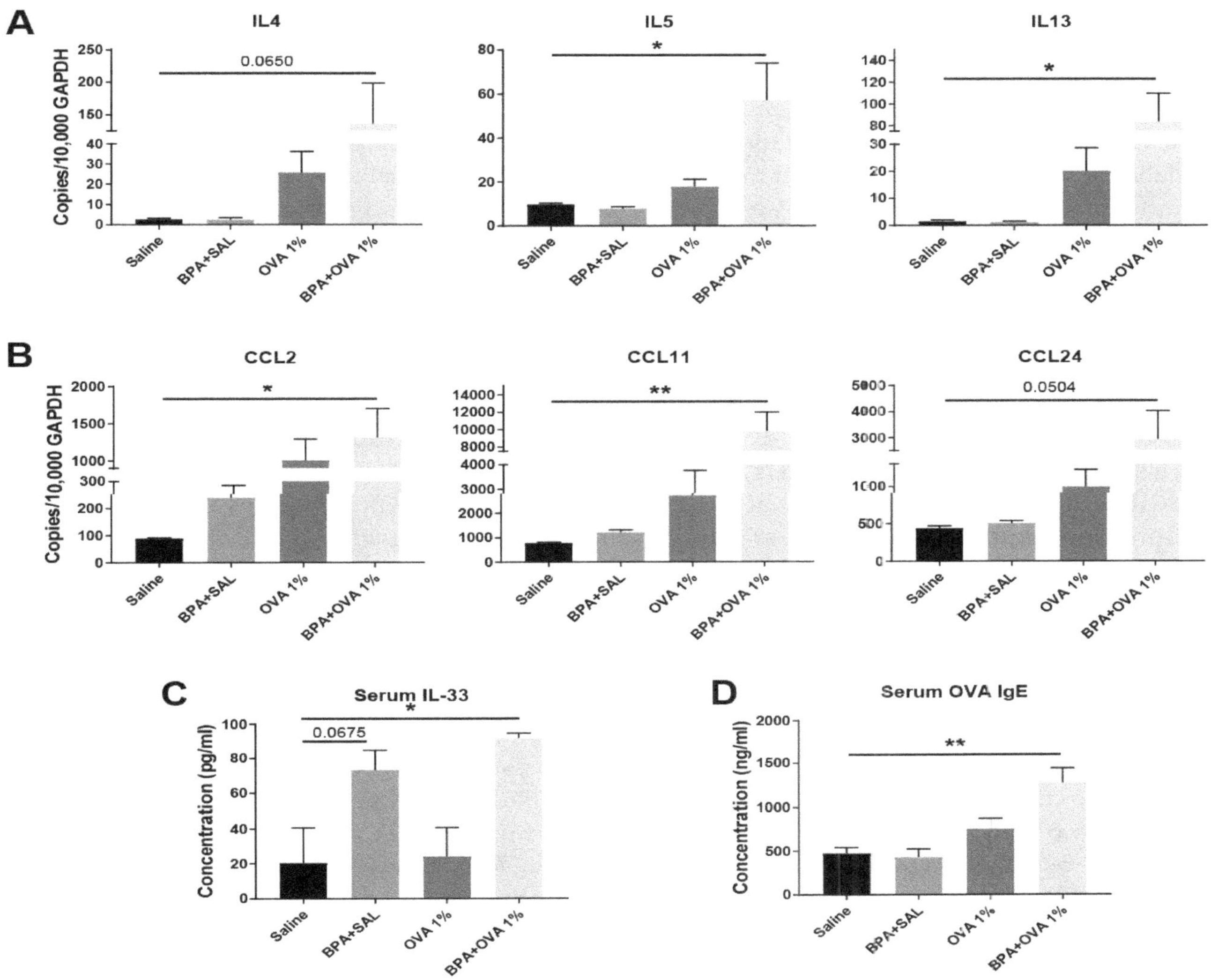

Figure 4. Chronic systemic BPA exposure induces allergic sensitization to innocuous OVA antigen exposure followed by the expression of Type 2 immune mediators. (**A**) Lung tissue expression of Type 2 cytokines by qPCR. (**B**) Lung tissue expression of chemokines by qPCR. (**C**) Serum protein levels of alarmin cytokine IL-33 by ELISA. (**D**) Serum levels of OVA-specific IgE antibodies by ELISA. N = 2 in saline group, N = 3-4 mice in treatment groups; all data shown from an experiment performed one time. *, $p < 0.05$, **, $p < 0.01$ by ANOVA.

4. Discussion

In this study, we tested whether xenoestrogen BPA, which is ubiquitous in the food and water supply of developed countries, promotes the endogenous systemic disruption of epithelial barriers and contributes to the initiation of allergic responses. With a total worldwide production capacity exceeding 6 billion pounds per year, BPA is one of the highest volume chemicals in commercial production today due to its widespread use in the production of plastics and flame retardants [14]. The ester bond linking BPA molecules in polycarbonates and resins undergoes hydrolysis, resulting in the release of low levels of free BPA into food, the water supply, and the environment. Measurements of unconjugated BPA in human blood, tissues, and urine in the United States, European Union, and Japan show higher than predicted levels, suggesting continuous exposure to significant amounts of BPA [14]. Normal functioning of the endocrine system is critical in the maintenance of multiple systemic homeostatic processes, including metabolism, normal neuroendocrine and immune function, and tissue homeostatic maintenance and renewal [28–30]. Sex steroids, in particular estrogens (aside from their function in reproduction and sexual development), are critical in maintaining systemic homeostasis in both sexes [19,28,31–33]. Given the centrality of hormones in the maintenance of systemic homeostasis, it is not surprising that epidemiological and experimental research studies link endocrine disruption by xenoestrogens to inflammatory diseases, cancer, metabolic syndrome, and neuroendocrine and reproductive abnormalities [34–36]. Mouse models suggest that BPA exacerbates allergic inflammation [37–40] and that maternal exposure to BPA enhances the development of allergic inflammation in offspring [15]. There are multiple epidemiological studies linking bisphenol exposures (typically measured in urine) to the development of asthma and other allergic conditions [41–43]. For example, higher postnatal urinary BPA concentrations were associated significantly with asthma in inner-city children [16]. The concentrations of BPA that we used in this study likely correspond only to high-end human exposures, since an acceptable daily human intake of BPA is typically 1000-fold below the NOAEL, and human serum levels of BPA range between 0.2 and 20 ng/mL [44]. However, our study was not aiming to represent daily human intake, but rather to add to the discovery of immune processes driven by "low-dose" BPA exposures typical for murine studies.

Tissue and epithelial homeostasis is maintained by balancing cell proliferation, differentiation, and death. It is well established that the nuclear receptor superfamily controls homeostasis by mediating the regulatory activities of many hormones, growth factors, and metabolites [45–48]. Estrogen receptors were shown to intricately interact with the WNT and Notch developmental pathways for the maintenance of epithelial homeostasis [21]. Consistent with this, we found that BPA could disrupt epithelium in a non-damaging manner via interfering with proliferation. Moreover, epithelial cells cultured with BPA expressed innate alarmin cytokine TSLP, which was also observed in study of BPA epithelial biology by Tajiki-Nishino et al. [37]. In support of these observations, it has been published that Notch-deficient keratinocytes fail to differentiate and release high levels of TSLP, which is critical to the development of allergic diseases [49]. More studies in the literature suggest that chronic BPA exposure could also affect the proliferation of epithelial basal progenitor cells [50]. Epithelial cells are known to produce innate cytokines in response to numerous stimuli [51]. The knockdown of filaggrin and E-cadherin induces the mRNA expression of TSLP through the epidermal growth factor receptor (EGFR) signaling pathways [52,53]. Importantly, Notch signaling and cellular receptors (protease-activated receptors (PARs), retinoic acid, and peroxisome proliferator-activated receptors (PPARs)) have regulatory activity for TSLP [49,51]. Studies of estrogen show similar effects to the results reported here for BPA, which is likely because both signal via a common pathway. In particular, estrogen has been demonstrated to induce the secretion of TSLP from human endometrial stromal cells in a dose-dependent manner [54]. Estrogen has also been shown to negatively regulate epithelial wound healing in multiple mouse and human studies [55–58]. Whether steroid hormones and xenoestrogens directly regulate TSLP and alarmin production by human epithelium warrants further investigation.

While evaluating in vivo epithelial barrier responses (skin, gut, airway) to systemic BPA exposure, we found that BPA significantly promoted the expression of Ccl1 and Ifnγ at more than one barrier site. Multiple mediators that are regulatory for the tissue innate immune system showed trending but not significant expression consistent with low-grade inflammatory response. Among them, chemokine Ccl1 is known to promote the recruitment of monocytes and eosinophils to tissue during the development of allergic inflammation [59]. Cxcl9, Cxcl10, and Cxcl11 are a family of interferon gamma-induced chemoattractant proteins stimulatory for the recruitment of monocytes, dendritic cells, and T cells to tissue. The induction of such responses is known to facilitate the inception of Type 2 sensitization [60]. Moreover, we found a significant increase in serum IL-33 protein levels after BPA exposure only. Such systemic action of BPA reported by us and others is consistent with the concept of a para-inflammatory response [61], which is likely mediated by its systemic interference with estrogen homeostatic signaling. Para-inflammation is a tissue adaptive response to persistent stress (distinct from direct injury and infection) to restore tissue functionality and homeostasis. It is thought to underlie the chronic inflammatory conditions associated with modern human diseases [62].

In our mouse experiments, such a systemically induced para-inflammatory state was sufficient to promote spontaneous, adjuvant-free sensitization as well as development of allergic inflammation. Although several previous studies examined the effect of oral and/or intratracheal BPA exposure on allergic responses in juvenile and adult mice, BPA was reported only as an exacerbating or aggravating factor in the development of allergic airway inflammation [37–40]. However, they parallel our results by showing the inflammatory-inducing potential of BPA in vivo via different exposure routes and the lack of necessity for standard adjuvants in these models. Our study, using a tolerogenic exposure protocol to low doses of highly purified OVA antigen, confirms that the ingestion of BPA is not only aggravating but is a sufficient factor to facilitate allergic sensitization. Thus, we would like to bring to attention that BPA may play an upstream role in sensitization via its ability to promote a para-inflammatory state, which warrants further mechanistic investigation. It is likely that multiple xenoestrogens, as well as other natural and systemic chemicals in our food supply, are capable of inducing similar systemic effects, possibly at different concentration ranges or exposure durations. Our study used bisphenol A as a prototypical xenoestrogen to emphasize the systemic inflammatory potential of endogenous endocrine dysregulation and suggest its potentially critical upstream role in promoting allergic responses.

5. Conclusions

The Endocrine disruption potential of BPA stems from its potential to interfere with epithelial homeostatic signals regulated by estrogen. We show that BPA exposure interferes with epithelial proliferation and triggers innate inflammatory responses from epithelial cells in vitro and systemically in vivo. Such systemic para-inflammatory response would present fertile ground for allergic sensitization, which we indeed observed in our brief study. Further mechanistic studies are needed to test conclusively whether endocrine disruption may play an upstream role in allergic sensitization via induction of a para-inflammatory state.

Author Contributions: S.B. conceived and designed the study. L.F.L. and S.B. performed experiments and contributed intellectually. L.F.L., M.E.C., and S.B. analyzed the data. M.E.C. and S.B. prepared the figures. L.F.L., M.E.C., and S.B. interpreted the results. The manuscript was written by S.B. and M.E.C. The final version of the manuscript was approved by S.B. All authors have read and agreed to the published version of the manuscript.

References

1. Van Ree, R.; Hummelshoj, L.; Plantinga, M.; Poulsen, L.K.; Swindle, E. Allergic sensitization: Host-immune factors. *Clin. Transl. Allergy* **2014**, *4*, 12. [CrossRef] [PubMed]
2. Jarvinen, K.M.; Konstantinou, G.N.; Pilapil, M.; Arrieta, M.C.; Noone, S.; Sampson, H.A.; Meddings, J.; Nowak-Wegrzyn, A. Intestinal permeability in children with food allergy on specific elimination diets. *Pediatr. Allergy Immunol.* **2013**, *24*, 589–595. [CrossRef] [PubMed]
3. Wolf, R.; Wolf, D. Abnormal epidermal barrier in the pathogenesis of atopic dermatitis. *Clin. Dermatol.* **2012**, *30*, 329–334. [CrossRef] [PubMed]
4. Xiao, C.; Puddicombe, S.M.; Field, S.; Haywood, J.; Broughton-Head, V.; Puxeddu, I.; Haitchi, H.M.; Vernon-Wilson, E.; Sammut, D.; Bedke, N.; et al. Defective epithelial barrier function in asthma. *J. Allergy Clin. Immunol.* **2011**, *128*, 549–556 e541-512. [CrossRef]
5. Perrier, C.; Corthesy, B. Gut permeability and food allergies. *Clin. Exp. Allergy* **2011**, *41*, 20–28. [CrossRef]
6. Fallon, P.G.; Sasaki, T.; Sandilands, A.; Campbell, L.E.; Saunders, S.P.; Mangan, N.E.; Callanan, J.J.; Kawasaki, H.; Shiohama, A.; Kubo, A.; et al. A homozygous frameshift mutation in the mouse Flg gene facilitates enhanced percutaneous allergen priming. *Nat. Genet.* **2009**, *41*, 602–608. [CrossRef]

7. Chan, L.S.; Robinson, N.; Xu, L. Expression of interleukin-4 in the epidermis of transgenic mice results in a pruritic inflammatory skin disease: An experimental animal model to study atopic dermatitis. *J. Invest. Dermatol.* **2001**, *117*, 977–983. [CrossRef]
8. Li, B.; Zou, Z.; Meng, F.; Raz, E.; Huang, Y.; Tao, A.; Ai, Y. Dust mite-derived Der f 3 activates a pro-inflammatory program in airway epithelial cells via PAR-1 and PAR-2. *Mol. Immunol.* **2019**, *109*, 1–11. [CrossRef]
9. Hiraishi, Y.; Yamaguchi, S.; Yoshizaki, T.; Nambu, A.; Shimura, E.; Takamori, A.; Narushima, S.; Nakanishi, W.; Asada, Y.; Numata, T.; et al. IL-33, IL-25 and TSLP contribute to development of fungal-associated protease-induced innate-type airway inflammation. *Sci. Rep.* **2018**, *8*, 18052. [CrossRef]
10. Schleimer, R.P.; Berdnikovs, S. Etiology of epithelial barrier dysfunction in patients with type 2 inflammatory diseases. *J. Allergy Clin. Immunol.* **2017**, *139*, 1752–1761. [CrossRef]
11. Bonds, R.S.; Midoro-Horiuti, T. Estrogen effects in allergy and asthma. *Curr. Opin. Allergy Clin. Immunol.* **2013**, *13*, 92–99. [CrossRef] [PubMed]
12. Rashid, H.; Alqahtani, S.S.; Alshahrani, S. Diet: A Source of Endocrine Disruptors. *Endocr. Metab. Immune Disord. Drug Targets* **2019**. [CrossRef] [PubMed]
13. Paterni, I.; Granchi, C.; Minutolo, F. Risks and benefits related to alimentary exposure to xenoestrogens. *Crit. Rev. Food Sci. Nutr.* **2017**, *57*, 3384–3404. [CrossRef] [PubMed]
14. Welshons, W.V.; Nagel, S.C.; vom Saal, F.S. Large effects from small exposures. III. Endocrine mechanisms mediating effects of bisphenol A at levels of human exposure. *Endocrinology* **2006**, *147*, S56–S69. [CrossRef] [PubMed]
15. Nakajima, Y.; Goldblum, R.M.; Midoro-Horiuti, T. Fetal exposure to bisphenol A as a risk factor for the development of childhood asthma: An animal model study. *Environ. Health* **2012**, *11*, 8. [CrossRef]
16. Donohue, K.M.; Miller, R.L.; Perzanowski, M.S.; Just, A.C.; Hoepner, L.A.; Arunajadai, S.; Canfield, S.; Resnick, D.; Calafat, A.M.; Perera, F.P.; et al. Prenatal and postnatal bisphenol A exposure and asthma development among inner-city children. *J. Allergy Clin. Immunol.* **2013**, *131*, 736–742. [CrossRef]
17. Houston, T.J.; Ghosh, R. Untangling the association between environmental endocrine disruptive chemicals and the etiology of male genitourinary cancers. *Biochem. Pharmacol.* **2019**, 113743. [CrossRef]
18. Verdier-Sevrain, S.; Bonte, F.; Gilchrest, B. Biology of estrogens in skin: Implications for skin aging. *Exp. Dermatol.* **2006**, *15*, 83–94. [CrossRef]
19. Morani, A.; Warner, M.; Gustafsson, J.A. Biological functions and clinical implications of oestrogen receptors alfa and beta in epithelial tissues. *J. Intern. Med.* **2008**, *264*, 128–142. [CrossRef]
20. Fu, X.D.; Simoncini, T. Extra-nuclear signaling of estrogen receptors. *IUBMB Life* **2008**, *60*, 502–510. [CrossRef]
21. Roarty, K.; Rosen, J.M. Wnt and mammary stem cells: Hormones cannot fly wingless. *Curr. Opin. Pharmacol.* **2010**, *10*, 643–649. [CrossRef] [PubMed]
22. Skandalis, S.S.; Afratis, N.; Smirlaki, G.; Nikitovic, D.; Theocharis, A.D.; Tzanakakis, G.N.; Karamanos, N.K. Cross-talk between estradiol receptor and EGFR/IGF-IR signaling pathways in estrogen-responsive breast cancers: Focus on the role and impact of proteoglycans. *Matrix Biol.* **2014**, *35*, 182–193. [CrossRef] [PubMed]
23. Zhang, Y.; Yi, B.; Zhou, X.; Wu, Y.; Wang, L. Overexpression Of ERbeta Participates In The Progression Of Liver Cancer Via Inhibiting The Notch Signaling Pathway. *Onco Targets Ther.* **2019**, *12*, 8715–8724. [CrossRef] [PubMed]
24. De Francesco, E.M.; Maggiolini, M.; Musti, A.M. Crosstalk between Notch, HIF-1alpha and GPER in Breast Cancer EMT. *Int. J. Mol. Sci.* **2018**, *19*, 2011. [CrossRef] [PubMed]
25. Hou, X.; Tan, Y.; Li, M.; Dey, S.K.; Das, S.K. Canonical Wnt signaling is critical to estrogen-mediated uterine growth. *Mol. Endocrinol.* **2004**, *18*, 3035–3049. [CrossRef] [PubMed]
26. Abdala Valencia, H.; Loffredo, L.F.; Misharin, A.V.; Berdnikovs, S. Phenotypic plasticity and targeting of Siglec-F(high) CD11c(low) eosinophils to the airway in a murine model of asthma. *Allergy* **2016**, *71*, 267–271. [CrossRef]
27. Bryce, P.J.; Geha, R.; Oettgen, H.C. Desloratadine inhibits allergen-induced airway inflammation and bronchial hyperresponsiveness and alters T-cell responses in murine models of asthma. *J. Allergy Clin. Immunol.* **2003**, *112*, 149–158. [CrossRef]
28. Foryst-Ludwig, A.; Kintscher, U. Metabolic impact of estrogen signalling through ERalpha and ERbeta. *J. Steroid Biochem. Mol. Biol.* **2010**, *122*, 74–81. [CrossRef]

29. Honeth, G.; Lombardi, S.; Ginestier, C.; Hur, M.; Marlow, R.; Buchupalli, B.; Shinomiya, I.; Gazinska, P.; Bombelli, S.; Ramalingam, V.; et al. Aldehyde dehydrogenase and estrogen receptor define a hierarchy of cellular differentiation in the normal human mammary epithelium. *Breast Cancer Res.* **2014**, *16*, R52. [CrossRef]
30. Wang, M.H.; Baskin, L.S. Endocrine disruptors, genital development, and hypospadias. *J. Androl.* **2008**, *29*, 499–505. [CrossRef]
31. Barros, R.P.; Gustafsson, J.A. Estrogen receptors and the metabolic network. *Cell Metab.* **2011**, *14*, 289–299. [CrossRef] [PubMed]
32. Faulds, M.H.; Zhao, C.; Dahlman-Wright, K.; Gustafsson, J.A. The diversity of sex steroid action: Regulation of metabolism by estrogen signaling. *J. Endocrinol.* **2012**, *212*, 3–12. [CrossRef] [PubMed]
33. Munoz-Cruz, S.; Togno-Pierce, C.; Morales-Montor, J. Non-reproductive effects of sex steroids: Their immunoregulatory role. *Curr. Top. Med. Chem.* **2011**, *11*, 1714–1727. [CrossRef] [PubMed]
34. Schug, T.T.; Janesick, A.; Blumberg, B.; Heindel, J.J. Endocrine disrupting chemicals and disease susceptibility. *J. Steroid Biochem. Mol. Biol.* **2011**, *127*, 204–215. [CrossRef]
35. Rochester, J.R. Bisphenol A and human health: A review of the literature. *Reprod. Toxicol.* **2013**, *42*, 132–155. [CrossRef]
36. Crews, D.; McLachlan, J.A. Epigenetics, evolution, endocrine disruption, health, and disease. *Endocrinology* **2006**, *147*, S4–S10. [CrossRef]
37. Tajiki-Nishino, R.; Makino, E.; Watanabe, Y.; Tajima, H.; Ishimota, M.; Fukuyama, T. Oral Administration of Bisphenol A Directly Exacerbates Allergic Airway Inflammation but Not Allergic Skin Inflammation in Mice. *Toxicol. Sci.* **2018**, *165*, 314–321. [CrossRef]
38. Koike, E.; Yanagisawa, R.; Win-Shwe, T.T.; Takano, H. Exposure to low-dose bisphenol A during the juvenile period of development disrupts the immune system and aggravates allergic airway inflammation in mice. *Int. J. Immunopathol. Pharmacol.* **2018**, *32*, 2058738418774897. [CrossRef]
39. He, M.; Ichinose, T.; Yoshida, S.; Takano, H.; Nishikawa, M.; Shibamoto, T.; Sun, G. Exposure to bisphenol A enhanced lung eosinophilia in adult male mice. *Allergy Asthma Clin. Immunol.* **2016**, *12*, 16. [CrossRef]
40. Yanagisawa, R.; Koike, E.; Win-Shwe, T.T.; Takano, H. Oral exposure to low dose bisphenol A aggravates allergic airway inflammation in mice. *Toxicol. Rep.* **2019**, *6*, 1253–1262. [CrossRef]
41. Mendy, A.; Salo, P.M.; Wilkerson, J.; Feinstein, L.; Ferguson, K.K.; Fessler, M.B.; Thorne, P.S.; Zeldin, D.C. Association of urinary levels of bisphenols F and S used as bisphenol A substitutes with asthma and hay fever outcomes. *Environ. Res.* **2019**, 108944. [CrossRef]
42. Youssef, M.M.; El-Din, E.; AbuShady, M.M.; El-Baroudy, N.R.; Abd El Hamid, T.A.; Armaneus, A.F.; El Refay, A.S.; Hussein, J.; Medhat, D.; Latif, Y.A. Urinary bisphenol A concentrations in relation to asthma in a sample of Egyptian children. *Hum. Exp. Toxicol.* **2018**, *37*, 1180–1186. [CrossRef]
43. Zhou, A.; Chang, H.; Huo, W.; Zhang, B.; Hu, J.; Xia, W.; Chen, Z.; Xiong, C.; Zhang, Y.; Wang, Y.; et al. Prenatal exposure to bisphenol A and risk of allergic diseases in early life. *Pediatr. Res.* **2017**, *81*, 851–856. [CrossRef] [PubMed]
44. Vandenberg, L.N.; Hauser, R.; Marcus, M.; Olea, N.; Welshons, W.V. Human exposure to bisphenol A (BPA). *Reprod. Toxicol.* **2007**, *24*, 139–177. [CrossRef] [PubMed]
45. Ordonez-Moran, P.; Munoz, A. Nuclear receptors: Genomic and non-genomic effects converge. *Cell Cycle* **2009**, *8*, 1675–1680. [CrossRef] [PubMed]
46. Schmuth, M.; Watson, R.E.; Deplewski, D.; Dubrac, S.; Zouboulis, C.C.; Griffiths, C.E. Nuclear hormone receptors in human skin. *Horm. Metab. Res.* **2007**, *39*, 96–105. [CrossRef]
47. McPherson, S.J.; Ellem, S.J.; Risbridger, G.P. Estrogen-regulated development and differentiation of the prostate. *Differentiation* **2008**, *76*, 660–670. [CrossRef]
48. Boonyaratanakornkit, V.; Edwards, D.P. Receptor mechanisms mediating non-genomic actions of sex steroids. *Semin. Reprod. Med.* **2007**, *25*, 139–153. [CrossRef]
49. Demehri, S.; Liu, Z.; Lee, J.; Lin, M.H.; Crosby, S.D.; Roberts, C.J.; Grigsby, P.W.; Miner, J.H.; Farr, A.G.; Kopan, R. Notch-deficient skin induces a lethal systemic B-lymphoproliferative disorder by secreting TSLP, a sentinel for epidermal integrity. *PLoS Biol.* **2008**, *6*, e123. [CrossRef]
50. Lobaccaro, J.M.; Trousson, A. Environmental estrogen exposure during fetal life: A time bomb for prostate cancer. *Endocrinology* **2014**, *155*, 656–658. [CrossRef]

51. Takai, T. TSLP expression: Cellular sources, triggers, and regulatory mechanisms. *Allergol. Int.* **2012**, *61*, 3–17. [CrossRef]
52. Heijink, I.H.; Kies, P.M.; Kauffman, H.F.; Postma, D.S.; van Oosterhout, A.J.; Vellenga, E. Down-regulation of E-cadherin in human bronchial epithelial cells leads to epidermal growth factor receptor-dependent Th2 cell-promoting activity. *J. Immunol.* **2007**, *178*, 7678–7685. [CrossRef]
53. Lee, K.H.; Cho, K.A.; Kim, J.Y.; Kim, J.Y.; Baek, J.H.; Woo, S.Y.; Kim, J.W. Filaggrin knockdown and Toll-like receptor 3 (TLR3) stimulation enhanced the production of thymic stromal lymphopoietin (TSLP) from epidermal layers. *Exp. Dermatol.* **2011**, *20*, 149–151. [CrossRef]
54. Chang, K.K.; Liu, L.B.; Li, H.; Mei, J.; Shao, J.; Xie, F.; Li, M.Q.; Li, D.J. TSLP induced by estrogen stimulates secretion of MCP-1 and IL-8 and growth of human endometrial stromal cells through JNK and NF-kappaB signal pathways. *Int. J. Clin. Exp. Pathol.* **2014**, *7*, 1889–1899.
55. Wang, S.B.; Hu, K.M.; Seamon, K.J.; Mani, V.; Chen, Y.; Gronert, K. Estrogen negatively regulates epithelial wound healing and protective lipid mediator circuits in the cornea. *FASEB J.* **2012**, *26*, 1506–1516. [CrossRef] [PubMed]
56. Mukai, K.; Nakajima, Y.; Asano, K.; Nakatani, T. Topical estrogen application to wounds promotes delayed cutaneous wound healing in 80-week-old female mice. *PLoS ONE* **2019**, *14*, e0225880. [CrossRef] [PubMed]
57. Hardman, M.J.; Ashcroft, G.S. Estrogen, not intrinsic aging, is the major regulator of delayed human wound healing in the elderly. *Genome Biol.* **2008**, *9*, R80. [CrossRef] [PubMed]
58. Mukai, K.; Nakajima, Y.; Urai, T.; Komatsu, E.; Nasruddin; Sugama, J.; Nakatani, T. 17beta-Estradiol administration promotes delayed cutaneous wound healing in 40-week ovariectomised female mice. *Int. Wound J.* **2016**, *13*, 636–644. [CrossRef]
59. Bishop, B.; Lloyd, C.M. CC chemokine ligand 1 promotes recruitment of eosinophils but not Th2 cells during the development of allergic airways disease. *J. Immunol.* **2003**, *170*, 4810–4817. [CrossRef]
60. Rowe, J.; Heaton, T.; Kusel, M.; Suriyaarachchi, D.; Serralha, M.; Holt, B.J.; de Klerk, N.; Sly, P.D.; Holt, P.G. High IFN-gamma production by CD8+ T cells and early sensitization among infants at high risk of atopy. *J. Allergy Clin. Immunol.* **2004**, *113*, 710–716. [CrossRef]
61. Chovatiya, R.; Medzhitov, R. Stress, inflammation, and defense of homeostasis. *Mol. Cell* **2014**, *54*, 281–288. [CrossRef] [PubMed]
62. Medzhitov, R. Origin and physiological roles of inflammation. *Nature* **2008**, *454*, 428–435. [CrossRef] [PubMed]

13

Optimizing Nutrition Assessment to Create Better Outcomes in Lung Transplant Recipients

Mara Weber Gulling [1], Monica Schaefer [1], Laura Bishop-Simo [1] and Brian C. Keller [2,*]

1 Nutrition Services, The Ohio State University Wexner Medical Center, Columbus, OH 43210, USA; Mara.Weber@osumc.edu (M.W.G.); Monica.Schaefer@osumc.edu (M.S.); Laura.Bishop-Simo@osumc.edu (L.B.-S.)

2 Division of Pulmonary, Critical Care & Sleep Medicine, The Ohio State University College of Medicine, Columbus, OH 43210, USA

* Correspondence: Brian.Keller2@osumc.edu

Abstract: Lung transplantation offers patients with end-stage lung disease an opportunity for a better quality of life, but with limited organ availability it is paramount that selected patients have the best opportunity for successful outcomes. Nutrition plays a central role in post-surgical outcomes and, historically, body mass index (BMI) has been used as the de facto method of assessing a lung transplant candidate's nutritional status. Here, we review the historical origins of BMI in lung transplantation, summarize the current BMI literature, and review studies of alternative/complementary body composition assessment tools, including lean psoas area, creatinine-height index, leptin, and dual x-ray absorptiometry. These body composition measures quantify lean body mass versus fat mass and may provide a more comprehensive analysis of a patient's nutritional state than BMI alone.

Keywords: lung transplantation; body mass index; nutrition; body composition; lean body mass; muscle mass; leptin; sarcopenia; creatinine-height index

---

Institutional lung transplant patient selection committees are faced with a daunting task: to accurately and expediently identify and predict candidates with a high likelihood of success following lung transplantation. The selection process involves a rigorous and comprehensive evaluation of the potential candidate's medical and surgical comorbidities, physical fitness and potential for improvement, and social and financial support. Also included in this assessment—though sometimes overlooked in its importance, particularly in the setting of critically ill patients—is nutritional status. In this review, we discuss the pre-transplant evaluation of nutritional status in patients with end-stage lung disease which, historically, has utilized the body mass index (BMI), and we discuss recent developments that may enhance our future ability to more finely characterize a candidate's preoperative nutritional status with the aim of better prognosticating outcomes after lung transplantation.

1. Lung Transplant Candidate Selection

Lung transplantation is the definitive treatment for end-stage lung disease and offers these patients the opportunity for better quality of life. Lung transplant rates continue to increase, with 2345 lung transplants performed in the USA in 2016. Yet, at the end of the year, 1395 candidates remained on the waiting list [1]. Despite the rise in numbers of transplants performed, survival outcomes after lung transplantation remain far lower than those of other solid organs, with a median survival of approximately 6 years [2]. Given the limited number of organs available and, in contrast, the large number of individuals awaiting transplantation, it is paramount that patients selected for transplant have the best potential for successful outcomes.

The Ohio State University Transplant Center follows a comprehensive lung transplant patient evaluation process based on the recommendations of The International Society for Heart & Lung Transplantation (ISHLT) [3]. Patients undergo an extensive review of their medical, surgical, family, social, medication, and allergy history. Pulmonary tests include chest radiography, chest computed tomography, quantitative lung perfusion, spirometry with lung volumes and diffusion capacity for carbon monoxide, 6-min walk test, and room air arterial blood gas testing. Cardiac and gastrointestinal testing includes echocardiogram and right/left heart catheterization and gastric emptying, esophageal pH testing, and esophageal manometry, respectively. Patients are screened for infectious diseases via survey and bloodwork, and health maintenance screenings are updated. Psychosocial evaluations are performed by social workers and/or psychologists/psychiatrists, and all potential candidates undergo a nutrition evaluation by a registered dietitian. Finally, a financial assessment, including insurance, is completed before the patient is brought to the patient selection committee.

Despite best efforts to select the most suitable candidates, there are areas for improvement. As described above, there are many facets to lung transplant candidate evaluation, including nutrition status. Within the realm of nutrition is a patient's body composition and state of nourishment. Use of historical as well as novel tools can facilitate a more objective assessment of a patient's body composition and nutrition status and potentially identify targets for early or aggressive intervention. Given that this area of medical science is young and developing, expert opinion has been the basis of much of the criteria available [4].

2. Nutrition Evaluation

When a patient is referred to our center, a preliminary nutrition screening is performed over the phone by a pre-transplant nurse coordinator who collects the patient's height and weight for the calculation of BMI. For the purpose of this article and the studies reviewed, BMI is calculated as weight (kg) divided by height^2 (m^2). Weight ranges are based on the World Health Organization (WHO) classification scheme: underweight (<18.5 kg/m^2); normal weight (18.5–24.9 kg/m^2); overweight (25–29.9 kg/m^2); and obese (>30 kg/m^2) [5].

A transplant pulmonologist completes an initial in-person assessment, and should the patient be deemed appropriate for full evaluation, additional consults and tests are arranged [6], including a full nutrition assessment with the transplant dietitian. The full nutrition evaluation has evolved and involves reviewing the history of present illness; past medical, surgical, and social histories; medication review; activity level, including review of 6-min walk test results; and diet history, including current diet, eating behaviors, current symptoms affecting oral intake, diabetes history, weight history, previous weight gain/loss attempts, food allergies, current and past use of oral nutrition supplement products, and a Nutrition Focused Physical Exam (hand grip currently not performed) [6]. Patients are then assigned a malnutrition diagnosis based on the 2012 Academy of Nutrition and Dietetics/American Society for Parental and Enteral Nutrition (AND/ASPEN) Guidelines [7], and an assessment is made of relative and absolute contraindications based on transplant center policy, transplant nutrition-related experience, and nutrition diagnosis. Finally, an individualized nutrition plan of care/goals, based on the patient and their readiness for change, resources available, severity of illness, and other factors, is developed. Additional support from other nutrition providers is utilized when possible, including comprehensive weight management services, nutrition care associated with pulmonary rehabilitation, and diabetes management, as well as other appropriate services dependent on patient needs and willingness/ability to participate.

Following completion of the pre-transplant assessment and testing, patients are presented at the Lung Transplant Patient Selection Committee for multidisciplinary team review. Relative and absolute contraindications are reviewed, including those that are pertinent from a nutrition perspective. Generally, much like the ISHLT Pulmonary Council, our center considers an absolute contraindication to lung transplant to be class II or III obesity (BMI $\geq$ 35 kg/m^2) [3]; obese individuals are, however, evaluated on a case by case basis and offered support to achieve a more desirable weight.

Relative contraindications associated with nutrition care include class I obesity (BMI > 30–34.9 kg/m^2), underweight BMI < 17 kg/m^2, cachexia, and malnutrition, as well as uncontrolled diabetes and osteoporosis [3]. For the purposes of this review, we focus on the use of BMI and malnutrition in the lung transplant evaluation and subsequent outcomes (Table 1).

Table 1. Summary of studies reviewed.

Author	Year	Study Type	Number of Patients	Nutrition Assessment	Results
Plöchl [8]	1996	Single center, retrospective	51	BMI	BMI in lowest quartile associated with ICU mortality in patients requiring >5-day ICU LOS
Schwebel [9]	2000	Single center, retrospective	78	CHI	Low lean body mass associated with more severe hypoxemia, reduced 6MWT, and higher mortality pre-transplant and longer post-transplant mechanical ventilation and ICU LOS
Madill [10]	2001	Single center, retrospective	251	BMI	Higher risk of post-transplant 90-day mortality in patients with BMI of ≤17 kg/m^2 or ≥25 kg/m^2
Kanasky [5]	2002	Single center, retrospective	85	BMI	3X increased risk of post-transplant mortality for obese (BMI > 30 kg/m^2) patients, but no difference between overweight (BMI 25–29.9 kg/m^2) and normal weight patients
Singer [11]	2014	Multicenter, retrospective	599	Leptin/DXA	Elevated leptin levels, but not BMI 30–34.9 kg/m^2, were associated with increased mortality
Weig [12]	2016	Single center, retrospective	103	LPA	Lower LPA associated with longer mechanical ventilation, need for tracheostomy, and ICU LOS

6MWT: 6-min walk test; BMI: body mass index; CHI: creatinine-height index; DXA: dual x-ray absorptiometry; ICU: intensive care unit; LOS: length of stay; LPA: lean psoas area.

3. BMI-Based Nutrition Assessment

The nutritional needs of the lung transplant population are immensely varied; individualized nutrition prescriptions are necessary to best serve each person, which can create challenges when studying this population. Broadly, transplants are provided for patients with four categories of lung disease: obstructive, suppurative, restrictive, and vascular [4]. As a result, transplant recipients and their nutritional needs can vary from young underweight cystic fibrosis (CF) patients to the older chronic obstructive pulmonary disease and pulmonary fibrosis patients that may be obese. Across the board, patients' candidacy still relies in part on weight status, usually in the form of BMI.

Interestingly, BMI itself dates back to the 19th century, when Belgian Adolphe Quetelet suggested the premise that "the transverse growth of man is less than the vertical" [qtd. in 13] and thus derived the equation weight (kg) divided by height (m) squared. It was not until much later that Ancel Keys coined the term "body mass index" with evidence to support the theory [13]. While BMI has long been the standard method of assessing nutrition status in potential candidates because of its ease and low cost, it was not always so. In fact, in the inaugural 1998 guidelines for selection of lung transplant candidates, ideal body weight (IBW) was recommended as the measure of nutritional status. Patients with IBW <70% or >130% were required to gain or lose weight, respectively, in order to move forward with transplant [14].

Historically, underweight and obese lung transplant recipients have been linked with poor post-surgical outcomes, though studies have been conflicting [12]. The utility of BMI in predicting lung transplant outcomes came to light with Plöchl's report of increased intensive care unit (ICU) mortality in lung transplant recipients whose BMI was in the lowest quartile [8], though no difference was observed in ICU length of stay (LOS). Following this, studies by Madill et al. and Kanasky et al. in the early 2000s were the first to demonstrate longer term adverse outcomes in lung transplantation at the extremes of nutrition status as measured by BMI [5,10]. In the first study, recipients with BMI <17 kg/m^2 or >25 kg/m^2 were associated with higher risk of death in the first 90 days compared to those with BMI between 20–25 kg/m^2 [10]. Recipients with BMI >27 kg/m^2 were even more at risk, with a 5-fold higher odds ratio of death compared to the reference group. In a single-center retrospective review of 85 patients, Kanasky et al. found that patients classified as obese (BMI ≥ 30 kg/m^2) prior to transplantation had markedly shorter post-transplant survival times (40% survival at 20 months for BMI ≥ 30 kg/m^2 versus nearly 70% survival at 50 months for BMI < 30 kg/m^2). Underweight patients (BMI < 18.5 kg/m^2) had better survival in the first 50 months post-transplant compared to normal (18.5–24.9 kg/m^2) or overweight (25–29.9 kg/m^2) recipients, with a late marked decline thereafter [5], a departure from Plöchl's findings. In contrast to Madill's earlier study, there was no difference in survival between normal and overweight recipients.

Based on these studies, BMI was eventually incorporated as a component of the lung allocation score, a method of prioritizing lung transplant candidates, introduced in 2005 [15], and BMI > 30 kg/m^2 was included as a relative contraindication to transplant in the 2006 update of lung transplant candidate selection guidelines [16]. In the most recent 2014 update to the guidelines, class II or III obesity (BMI ≥ 35 kg/m^2) is now considered an absolute contraindication to lung transplant, while class I obesity (BMI 30–34.9 kg/m^2) remains a relative contraindication [3].

However, as newer methods for measuring body composition are developed, BMI's role as the sole measure of nutrition status in lung transplant candidates is now being questioned. Inconsistencies among the aforementioned studies may be due to BMI's inability to discriminate different body compositions (adipose tissue mass and muscle mass). Consequently, the use of BMI alone can place patients in a gray area when determining their transplant candidacy, especially for those who are asked to gain or lose weight prior to transplant listing, a difficult task in patients with end-stage lung disease. Therefore, use of alternative and complementary modalities to BMI may better delineate a candidate's nutrition status.

4. Creating Better Outcomes through Use of BMI Alternatives

Body composition can be computed a number of different ways, including, but not limited to, computed tomography (CT), magnetic resonance imaging (MRI), dual x-ray absorptiometry (DXA), and bioimpedance analysis (BIA). Both CT and MRI are considered the gold standards for estimating muscle mass in research [17]. Unfortunately, there are drawbacks (e.g., exposure to radiation, higher cost, and availability of equipment) to using these gold standard methods routinely in the clinic that may contribute to the continued use of BMI as a means of assessing candidates [18]. While BMI is most frequently used in the assessment of lung transplant candidates, our notion that body composition may produce better outcomes is not considered novel. Several studies, including those highlighted below, analyzed body composition through CT, DXA, as well as creatinine-height index (CHI), and measured leptin levels.

4.1. Lean Psoas Area

Sarcopenia is defined by decreased muscle mass and either low peripheral muscle strength or function and becomes more prevalent with aging [18]. Assessment of muscle tone therefore becomes that much more essential, particularly in lung transplant candidates, a population that has steadily increased in age [19]. Moreover, sarcopenia affects people of all weight classes. Core muscle size, estimated by lean psoas area (LPA) using CT scans, was evaluated as a predictor of postoperative outcomes in lung transplant recipients. LPA, not BMI, was associated with shorter duration of mechanical ventilation, reduced need for tracheostomy, and shorter ICU LOS [12]. Six-minute walk distance increased with increasing LPA and decreased with increasing BMI. Sarcopenia (measured as low LPA) was present in one-third of normal weight and one-fourth of overweight patients. On the other hand, half of the underweight population had normal or high LPA. While further studies are needed, it is likely that transplant outcomes will be less favorable in sarcopenic patients with normal or elevated BMI due to BMI's inability to account for body composition.

4.2. Leptin and DXA

In contrast to the aforementioned BMI studies, Singer et al. found that class I obesity (BMI 30–34.9) was not associated with one-year mortality after lung transplant [11]. However, using DXA and measured leptin levels, the authors identified a linkage between body composition and survival. Leptin, a satiety hormone produced by adipose cells, is required for energy balance [20]. Mutations in *LEP*, the gene encoding leptin, led to altered metabolism and the development of obesity [20]. Compared to BMI, leptin levels correlate more strongly with percent body fat [21]. In lung transplant recipients, higher preoperative plasma leptin levels were associated with increased one-year mortality in patients not requiring intraoperative cardiopulmonary bypass support. Body composition analysis with DXA identified obesity in 51% of patients with a normal BMI. Conversely, sarcopenia was noted in 46% of patients by DXA, whereas only 5% of patients were classified as underweight by BMI alone. This data suggests that nutrition analysis by BMI alone may be insufficient. For patients classified as underweight based on BMI, body composition analysis may have mitigated the need for pre-transplant weight gain and, thus, delay in transplant listing. The reverse is also true; patients with sarcopenic obesity could be educated on muscle mass maintenance rather than strict weight loss, which, in turn, may improve outcomes such as shortening post-transplant hospital LOS [22].

4.3. Creatinine-Height Index

The creatinine-height index (CHI) was developed in the 1970s as a measure of protein nutrition and lean muscle mass [23] and is calculated as:

$$\text{CHI} = \frac{\text{24 h urinary creatinine of subject}}{\text{expected 24 h urinary creatinine of person of same height and sex}} \times 100.$$

Comparing CHI and percent ideal body weight (IBW), Schwebel et al. noted that nutritional depletion was prevalent in lung transplant candidates and was a risk factor for higher mortality. In this study, 72% had some form of nutritional depletion, which included patients with weights <90% and ≥90% of IBW. Furthermore, lower 6-min walk distance and more severe hypoxemia were observed in individuals with a higher percent IBW but poorer lean body mass as estimated by CHI, even more so than those with low weight and low lean body mass. Therefore, lean body mass depletion is not exclusively tied to decreased body weight. This research supports the use of supplemental measures, like CHI, to more precisely assess nutritional status and ultimately predict post-transplant outcomes. The authors hypothesized that improving nutritional status pre-transplant might improve body composition quality and therefore reduce ICU LOS and overall costs [9].

5. Optimizing Nutrition in Lung Transplant Candidates

5.1. Outcomes in Relation to Nutritional State

With the understanding that nutrition, with time, can improve patient health before, during, and after transplantation, the role of the dietitian at each stage is essential. Unfortunately, disease states can progress quickly, and sometimes a patient's nutrition status may be less than ideal prior to surgery despite nutritional intervention. Following transplant, similar issues may be seen. Complications during the perioperative period or longer term can have detrimental effects on patient health. In the acute perioperative phase, nutrition's role includes promoting wound healing, preventing infection, and meeting a patient's macronutrient needs given their catabolic state. Further beyond transplant, nutrition's role shifts but continues to be paramount, assisting in healthy weight maintenance, aiding in blood glucose control, preventing chronic metabolic diseases, and reducing potential complications like graft rejection [24].

For those diagnosed with malnutrition, addressing weight loss and loss of lean body mass is imperative. A potential linkage between the degree of malnutrition and airflow obstruction has been reported [25]. Loss of lean body mass has been associated with a greater loss in lung function, reduced distance on 6-min walk test, and worsened hypoxemia [9,26]. Additionally, these patients are likelier to experience prolonged ICU LOS, days on mechanical ventilation, and increased mortality [8,10,12,27]. Similarly, pre-transplant serum prealbumin, a marker of both inflammation and nutrition status, has been linked to outcomes in lung transplant recipients, with low prealbumin levels (<18 g/dL) associated with a threefold higher risk of death than levels above 18 g/dL [27].

5.2. Weight Gains and Losses

For patients at the upper end or just above a program's maximally acceptable BMI, weight loss is likely to be recommended prior to transplant listing. Weight loss improves survival and perioperative morbidity and leads to reduced ICU LOS and duration of mechanical ventilation [28]. As previously mentioned, obese patients are at higher risk for complications, however, strict weight loss may not guarantee better outcomes, especially if it means a loss of muscle mass [11]. Rather, emphasis on healthful weight loss (loss of fat mass rather than muscle mass, an endeavor that takes a great deal of time, which may be limiting in lung transplant candidates) would prove to be more beneficial regarding post-transplant outcomes.

In the immediate postoperative period, patients experience a decline in weight and BMI despite the best efforts of dietary staff to improve their nutritional state pre-transplant. The postoperative catabolic state and potential intestinal absorption concerns following the initiation of anti-rejection medications may play an important role in this weight loss, such that oral intake alone may be insufficient in meeting nutritional needs, especially in patients severely malnourished prior to transplant [29]. This is important because postoperative malnutrition impacts morbidity and mortality through effects on immune cell and skeletal muscle function and impaired wound healing [30], leading to a 3-fold increased risk of nosocomial infection [29].

Beyond the immediate postoperative period, a median weight gain of 10% is anticipated [31]. While not an exhaustive list, weight gain after transplant may be a result of corticosteroid use, increased leptin levels, decreased resting energy expenditure, and reduced production of cachexia-associated cytokines [31]. While steroid use in transplant patients may contribute to weight gain, due to dose tapering, this weight gain may not contribute as much as anticipated [31,32]. The most substantial weight gain occurs during the first year, and patients with successful early post-transplant weight gain demonstrate better survival [31]. CF patients and younger patients also tend to gain more weight [31,33]. The reasons for this are still not clear, but may be due to better early lung allograft function, fewer pro-inflammatory cytokines, decreased work of breathing, or enhanced immunosuppressive efficacy.

5.3. Opportunities for Further Research

More studies are necessary to better define the role of pre-transplantation weight loss, nutrition counseling, and body composition on lung transplant outcomes, including survival and quality of life [28]. In addition to nutrition counseling, to best maintain muscle mass during intended periods of weight loss, candidates benefit from pulmonary rehabilitation (pre-habilitation) at regular intervals. However, the impact of pre-habilitation on nutrition status remains understudied. Some patients experience unintentional weight loss while awaiting transplant. How this might affect transplant outcomes compared to intentional weight loss is unknown. Lastly, even though nutrition counseling is provided, given the time patients may remain on the waiting list, the optimal frequency of nutrition consultations to best achieve and maintain a healthy nutritional state in patients awaiting transplant is unclear.

6. Conclusions

In this short review, we sought to review the use of BMI as a metric of nutrition status in the evaluation of potential lung transplant recipients. Because of its low cost, ease of use, and studies linking outcomes to BMI extremes, BMI ranges are currently utilized in published guidelines as absolute or relative contraindications to lung transplant. However, the use of BMI alone to assess nutrition status may lead to miscalculation of a candidate's true nutrition status. Body composition analysis through DXA, CHI, lean psoas area, or measured leptin levels can augment BMI through the identification of sarcopenia in overweight/obese patients or higher than anticipated lean muscle mass in underweight patients. Further, repeated measures in patients awaiting transplant can help to determine the success of pre-transplant nutritional interventions.

The role of the dietitian is critical in the multidisciplinary review of potential lung transplant candidates. Dietitians provide diet education and healthy weight loss counseling in overweight and obese patients, with emphasis on slow steady loss in coordination with pulmonary pre-habilitation services to prevent muscle wasting. In underweight patients, dietitians develop a strategy for healthfully gaining weight. They may provide oral nutrition supplements or suggest the initiation of nutrition support (enteral or parenteral) should it be deemed essential. With adequate time, as a result, patients may lose unwanted fat, gain muscle tone, and improve their overall nutrition status and candidacy for transplant. Similar measures can be taken following transplant to improve or maintain nutritional status with the goal of optimizing post-transplant outcomes.

Author Contributions: Project conceptualization: M.W.G., M.S., L.B.-S., and B.C.K.; writing—original draft preparation: M.W.G., M.S., and L.B.-S.; writing—review and editing: M.W.G., M.S., L.B.-S., and B.C.K.; supervision: B.C.K.; project administration: B.C.K.

References

1. Valapour, M.; Lehr, C.J.; Skeans, M.A.; Smith, J.M.; Carrico, R.; Uccellini, K.; Lehman, R.; Robinson, A.; Israni, A.K.; Snyder, J.J.; et al. OPTN/SRTR 2016 Annual Data Report: Lung. *Am. J. Transplant.* **2018**, *18* (Suppl. 1), 363–433. [CrossRef]
2. Clausen, E.S.; Frankel, C.; Palmer, S.M.; Snyder, L.D.; Smith, P.J. Pre-transplant weight loss and clinical outcomes after lung transplantation. *J. Heart Lung Transplant.* **2018**, *37*, 1443–1447. [CrossRef]
3. Weill, D.; Benden, C.; Corris, P.A.; Dark, J.H.; Davis, R.D.; Keshavjee, S.; Lederer, D.J.; Mulligan, M.J.; Patterson, G.A.; Singer, L.G.; et al. A consensus document for the selection of lung transplant candidates: 2014—An update from the Pulmonary Transplantation Council of the International Society for Heart and Lung Transplantation. *J. Heart Lung Transplant.* **2015**, *34*, 1–15. [CrossRef]
4. Jomphe, V.; Lands, L.C.; Mailhot, G. Nutritional Requirements of Lung Transplant Recipients: Challenges and Considerations. *Nutrients* **2018**, *10*. [CrossRef]
5. Kanasky, W.F.; Anton, S.D.; Rodrigue, J.R.; Perri, M.G.; Szwed, T.; Baz, M.A. Impact of Body Weight on Long-term Survival After Lung Transplantation. *Chest* **2002**, *121*, 401–406. [CrossRef]
6. Hasse, J.M. Nutrition Assessment and Support of Organ Transplant Recipients. *J. Parenter. Enter. Nutr.* **2001**, *25*, 120–131. [CrossRef]
7. White, J.V.; Guenter, P.; Jensen, G.; Malone, A.; Schofield, M. Consensus Statement: Academy of Nutrition and Dietetics and American Society for Parenteral and Enteral Nutrition. *J. Parenter. Enter. Nutr.* **2012**, *36*, 275–283. [CrossRef]
8. Plöchl, W.; Pezawas, L.; Hiesmayr, M.; Artemiou, O.; Grimm, M.; Klepetko, W. Nutritional status, ICU duration and ICU mortality in lung transplant recipients. *Intensive Care Med.* **1996**, *22*, 1179–1185. [CrossRef]
9. Schwebel, C.; Pin, I.; Barnoud, D.; Devouassoux, G.; Brichon, P.Y.; Chaffanjon, P.; Chavanon, O.; Sessa, C.; Blin, D.; Guignier, M.; et al. Prevalence and conseqences of nutritional depletion in lung transplant candidates. *Eur. Respir. J.* **2000**, *16*, 1050–1055. [CrossRef]
10. Madill, J.; Gutierrez, C.; Grossman, J.; Allard, J.; Chan, C.; Hutcheon, M.; Keshavjee, S.H. Nutritional assessment of the lung transplant patient: Body mass index as a predictor of 90-day mortality following transplantation. *J. Heart Lung Transplant.* **2001**, *20*, 288–296. [CrossRef]

11. Singer, J.P.; Peterson, E.R.; Snyder, M.E.; Katz, P.P.; Golden, J.A.; D'Ovidio, F.; Bacchetta, M.; Sonett, J.R.; Kukreja, J.; Shah, L.; et al. Body composition and mortality after adult lung transplantation in the United States. *Am. J. Respir. Crit. Care Med.* **2014**, *190*, 1012–1021. [CrossRef]
12. Weig, T.; Milger, K.; Langhans, B.; Janitza, S.; Sisic, A.; Kenn, K.; Irlbeck, T.; Pomschar, A.; Johnson, T.; Irlbeck, M.; et al. Core Muscle Size Predicts Postoperative Outcome in Lung Transplant Candidates. *Ann. Thorac. Surg.* **2016**, *101*, 1318–1325. [CrossRef]
13. Blackburn, H.; Jacobs, D. Commentary: Origins and evolution of body mass index (BMI): Continuing saga. *Int. J. Epidemiol.* **2014**, *43*, 665–669. [CrossRef]
14. American Society for Transplant Physicians; American Thoracic Society; European Respiratory Society; International Society for Heart and Lung Transplantation. International Guidelines for the Selection of Lung Transplant Candidates. *Am. J. Respir. Crit. Care Med.* **1998**, *158*, 335–339. [CrossRef]
15. Egan, T.M.; Murray, S.; Bustami, R.T.; Shearon, T.H.; McCullough, K.P.; Edwards, L.B.; Coke, M.A.; Garrity, E.R.; Sweet, S.C.; Heiney, D.A.; et al. Development of the New Lung Allocation System in the United States. *Am. J. Transplant.* **2006**, *6*, 1212–1227. [CrossRef]
16. Orens, J.B.; Estenne, M.; Arcasoy, S.; Conte, J.V.; Corris, P.; Egan, J.J.; Egan, T.; Keshavjee, S.; Knoop, C.; Kotloff, R.; et al. International Guidelines for the Selection of Lung Transplant Candidates: 2006 Update—A Consensus Report From the Pulmonary Scientific Council of the International Society for Heart and Lung Transplantation. *J. Heart Lung Transplant.* **2006**, *25*, 745–755. [CrossRef]
17. Cruz-Jentoft, A.J.; Baeyens, J.P.; Bauer, J.M.; Boirie, Y.; Cederholm, T.; Landi, F.; Martin, F.C.; Michel, J.P.; Rolland, Y.; Schneider, S.M.; et al. Sarcopenia: European consensus on definition and diagnosis: Report of the European Working Group on Sarcopenia in Older People. *Age Ageing* **2010**, *39*, 412–423. [CrossRef]
18. Rozenberg, D.; Wickerson, L.; Singer, L.G.; Mathur, S. Sarcopenia in lung transplantation: A systematic review. *J. Heart Lung Transplant.* **2014**, *33*, 1203–1212. [CrossRef]
19. Chambers, D.C.; Cherikh, W.S.; Goldfarb, S.B.; Hayes, D., Jr.; Kucheryavaya, A.Y.; Toll, A.E.; Khush, K.K.; Levvey, B.J.; Meiser, B.; Rossano, J.W.; et al. The International Thoracic Organ Transplant Registry of the International Society for Heart and Lung Transplantation: Thirty-fifth adult lung and heart-lung transplant report-2018; Focus theme: Multiorgan Transplantation. *J. Heart Lung Transplant.* **2018**, *37*, 1169–1183. [CrossRef]
20. Wasim, M.; Awan, F.R.; Najam, S.S.; Khan, A.R.; Khan, H.N. Role of Leptin Deficiency, Inefficiency, and Leptin Receptors in Obesity. *Biochem. Genet.* **2016**, *54*, 565–572. [CrossRef]
21. Considine, R.V.; Sinha, M.K.; Heiman, M.L.; Kriauciunas, A.; Stephens, T.W.; Nyce, M.R.; Ohannesian, J.P.; Marco, C.C.; McKee, L.J.; Bauer, T.L.; et al. Serum Immunoreactive-Leptin Concentrations in Normal-Weight and Obese Humans. *N. Engl. J. Med.* **1996**, *334*, 292–295. [CrossRef]
22. Capel, E.M.; O'Driscoll, M.; Tierney, A.; Snell, G. Pre-Lung Transplant Body Composition and Associations with Post Transplant Outcomes. *J. Heart Lung Transplant.* **2016**, *35*, S49. [CrossRef]
23. Datta, D.; Foley, R.; Wu, R.; Grady, J.; Scalise, P. Can Creatinine Height Index Predict Weaning and Survival Outcomes in Patients on Prolonged Mechanical Ventilation After Critical Illness? *J. Intensive Care Med.* **2018**, *33*, 104–110. [CrossRef]
24. Zeltzer, S.M.; Taylor, D.O.; Tang, W.H.W. Long-term dietary habits and interventions in solid-organ transplantation. *J. Heart Lung Transplant.* **2015**, *34*, 1357–1365. [CrossRef]
25. Sahebjami, H.; Doers, J.T.; Render, M.L.; Bond, T.L. Anthropometric and pulmonary function test profiles of outpatients with stable chronic obstructive pulmonary disease. *Am. J. Med.* **1993**, *94*, 469–474. [CrossRef]
26. Tynan, C.; Hasse, J.M. Current Nutrition Practices in Adult Lung Transplantation. *Nutr. Clin. Pract.* **2004**, *19*, 587–596. [CrossRef]
27. González-Castro, A.; Llorca, J.; Suberviola, B.; Díaz-Regañón, G.; Ordóñez, J.; Miñambres, E. Influence of Nutritional Status in Lung Transplant Recipients. *Transplant. Proc.* **2006**, *38*, 2539–2540. [CrossRef]
28. Chandrashekaran, S.; Keller, C.A.; Kremers, W.K.; Peters, S.G.; Hathcock, M.A.; Kennedy, C.C. Weight loss prior to lung transplantation is associated with improved survival. *J. Heart Lung Transplant.* **2015**, *34*, 651–657. [CrossRef]
29. Boura, S.; Severac, F.; Alali, O.; Kessler, R.; Renaud-Picard, B. Optimization of nutritional management of patients awaiting lung transplant at the Strasbourg University Hospitals. *Clin. Nutr. Exp.* **2019**. [CrossRef]
30. Chamogeorgakis, T.; Mason, D.P.; Murthy, S.C.; Thuita, L.; Raymond, D.P.; Pettersson, G.B.; Blackstone, E.H. Impact of nutritional state on lung transplant outcomes. *J. Heart Lung Transplant.* **2013**, *32*, 693–700. [CrossRef]

31. Singer, L.G.; Brazelton, T.R.; Doyle, R.L.; Morris, R.E.; Theodore, J.; International Lung Transplant Database Study Group. Weight gain after lung transplantation. *J. Heart Lung Transplant.* **2003**, *22*, 894–902. [CrossRef]
32. Madill, J.; Maurer, J.R.; de Hoyos, A. A comparison of preoperative and postoperative nutritional states of lung transplant recipients. *Transplantation* **1993**, *56*, 347–350. [CrossRef] [PubMed]
33. Hollander, F.M.; van Pierre, D.D.; de Roos, N.M.; van de Graaf, E.A.; Iestra, J.A. Effects of nutritional status and dietetic interventions on survival in Cystic Fibrosis patients before and after lung transplantation. *J. Cyst. Fibros.* **2014**, *13*, 212–218. [CrossRef] [PubMed]

Permissions

All chapters in this book were first published by MDPI; hereby published with permission under the Creative Commons Attribution License or equivalent. Every chapter published in this book has been scrutinized by our experts. Their significance has been extensively debated. The topics covered herein carry significant findings which will fuel the growth of the discipline. They may even be implemented as practical applications or may be referred to as a beginning point for another development.

The contributors of this book come from diverse backgrounds, making this book a truly international effort. This book will bring forth new frontiers with its revolutionizing research information and detailed analysis of the nascent developments around the world.

We would like to thank all the contributing authors for lending their expertise to make the book truly unique. They have played a crucial role in the development of this book. Without their invaluable contributions this book wouldn't have been possible. They have made vital efforts to compile up to date information on the varied aspects of this subject to make this book a valuable addition to the collection of many professionals and students.

This book was conceptualized with the vision of imparting up-to-date information and advanced data in this field. To ensure the same, a matchless editorial board was set up. Every individual on the board went through rigorous rounds of assessment to prove their worth. After which they invested a large part of their time researching and compiling the most relevant data for our readers.

The editorial board has been involved in producing this book since its inception. They have spent rigorous hours researching and exploring the diverse topics which have resulted in the successful publishing of this book. They have passed on their knowledge of decades through this book. To expedite this challenging task, the publisher supported the team at every step. A small team of assistant editors was also appointed to further simplify the editing procedure and attain best results for the readers.

Apart from the editorial board, the designing team has also invested a significant amount of their time in understanding the subject and creating the most relevant covers. They scrutinized every image to scout for the most suitable representation of the subject and create an appropriate cover for the book.

The publishing team has been an ardent support to the editorial, designing and production team. Their endless efforts to recruit the best for this project, has resulted in the accomplishment of this book. They are a veteran in the field of academics and their pool of knowledge is as vast as their experience in printing. Their expertise and guidance has proved useful at every step. Their uncompromising quality standards have made this book an exceptional effort. Their encouragement from time to time has been an inspiration for everyone.

The publisher and the editorial board hope that this book will prove to be a valuable piece of knowledge for researchers, students, practitioners and scholars across the globe.

List of Contributors

Lieve van Brakel, Ronald P. Mensink and Jogchum Plat
Department of Nutrition and Movement Sciences, NUTRIM (School of Translational Research in Metabolism), Maastricht University Medical Center, 6200 MD Maastricht, The Netherlands

Geertjan Wesseling
Department of Respiratory Medicine, Maastricht University Medical Center, 6200 MD Maastricht, The Netherlands

Patrick Holford
Institute for Optimum Nutrition, Ambassador House, Richmond TW9 1SQ, UK

Anitra C. Carr
Nutrition in Medicine Research Group, Department of Pathology & Biomedical Science, University of Otago, Christchurch 8140, New Zealand

Thomas H. Jovic, Stephen R. Ali and Iain S. Whitaker
Reconstructive Surgery & Regenerative Medicine Research Group, Institute of Life Sciences, Swansea University Medical School, Swansea University, Swansea SA2 8PY, UK
Welsh Centre for Burns & Plastic Surgery, Morriston Hospital, Swansea SA6 6NL, UK

Paul E. Marik
Division of Pulmonary and Critical Care Medicine, Eastern Virginia Medical School, Norfolk, VA 23507, USA

A. David Smith
Department of Pharmacology, University of Oxford, Oxford OX1 3QT, UK

Emilia Vassilopoulou and Lemonica Koumbi
Department of Nutritional Sciences and Dietetics, International Hellenic University, 57400 Thessaloniki, Greece

George N. Konstantinou
Department of Allergy and Clinical Immunology, 424 General Military Training Hospital, 57400 Thessaloniki, Greece

Anastasia Dimitriou and Nikolaos G. Papadopoulos
Allergy Department, 2nd Pediatric Clinic, University of Athens, 11528 Athens, Greece

Yannis Manios
Department of Nutrition and Dietetics, Harokopio University of Athens, 70 El. Venizelou Avenue, 17671 Kallithea, Greece

Alex Pizzini, Thomas Sonnweber, Guenter Weiss and Ivan Tancevski
Department of Internal Medicine II, Infectious Diseases, Pneumology, Rheumatology, Medical University of Innsbruck, 6020 Innsbruck, Austria

Lukas Lunger
Department of Urology, Klinikum rechts der Isar, Technische Universität München, 81675 Munich, Germany

María Callejo and Francisco Perez-Vizcaino
Department of Pharmacology and Toxicology, School of Medicine, Universidad Complutense de Madrid, 28040 Madrid, Spain
CIBER Enfermedades Respiratorias, Ciberes, 28029 Madrid, Spain
Instituto de Investigación Sanitaria Gregorio Marañón (IISGM), 28007 Madrid, Spain

Joan Albert Barberá
CIBER Enfermedades Respiratorias, Ciberes, 28029 Madrid, Spain
Department of Pulmonary Medicine, Hospital Clínic-Institut d'Investigacions Biomèdiques August Pi I Sunyer (IDIBAPS), Universitat de Barcelona, 08036 Barcelona, Spain

Juan Duarte
Department of Pharmacology, School of Pharmacy, Universidad de Granada, 18071 Granada, Spain
CIBER Enfermedades Cardiovasculares, CiberCV, 28029 Madrid, Spain
Instituto de Investigación Biosanitaria (ibs.Granada), 18012 Granada, Spain
Centro de Investigaciones Biomédicas (CIBM), 18016 Granada, Spain

Rodrigo Rodrigues e-Lacerda, Caio Jordão Teixeira, Edson Antunes and Gabriel Forato Anhê
Department of Pharmacology, Faculty of Medical Sciences, State University of Campinas, 13083-881 Campinas, SP, Brazil

Silvana Bordin
Department of Physiology and Biophysics, Institute of Biomedical Sciences, University of Sao Paulo, 05508-900 Sao Paulo, SP, Brazil

Fiammetta Piersigilli, Bénédicte Van Grambezen and Catheline Hocq
Division of Neonatology, St-Luc University Hospital, Catholic University of Louvain, Brussels 1200, Belgium

Olivier Danhaive
Division of Neonatology, St-Luc University Hospital, Catholic University of Louvain, Brussels 1200, Belgium
Department of Pediatrics, Benioff Children's Hospital, University of California San Francisco, San Francisco, CA 94158, USA

Shaun Eslick, Peter G. Gibson and Lisa G. Wood
Priority Research Centre for Healthy Lungs, Hunter Medical Research Institute, The University of Newcastle, New Lambton Heights, NSW 2305, Australia

Megan E. Jensen
Priority Research Centre Grow Up Well, Hunter Medical Research Institute, School of Medicine and Public Health, The University of Newcastle, New Lambton Heights, NSW 2305, Australia

Clare E. Collins
Priority Research Centre in Physical Activity and Nutrition, Faculty of Health and Medicine, The University of Newcastle, Callaghan, NSW 2308, Australia

Jodi Hilton
Pediatric Respiratory and Sleep Medicine, John Hunter Children's Hospital, New Lambton Heights, NSW 2305, Australia

Isobel Stoodley
Priority Research Centre for Healthy Lungs, Hunter Medical Research Institute, Newcastle, NSW 2305, Australia
School of Health Sciences, University of Newcastle, Callaghan, NSW 2308, Australia

Lesley Macdonald-Wicks
School of Health Sciences, University of Newcastle, Callaghan, NSW 2308, Australia

Manohar Garg
School of Biomedical Science and Pharmacy, University of Newcastle, Callaghan, NSW 2308, Australia

Hayley Scott, Bronwyn Berthon and Lisa Wood
Priority Research Centre for Healthy Lungs, Hunter Medical Research Institute, Newcastle, NSW 2305, Australia
School of Biomedical Science and Pharmacy, University of Newcastle, Callaghan, NSW 2308, Australia

Juan Fandiño, Laura Toba, Lucas C. González-Matías, Yolanda Diz-Chaves and Federico Mallo
Laboratory of Endocrinology (LabEndo), The Biomedical Research Centre (CINBIO), University of Vigo, Campus Universitario de Vigo (CUVI), 36310 Vigo, Spain

Egeria Scoditti and Marika Massaro
National Research Council (CNR), Institute of Clinical Physiology (IFC), 73100 Lecce, Italy

Sergio Garbarino
Department of Neuroscience, Rehabilitation, Ophthalmology, Genetics and Maternal/Child Sciences, University of Genoa, 16132 Genoa, Italy

Domenico Maurizio Toraldo
Rehabilitation Department, Cardio-Respiratory Care Unit, "V Fazzi" Hospital, ASL Lecce, 73100 Lecce, Italy

Lucas Fedele Loffredo, Mackenzie Elyse Coden and Sergejs Berdnikovs
Division of Allergy and Immunology, Department of Medicine, Northwestern University Feinberg School of Medicine, Chicago, IL 60611, USA

Mara Weber Gulling, Monica Schaefer and Laura Bishop-Simo
Nutrition Services, The Ohio State University Wexner Medical Center, Columbus, OH 43210, USA

Brian C. Keller
Division of Pulmonary, Critical Care & Sleep Medicine, The Ohio State University College of Medicine, Columbus, OH 43210, USA

Index

www.ingramcontent.com/pod-product-compliance
Lightning Source LLC
LaVergne TN
LVHW082143200926
848484LV00008B/2099
* 9 7 9 8 8 8 7 4 0 4 3 6 3 *